Reproductive Health in Developing Countries

Expanding Dimensions, Building Solutions

Amy O. Tsui, Judith N. Wasserheit, and John G. Haaga, *Editors*

Panel on Reproductive Health

Committee on Population

Commission on Behavioral and Social Sciences and Education

National Research Council

NATIONAL ACADEMY PRESS
Washington, D.C.   1997

NATIONAL ACADEMY PRESS • 2101 Constitution Ave., N.W. • Washington, D.C. 20418

NOTICE: The project that is the subject of this report was approved by the Governing Board of the National Research Council, whose members are drawn from the councils of the National Academy of Sciences, the National Academy of Engineering, and the Institute of Medicine. The members of the committee responsible for the report were chosen for their special competences and with regard for appropriate balance.

This report has been reviewed by a group other than the authors according to procedures approved by a Report Review Committee consisting of members of the National Academy of Sciences, the National Academy of Engineering, and the Institute of Medicine.

This activity was funded by a cooperative agreement with the Office of Population of the U.S. Agency for International Development and by grants from the Andrew W. Mellon Foundation and the William and Flora Hewlett Foundation. Any opinions, findings, conclusions, or recommendations expressed in this publication are those of the author(s) and do not necessarily reflect the view of the organizations or agencies that provided support for this project.

Library of Congress Cataloging-in-Publication Data

Reproductive health in developing countries : expanding dimensions, building solutions /
    Amy O. Tsui, Judith N. Wasserheit, and John G. Haaga, editors ; Panel on Reproductive
    Health, Committee on Population, Commission on Behavioral and Social Sciences and
    Education, National Research Council.
       p. cm.
    Includes bibliographical references and index.
    ISBN 0-309-05644-6 (cloth)
      1. Gynecology—Social aspects—Developing countries. 2. Human reproduction—
    Social aspects—Developing countries. 3. Hygiene, Sexual—Developing countries.
    I. Tsui, Amy Ong. II. Wasserheit, Judith N. III. Haaga, John, 1953- . IV. National
    Research Council (U.S.). Panel on Reproductive Health.
    RG103.R453 1997
    614.5′992′091724—dc21
                                      97-4867
                                          CIP

Reproductive Health in Developing Countries: Expanding Dimensions, Building Solutions is available for sale from
National Academy Press
2101 Constitution Avenue, N.W.
Washington, D.C. 20418
Call 800-624-6242 or 202-334-3313 (in the Washington Metropolitan Area).

This report is also available on line at **http://www.nap.edu**

Printed in the United States of America

José Luis Bobadilla

1955-1996

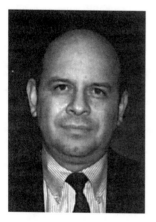

This volume is dedicated to our colleague José Luis Bobadilla, who died as it neared completion.

José Luis had an exceptionally active career as scholar, teacher, and policy adviser. He was a leading researcher on the neglected field of perinatal mortality in developing countries, and one of the first to document the harmful effects of inappropriate use of obstetric interventions. Much of his work dealt with evaluations of the effectiveness of antenatal, obstetric, and neonatal health care. In recent years he was a leader in both developing and applying new ways to use mortality and disability statistics and cost-effectiveness analysis for health planning in developing countries.

José Luis was a particularly energetic and constructive member of the National Research Council's Committee on Population and of the Panel on Reproductive Health. He combined an ability to carry out research and an ability to discern the important points for health policy in a way that very few can equal. His tragically early death was mourned by his friends all over the world, in many different institutions and policy and research networks. We particularly remember him as a friend who always steered the discussion toward the goal: to make a difference in public health.

Ronald D. Lee, *Chair*, Committee on Population

The National Academy of Sciences is a private, nonprofit, self-perpetuating society of distinguished scholars engaged in scientific and engineering research, dedicated to the furtherance of science and technology and to their use for the general welfare. Upon the authority of the charter granted to it by the Congress in 1863, the Academy has a mandate that requires it to advise the federal government on scientific and technical matters. Dr. Bruce M. Alberts is president of the National Academy of Sciences.

The National Academy of Engineering was established in 1964, under the charter of the National Academy of Sciences, as a parallel organization of outstanding engineers. It is autonomous in its administration and in the selection of its members, sharing with the National Academy of Sciences the responsibility for advising the federal government. The National Academy of Engineering also sponsors engineering programs aimed at meeting national needs, encourages education and research, and recognizes the superior achievements of engineers. Dr. William A. Wulf is president of the National Academy of Engineering.

The Institute of Medicine was established in 1970 by the National Academy of Sciences to secure the services of eminent members of appropriate professions in the examination of policy matters pertaining to the health of the public. The Institute acts under the responsibility given to the National Academy of Sciences by its congressional charter to be an adviser to the federal government and, upon its own initiative, to identify issues of medical care, research, and education. Dr. Kenneth I. Shine is president of the Institute of Medicine.

The National Research Council was organized by the National Academy of Sciences in 1916 to associate the broad community of science and technology with the Academy's purposes of furthering knowledge and advising the federal government. Functioning in accordance with general policies determined by the Academy, the Council has become the principal operating agency of both the National Academy of Sciences and the National Academy of Engineering in providing services to the government, the public, and the scientific and engineering communities. The Council is administered jointly by both Academies and the Institute of Medicine. Dr. Bruce M. Alberts and Dr. William A. Wulf are chairman and vice chairman, respectively, of the National Research Council.

Preface

The Panel on Reproductive Health in Developing Countries was established in 1994 under the auspices of the Committee on Population of the National Research Council. This volume is its final report.

The Committee on Population has been involved for many years in the study of reproductive health issues in developing countries. Previous reports have dealt with particular reproductive health issues, often with a focus on Africa:

- the effects of contraception and reproductive patterns on women's and children's health;
- organization of family planning programs;
- developing new contraceptives and introducing new contraceptive technology into programs;
- adolescent fertility and contraceptive use in Africa; and
- the AIDS epidemic in Africa.

In addition to these major studies, the committee has organized workshops on issues in family planning, health, and mortality in developing countries and published short summaries and collections of papers on these topics.

The Panel on Reproductive Health builds on this work and the work of related committees of the Institute of Medicine. The idea for the panel was discussed by the committee and its sponsors during the period of preparations for the 1994 International Conference on Population and

Development (ICPD) in Cairo, Egypt. The ICPD Programme of Action, signed by representatives of more than 180 governments, set a new agenda for family planning and other health and social programs in developing countries. The task for the panel was to delineate the magnitude and patterns of reproductive health problems and to review what is known about the effectiveness of interventions designed to deal with them.

The committee was especially fortunate to be able to call on Amy Tsui of the University of North Carolina at Chapel Hill and Judith Wasserheit of the U.S. Centers of Disease Control and Prevention to cochair the panel. The members of the panel brought to the task an array of disciplinary backgrounds—medicine, economics, sociology, psychology, biology, anthropology, and biostatistics—and geographic perspectives, spanning Asia, the Middle East, Africa, and Latin America. They met five times over the course of 2 years, listening to evidence and arguments, drafting and redrafting the report, and debating their conclusions. We are grateful for all their efforts.

The committee was also fortunate to have the services of the study director, John Haaga, who worked closely with the cochairs in drafting and editing report chapters and coordinating the contributions of various panel members, as well as planning meetings, supervising staff, and commissioning background work. With the cochairs, he accomplished a prodigious amount of synthesis and revision.

Carole Jolly of the Committee on Population staff, assisted by Susan Shuttleworth, organized the panel and its early work, and served very efficiently as its first program officer until she moved overseas with her family. Joel Rosenquist organized meetings and handled the production of numerous drafts, with efficiency and good humor. Trish DeFrisco very capably took over his responsibilities at key points when Joel was occupied with another panel; the two of them worked well as a team. Eugenia Grohman skillfully edited the report and made numerous valuable contributions to the project.

The committee is grateful as well to the sponsors of this project: The U.S. Agency for International Development, the Andrew W. Mellon Foundation, and the William and Flora Hewlett Foundation. We would particularly like to thank Ellen Starbird, Carolyn Makinson, and Joseph Speidel for their encouragement and intellectual contributions to the charge to the panel.

The panel's work drew on the efforts of a great many people. Kevin O'Reilly and Monir Islam of the World Health Organization wrote a background paper on interventions for prevention of sexually transmitted diseases, especially HIV/AIDS, that was very useful in the preparation of this report. Rae Galloway of John Snow International wrote a background paper on the determinants and consequences of micronutrient malnutrition, which contributed to the panel's work on safe pregnancy and delivery. Cate Johnson of the U.S. Agency for International Development wrote an informative background paper for the panel on protein-energy malnutrition. Gustavo Angeles of the Carolina Population Center, University of North Carolina, analyzed data from the Demographic and Health Surveys on fertility intentions and on service availability. Suzanne Cohen of the University of North Carolina at Chapel Hill assisted in preparing case study material on national implementation of reproductive health programs. Sarah Verbiest and Jessica Lee of the same university provided research assistance on reproductive health services of nongovernmental organizations. Jennifer Johnson-Kuhn of Northwestern University helped review literature on abortion and family planning. Peter Cowley and Melissa Gamponia revised spreadsheet cost models and advised panel members and staff on illustrative cost studies (discussed in Chapter 7 and Appendix C). Nancy Crowell and Katherine Darke of the National Research Council Staff wrote background notes and commented on drafts dealing with violence and female genital mutilation. The participants in a workshop on reproductive health interventions organized by the panel wrote and discussed background papers that were very useful in preparing several parts of this report.

We are grateful to all those who have given their talents and energy to this effort, and we sincerely hope that the result will contribute to the improvement of reproductive health.

Ronald D. Lee, *Chair*
Committee on Population

Contents

Reproductive Health in Developing Countries

Summary

In 1994 representatives of more than 180 nations met at the International Conference on Population and Development (ICPD) and approved a Programme of Action to improve reproductive health. To help in the process of defining, implementing, and evaluating strategies to carry out the ICPD program at the request of the U.S. Agency for International Development, the Committee on Population of the National Research Council organized the Panel on Reproductive Health in Developing Countries to: (1) examine the magnitude and severity of reproductive health problems in developing countries; (2) assess the likely costs and effectiveness of interventions to improve reproductive health; and (3) recommend priorities for programs and research.

The panel began with the vision of reproductive health embodied in the ICPD:

- Every sex act should be free of coercion and infection.
- Every pregnancy should be intended.
- Every birth should be healthy.

No population in the world has yet met these goals. Problems are particularly acute in developing countries:

- Between 20 and 40 percent of births are unwanted or mistimed, posing hardships for families and jeopardizing the health of millions of women and children.

1

• An estimated 50 million induced abortions are performed each year, with some 20 million of these performed in unsafe circumstances or by untrained providers.

• Almost 600,000 women each year die due to pregnancy-related causes, 99 percent of them in developing countries. Approximately 7.6 million infants die in the perinatal period each year.

• There are more than 333 million new cases of curable sexually transmitted diseases worldwide each year. Largely as a result of these infections, a high proportion of couples in some regions cannot conceive the children they want. Among those who have sexually transmitted infections who do achieve pregnancy, between 30 and 70 percent will transmit the infection to their infants, and many will deliver prematurely or suffer a miscarriage or stillbirth.

• Nearly 22 million people are estimated to be infected with the human immunodeficiency virus (HIV, the virus that causes AIDS), of whom 14 million are in sub-Saharan Africa, with rapidly increasing numbers of infected persons in South and Southeast Asia. The risk of transmission of HIV through heterosexual contact is increased two- to five-fold by infection with other sexually transmitted diseases (STDs).

Although a great deal of research and experimentation with programs need to be done, there are measures available now that could have an effect on these interrelated problems. We recommend a multisectoral approach involving public services, the private sector, and policy changes. Even poor countries could make progress on the major reproductive health problems with well targeted efforts and the support of the international community.

HEALTHY SEXUALITY

Healthy sexuality is a vital component of reproductive health, both in its own right as an aspect of emotional and mental well-being and as a determinant of other aspects of reproductive health. Healthy sexuality should include the concept of volition and informed decision-making. Cultures differ in norms about sexuality, particularly those concerning sexual behavior of young people before marriage and women's rights to refuse unwanted sexual relations within marriage or to initiate sexual relations. But many serious health problems are caused by behavior that violates norms that are shared across cultures, such as those against sexual violence and sexual exploitation of children.

Sexuality education and communication are needed to contribute to changing norms and behavior to build images of responsible sexual behavior. Sexuality education programs do not currently reach most young people and adults, and programs that do exist often provide little more than information about reproduction, contraception, and STDs. Evidence, albeit mainly from developed countries, suggests that well-designed sexuality education can reduce risky sexual behaviors. Curricula should include components on gender roles, self-esteem, decision making, sexual and domestic violence, and communication and negotiation skills. Information alone is seldom sufficient to produce changes in health-related behaviors. Programs will also need to be developed or strengthened to provide specific skills to health care providers and to individuals to improve sexual health.

Sexual violence and coercion are widespread problems and have serious health consequences. High priorities in every society should be identification and removal of barriers to victims' access to the law enforcement system and creation of support services for victims. Laws against sexual and domestic violence need to be enacted, and existing laws enforced. Health services have an important role in both providing counseling and treating the victims of violence. Nongovernmental organizations may have an advantage in provision of services, but government support and reforms are needed as well.

In addition to direct policies aimed at sexual violence, measures to increase women's autonomy—through higher education, opportunities for financial independence, laws guaranteeing inheritance rights and rights on the dissolution of marriage—are also likely to reduce women's vulnerability to coercion and violence.

Where female genital mutilation is common, reproductive health strategies should include, at a minimum, measures to educate the public and formal and informal health care providers about its harmful effects on women's health and to enforce existing bans on the practice. Female genital mutilation is performed on some 2 million girls each year, primarily in Africa and the Middle East. There are several variants of the practice, which is typically intended as a restraint on sexual behavior. It is usually carried out in unhygienic circumstances, most often without anesthesia, and puts girls at high risk of infection and later sexual and genitourinary problems.

INFECTION-FREE SEX AND REPRODUCTION

Reproductive tract infections (RTIs) include:

- sexually transmitted diseases,
- endogenous infections that result from overgrowth of organisms normally present in the reproductive tract (such as bacterial vaginosis and candidiasis), and
- iatrogenic infections due to medical procedures.

These infections can have severe consequences, including enhanced HIV transmission, infertility, ectopic pregnancy, and genital neoplasia. Nearly every pathogen that is sexually transmitted can also be passed on to the fetus or infant, often with tragic consequences such as AIDS, fetal wastage, premature birth, permanent neurological impairment, or blindness.

To control STDs, we recommend a two-pronged approach to eliminate symptoms and reduce complications for individuals and to interrupt transmission of infections within a population. First, family planning, prenatal and general health services should include capability for management of symptomatic RTIs, since clinical encounters offer opportunities to treat infections among women who would not come into contact with specialized STD treatment settings. Second, services should be designed to meet the special needs of individuals whose behaviors are critical to sustaining STD transmission in communities, such as commercial sex workers and men with multiple sex partners.

Primary prevention of STDs requires changes in personal behaviors, supported by changes in community norms. For the general population, interventions should:

- increase knowledge of the symptoms, signs, and consequences of STDs,
- encourage delay in initiation of sex among adolescents,
- promote use of condoms and other barrier methods among those who are sexually active in relationships that are not mutually monogamous, and
- identify sources of quality care for suspected infections.

The campaigns that appear most successful have used a range of media, have been designed with attention to local cultural norms, and have employed audience segmentation and professional production and pretesting. Condom social marketing programs have used a range of print and broadcast media, widespread distribution, and point-of-purchase advertising to increase condom sales, even in some of the world's poorest countries. Mass media campaigns can be a valuable channel for these efforts, but alone are likely to be insufficient to catalyze widespread behavior change.

Family planning, prenatal, and primary health care facilities should ensure that symptomatic individuals can obtain appropriate management of STDs. Particularly in settings where resources are very limited, the highest priority for RTI clinical services should be the case management of STDs both because these infections most frequently result in severe complications for individuals and because, unlike other RTIs, they can spread through communities. Standardized case management using currently available tools should be a routine responsibility of family planning and other reproductive health services. Management of STDs can and should be offered by every facility, program, or country that wishes to improve reproductive health. At a minimum, family planning and primary health care facilities should ensure that symptomatic women and men can obtain appropriate management of genital ulcers, discharge syndromes, and pelvic inflammatory disease.

The use of locally adapted versions of standardized algorithms for syndromic management developed by the World Health Organization should help achieve this goal. These algorithms do not require laboratory support and perform well for genital ulcers in both sexes and for urethritis in men. Unfortunately, the algorithms perform less well for the syndromes that are most common among women—vaginal discharge and lower abdominal pain. The performance of these algorithms may be improved using locally appropriate means to assess behavioral risk factors.

Treatment of sex partners and risk reduction counseling for infected individuals and their partners are essential to the success of STD clinical prevention services. Treatment protocols at all levels must be developed and periodically revised in light of local disease and antibiotic resistance patterns. Sentinel surveillance or special studies of etiologies of STD syndromes and antibiotic resistance patterns are needed to guide these decisions.

STD screening, regardless of symptom status, and treatment as appropriate should be provided for sex workers. Screening services require the commitment of resources for etiologic laboratory testing and for targeted outreach activities. Together with treatment of symptomatic men, STD detection and treatment among sex workers are central to limiting the spread of STDs in the community. Over time the primary and secondary prevention efforts aimed at these groups should help reduce the STD burden among clients attending family planning and other health facilities. Targeted health promotion efforts should aim at reduction in number of sex partners and risky sexual practices, together with promotion of condoms and other barrier methods, and early health care seeking. Peer counseling and skill building should be tested in more settings in developing countries.

Prenatal and delivery care should include syphilis screening and treatment during pregnancy and newborn prophylaxis for gonococcal eye infections. These are simple, inexpensive interventions that are highly cost-effective in most parts of the developing world.

Prevention of endogenous infection requires efforts to improve women's and men's knowledge of reproductive physiology, menstrual and personal hygiene, health-seeking behavior, and adherence with prescribed therapy. Efforts should focus on reducing use of harmful intravaginal substances (i.e., douches and desiccants) and on curtailing inappropriate use of broad-spectrum, systemic antibiotics. The latter will require changing prescribing practices of both traditional and allopathic health care providers, pharmacists, and family members. Family planning and other health services should use simple, inexpensive tests of vaginal secretions for symptomatic women and provide appropriate management of endogenous RTIs.

Infection prevention, consisting of simple measures such as hand washing, appropriate use of gloves, and adequate sterilization of instruments, should be a minimum standard. Prevention of iatrogenic infection requires improvement in overall quality of reproductive health services, particularly transcervical procedures. One of the most effective ways to prevent iatrogenic RTIs is to reduce the number of unsafe abortions by improving the supply of contraceptive services, promoting the use of emergency contraception, and decriminalizing abortions.

INTENDED BIRTHS

In developing countries outside sub-Saharan Africa, between one-tenth and one-third of all recent births are reported as unwanted, and the same percentages are reported to be the result of mistimed conceptions. In Africa these percentages are typically lower, but since fertility rates are high, the proportion of women and families affected by unintended pregnancies is as high as elsewhere.

Reducing unwanted pregnancies promotes maternal health mainly by reducing the number of times that a woman is exposed to the risks of pregnancy and childbearing in poor environments. Children's health is also affected: unintended pregnancies are disproportionately in high-risk categories, and lower fertility results in increased family and social investments in health care, schooling, and nutrition for the planned children.

To meet existing and growing unmet need for contraception, access to contraceptive services should be expanded through clinical and nonclinical channels, including postpartum care and STD prevention services. Reducing unmet need for family planning through safe access to a range of contraceptive methods is a high priority for reproductive health programs. A basic task for family planning and health programs is to support informed choice by clients. Information, education, and communication programs and improvements in counseling are still needed, even where family planning programs are well established, because of gaps in the knowledge of providers, clients, and potential clients about how to use contraceptives and the advantages and disadvantages of the methods available.

Use of contraceptive pills for emergency contraception appears safe and effective for women who have unprotected mid-cycle intercourse. Information on the techniques should be provided widely to health care and family planning staff and those who may need it.

Unsafe abortion remains a leading cause of maternal death. Access to safe means for abortion care, including early intervention to treat abortion complications, is needed to reduce the numbers of deaths. Even where abortion is legal, services are often low in quality, stigmatized, and access is difficult, making abortion needlessly dangerous. In those countries governments should ensure (through direct provision or regulation) adequate equipment and training for manual vacuum aspiration in the first trimester of pregnancy. Where medical supervision and surgical backup are feasible for medical abortions, the option should be available for first-trimester abortions. Health care and family planning providers will require training on medical abortion and contraindications. Where abortions are illegal, health services should ensure that women who have had septic and incomplete abortions are treated appropriately and promptly. Where the prevalence of infertility is high, as in much of Africa, measures to reduce infertility should be a high priority, including programs to control STDs, provision of aseptic abortion, and early treatment of septic abortion.

HEALTHY PREGNANCY AND CHILDBEARING

The major direct causes of maternal deaths in the developing world are hemorrhage, sepsis, obstructed and prolonged labor, septic abortion, and hypertensive disorders of pregnancy. Even among survivors, consequences of these conditions can be severe. It makes sense to consider maternal and perinatal health together, because both mother and child are affected by the direct causes of death and disability and because the interventions designed to promote maternal and perinatal health often overlap or are operationally linked.

Priority should be given to providing women with essential care for obstetric complications, in particular by establishing or strengthening obstetric units at hospitals. The quality and appropriateness of skills for the management of labor should be upgraded and maintained. The major causes of maternal mortality cannot be predicted or prevented well enough during pregnancy to allow reliance on primary prevention and screening for high risk. Many previous efforts to reduce maternal mortality in developing countries have foundered because they relied solely on attempts to train traditional birth attendants, screen high-risk pregnancies, and refer women to expensive, distant, and ineffective sources of treatment. Improvements in maternal death rates will require access to facilities and trained providers and equipment in facilities that can carry out essential care of obstetric complications.

Most births in developing countries take place outside health facilities, so the most effective strategy is to ensure that complications of pregnancy and delivery are recognized once they occur and that women are taken to a facility where essential care of obstetric complications of adequate quality is provided. This strategy has four elements: First, a life-threatening complication must be recognized by the woman, her family, traditional birth attendant, or others in attendance. Second, those in attendance have to decide to seek appropriate care and then, third, get the woman to an adequate facility in time. Barriers to access currently include distance, the cost or lack of transport, cost of the services, geographical or weather constraints, and perceived poor quality or attitude of the providers. Lastly, care for obstetric complications and neonatal care in the facility have to be adequate. The few existing studies of the quality of maternity care identify major deficiencies; many preventable maternal deaths are due to inappropriate or delayed care in health facilities.

Most efforts to improve quality of care have focused on training— for example, training midwives in life-saving skills and interpersonal communication. Training of one cadre of workers is not enough to sustain improved practices. Programs must also train those to whom midwives are supposed to refer women and devise policies that allow trainees to put their new skills to use and improve management and supervision, information systems, logistics, and supplies.

Protocols for the management of obstetric and neonatal complications are useful for medical care providers to guide and coordinate their actions, know their limits and next steps. In cities in some middle-income countries, obstetric care can be too interventionist, with potential harm for the health of mothers and infants and wasting resources. Inappropriately aggressive care in urban areas often coexists with a lack of access to obstetric care in rural areas and for the poor.

Some obstetric problems may be managed or stabilized by trained midwives or other providers at a peripheral level (antibiotics for infections, sedatives for eclamptic patients) prior to referral to a site with more complete essential care of obstetric complications. How to do this effectively and for which complications are important topics for operational research.

Interventions are needed to improve community awareness of, support for, and involvement in the transportation of women with obstetric complications to facilities that can deliver essential care. Families (and those who influence them) need to know signs of obstetric complications and where to seek care.

Reproductive health services need to include information and education programs about early recognition of signs and symptoms of obstetric complications and when and where to seek needed help. These campaigns can draw a wide variety of media, including mass communication, face-to-face communication as part of child survival or family planning programs, and existing prenatal care.

Appropriate prenatal care should include screening and treatment for syphilis, for anemia, and detection and management of pregnancy-induced hypertension. Delivery care should include neonatal prophylaxis for ophthalmia neonatorum. Postpartum care should include contraceptive counseling. Prenatal, delivery, and neonatal care provide multiple opportunities to promote reproductive health, many of which are missed opportunities when services are fragmented. Prenatal care of some kind now reaches the majority of pregnant women in developing countries and should be used to provide more effective interventions to improve both maternal and perinatal health.

PROGRAM DESIGN AND IMPLEMENTATION

Even in countries where fertility decline has already begun, the momentum of population growth ensures that there will be significant increases in the number of women aged 15-49 and rapid increases in the number of young people during the next several years. Just to keep up present inadequate levels of services would require substantial growth in absolute terms; to expand and improve services will require both increased resources and skilled management.

Although no one configuration of reproductive health services will serve all needs, a number of potentially effective clinical and nonclinical interventions can be implemented now at different levels of the health care system.

For some aspects of reproductive health, there is a good deal of experience with different types of service delivery and different scales of operation. But development of comprehensive reproductive health services will require experimentation. Research on the determinants of organizational effectiveness in provision of reproductive health care is urgently needed.

Reproductive health services should concentrate on strengthening coordination, referral, and linkage among three principal service domains of reproductive health programs: STD prevention and management; pregnancy and contraceptive services; and delivery care for both mothers and newborns.

Whether to integrate services at different levels cannot be decided in the abstract. Functional integration may increase the convenience of services for clients, increase the likelihood that their particular needs will be diagnosed and met, and minimize "down time" for multipurpose providers. Its disadvantages come when providers are overloaded or insufficiently trained and supervised for some of their functions.

Examples of successful functional integration of reproductive health services already exist, particularly in provision of information and counseling. HIV/AIDS information and prevention messages have been incorporated into some family planning information, education, and communication efforts. Provision of information about STDs and about danger signs in pregnancy and labor, and where to go for help, should likewise be added to the duties of every service provider who comes into contact with adult women and their families.

There are also examples of successful linkage of different reproductive health services at the clinic level. In many countries, linkage with child health services is a major convenience for mothers or legitimizes what would otherwise be an embarrassing clinic visit or one considered not worth the cost.

Administrative integration in public systems is often difficult to impose. Its advantages are that it allows coordination and setting of priorities across services and that it spreads the cost of overhead services across many programs. The disadvantages are that particular functions may be neglected and managers may not feel accountable for their successful performance.

Effective reproductive health programs will require a focused and measurable set of objectives, adequate resources, and, sometimes, generation of demand for their services. Reproductive health is most likely to succeed if objectives are focused and managers held accountable for their achievement. Implementation of effective reproductive health programs will require significant and continuous building of local capacity in systems such as training, supervision, and management; procurement and distribution of supplies; information, education, and communication efforts; and record-keeping and evaluation.

Both public- and private-sector organizations have an important role to play in increasing awareness of reproductive health services and how and when to use them—particularly recognition and treatment of RTIs and pregnancy complications. Research is needed on the determinants of demand for specific components of reproductive health services, especially how women and men come to believe treatment is needed and what motivates them to seek care in various settings.

COSTS, FINANCING, AND SETTING PRIORITIES

Financial, managerial and administrative resources for health are tightly constrained in low-income countries. Recommendations for reproductive health must be considered in light of such overall resource constraints.

Reproductive health services are among the most cost-effective health investments available to both low- and middle-income countries. More research is needed at a country level on costs, as well as evaluations of effectiveness of operational scale programs. Cost-effectiveness estimates are imprecise, but even allowing for a wide margin for error, many reproductive health interventions rank high in comparison with other potential health sector investments and should receive greater priority in health sector budgets. Analyses using cost models developed for related interventions show that costs of a package of basic interventions, relative to current health care spending, can range from modest, in moderate-income settings, to significant, in low-income settings. Cost estimates vary greatly, depending on the salary costs and the degree to which personnel and infrastructure are fully utilized and are shared with other health services. Per capita costs can be high when expensive facilities are underutilized, as is often the case. Improvements in quality of services and communicating information about their availability and benefits may help achieve operation at efficient scale.

Both costs and effectiveness will change over time, as service delivery organizations learn by doing and as increased demand for services changes the scale of operations. Cost-effectiveness studies are not a once-and-for-all effort to describe the best set of services, but a framework for continuous evaluation and redirection as reforms are introduced.

Public-sector financing need not preclude private-sector provision of reproductive health services. Subsidies should be targeted to the poor, especially in middle-income countries and for well-established services. Improvements in reproductive health are probably best achieved by a mix of public and private finance and provision, as well as other government instruments, such as mandates and regulation.

User fees are increasingly common in developing countries. While they can generate resources and spur efficiency, user fees should be implemented with caution and accompanied by monitoring and evaluation. Many of the services called for in this report are not only of community benefit rather than only individual benefit, but are also new and unfamiliar to their intended clients. Efforts to make them self-sufficient too quickly could stifle attempts to build demand. Safeguards are needed to protect access to services for the poor and services with significant public health benefits.

1

Introduction

In 1994 representatives of nearly 180 countries at the International Conference on Population and Development (ICPD) adopted a Programme of Action, a crucial section of which included a definition of reproductive health (United Nations, 1994):

> Reproductive health is a state of complete physical, mental and social well-being and not merely the absence of disease or infirmity, in all matters relating to the reproductive system and its processes. Reproductive health therefore implies that people are able to have a satisfying and safe sex life and that they have the capability to reproduce and the freedom to decide if, when, and how often to do so. Implicit in this last condition are the right of men and women to be informed and to have access to safe, effective, affordable and acceptable methods of family planning of their choice, as well as other methods of their choice for the regulation of fertility which are not against the law, and the right of access to appropriate health-care services that enable women to go safely through pregnancy and childbirth and provide couples with the best chance of having a healthy infant. . . . It also includes sexual health, the purpose of which is the enhancement of life and personal relations, and not merely counselling and care related to reproduction and sexually transmitted diseases.

Linking fertility regulation to other positive goals of reproductive health was seen as a call for change in the focus of population policy and for commitment of resources to meet previously neglected health needs. The Programme of Action entails both expansion and reform of health services, as well as action by sectors other than health to create the supportive environment for improvements in reproductive health. Implementing the Programme of Action will require improvements in the quality and range of existing services, as well as basic and applied research on new services. It will also require information on the magnitude of reproductive health problems, the effectiveness and feasibility of alternate actions to overcome the problems, and the resources needed to do so.

To aid in this process, the U.S. Agency for International Development, the Andrew W. Mellon Foundation, and the William and Flora Hewlett Foundation asked the Committee on Population of the National Research Council to: (1) assess the magnitude and severity of reproductive health problems in developing countries, (2) assess the likely costs and effectiveness of interventions to improve reproductive health, and (3) recommend priorities for programs and research. To carry out this task, the Research Council formed the Panel on Reproductive Health in Developing Countries.

THE PANEL'S FRAMEWORK

To organize our research and presentation, the panel adopted the ICPD's vision of reproductive health:

1. Every sex act should be free of coercion and infection.
2. Every pregnancy should be intended.
3. Every birth should be healthy.

This vision is also consonant with other widely used definitions of reproductive health (see Fathalla, 1988; Germain and Antrobus, 1989).

No population in the world has attained the state of health described by the ICPD definition quoted above nor fully realized the vision adopted by the panel. By stating the goals positively, rather than in terms of reduction in morbidity, mortality, and other forms of suffering, we emphasize health and a broad focus. We consider social and behavioral change and policy changes, as well as programs targeted directly against particular causes of illness and death. Improving reproductive health involves social and cultural influences and the behavior of individuals and their families, at least as much as delivery of services by public and private agencies to their clients.

This report should be useful for those who design reproductive health programs in developing countries, set priorities for funding them, and conduct or fund research to improve programs. The geographic focus of this report is primarily the low- and middle-income countries of Asia, the Pacific islands, Africa, Latin America, and the Caribbean basin. However, many of the conclusions and recommendations are also relevant to the formerly socialist countries in transition to market economies and to high-income countries.

Reproductive health overlaps with, but is not the same as, women's health. Reproductive health includes the health of men; reproductive rights include men's rights. However, the programmatic discussion in the following chapters deals more with women than with men, for several reasons. For example, sexually transmitted diseases are more often recognized and treated among men than among women, and the challenge for policy is to design services that reach women effectively and appropriately. Sexual violence and circumcision are more serious threats to health for women than for men. Abortion, pregnancy care, and safe delivery all have more direct effect on women's health than on men's, although men's views and behavior affect these aspects of reproductive health. Most problems and interventions we discuss below cannot simply be classified as women's health or men's health. Prevention of sexual coercion, condom use for prevention of sexually transmitted diseases (STDs), prevention of infertility, provision of contraceptive methods, and communication of information for health promotion are all measures to improve the sexual and reproductive health of both women and men. And pregnancy and delivery care, education in general, and sexuality education can improve the health and development of all children.

THE CHALLENGES

Many of the barriers to achieving reproductive health in developing countries described in this report exist in developed countries as well, but the problems are particularly acute in the developing countries.

Nearly 90 percent of all the births in the world occur in developing countries—115 million births per year. These 115 million births are the outcomes of about 180 million pregnancies. A significant proportion of these births—about one-fifth—are unintended. An estimated 50 million induced abortions are performed each year, with some 20 million of these performed in unsafe circumstances or by untrained providers. There are estimated to be more than 333 million new cases of curable sexually transmitted diseases worldwide each year. Partly as a result of these infections, an unknown, but in some countries tragically high, number of couples cannot have the children they want. Almost 600,000 women each year die from pregnancy-related causes (complications of pregnancy, delivery, puerperium, or abortion), 99 percent of them in developing countries. About 1 in 48 women in developing countries dies from these causes, compared with only about 1 in 1,800 women in developed countries.

Some 7.6 million infants die in the perinatal period each year. Far larger numbers of women and their children survive the reproductive process but with disabilities that may profoundly affect their lives. The imprecision of such estimates, and the lack of any statistics for some of the problems discussed in this report, are due in part to the lack of past attention to research and measurement of these problems.

Gaps in knowledge of the extent of problems are also due to inadequate health services at crucial stages of reproduction. Millions of women do not receive adequate delivery care. Their deaths, the vast majority of which are preventable, are due to lack of contact with health care providers, or late contact, or inadequate action after contact. Millions of women and men do not have the knowledge about, or access to, family planning and safe abortion that would help them make and implement informed choices about fertility. Millions of people lack knowledge about, or access to, services that would help them avoid infections that can permanently affect their health, including their fertility.

One immediate challenge for reproductive health is the sheer growth in the size of the populations to be served. Even in countries in which declines in fertility have begun, there will still be rapid increases in the number of women aged 15-49 and in the number of young people during the next few years.

The challenge is particularly daunting for countries with poorly developed family planning services—those with very low prevalence of modern contraception. All of these countries are projected to have increases of 50 percent from 1995 to 2010 in their population of women aged 15-49; see Table 1-1. (The population of men in these high-fertility years, not shown in Table 1-1, will also increase by almost exactly the same proportions as the population of women.) Just to continue present *inadequate* levels of services would require very rapid growth in absolute terms; to expand and improve the quality and range of services will require both increased resources and skilled management.

In countries in which health and family planning services are better established (again, the proxy measure is the contraceptive prevalence rate), less effort will be required to match the expected growth rate of the populations to be served. In Colombia, for example, the number of adult women will increase by less than one-fourth over the 15-year span, and the number of young people by one-tenth. In Thailand, the number of young people will actually decrease. This does not mean that Colombia and Thailand do not need resources and policy attention for reproductive health: The epidemic of AIDS and other STDs, the need to improve quality of other reproductive health programs, and the need to reach previously underserved populations present major challenges. However, these

TABLE 1-1 Projected Increases in Number of Women Aged 15-49, Number of Persons Aged 15-24, and Percentage of Population Living in Cities, Selected Countries, 1995-2010

Country	% Increase in Number of Women Aged 15-49	% Increase in Population Aged 15-24	% Urban	
			1995	2010
Low Contraceptive Prevalence (<20%)				
Ghana	62	63	36	47
Nigeria	59	64	39	51
Pakistan	65	68	35	45
Tanzania	58	55	24	36
Zambia	56	58	43	50
Medium Contraceptive Prevalence (20-45%)				
Bangladesh	46	20	18	28
Bolivia	45	37	61	72
Cameroon	60	52	45	57
India	34	24	27	34
Kenya	66	56	28	39
Zimbabwe	49	48	32	44
High Contraceptive Prevalence (>45%)				
Indonesia	26	3	35	50
Colombia	22	10	73	79
Thailand	10	−13	20	27

SOURCE: United Nations (1995a, 1995b); medium variant projections.

tasks can be undertaken against a background of relatively stable population growth.

Rapid urbanization is the other demographic change that is affecting the populations that are the focus of this report. In all the countries shown in Table 1-1, the urban population is growing much more rapidly than the rural population, due to migration, natural increase, and the reclassification of growing towns as cities. In some ways the increasing concentration of populations should make the provision of high-quality reproductive health services easier, particularly for services such as clinical contraception and safe delivery care, which have always been hard to deliver among dispersed populations. But many programs will have to adapt models of community-based services that were developed for largely rural societies for urban populations.

SCOPE OF THE REPORT

The panel's work builds in many ways on the report of the Committee on Population's Working Group on Health Effects of Contraception and Reproduction (National Research Council, 1989), which strengthened the scientific understanding of associations of fertility patterns and family planning with infant and maternal health.

Like the former working group, the panel attaches particular significance to the view that reproductive health concerns the entire life-cycle. Some reproductive health problems have their origins in insufficient investment in nutrition, health care, and education early in childhood and adolescence. Gender inequities in these investments by parents and society at large have long-lasting, harmful effects. Some reproductive health problems have consequences for women's health during and after menopause. Reproductive health is thus not confined to what are considered the "reproductive years."

The panel neither adopted nor rejected the framework of reproductive rights that guided much of the discussion before and during the ICPD, nor did we adopt the approach of defining rights to health care, education, or other basic needs.[1] The human rights approach can be very important as a way to define international agreement and hold governments accountable for their actions or inactions. But our aim is more modest: given considerable agreement about the goals, as shown by the willingness of nearly 180 governments to sign the ICPD Programme of Action, what can we say about practical next steps that can be taken within 5-10 years to bring all countries closer to the goals? Though we do not define a single minimum package of reproductive health interventions, we argue that there are steps that can be taken in all settings, even where rights to health care, and many other rights, are realized only very imperfectly.

Several topics implied by a broad definition of reproductive or sexual health are not encompassed in the framework used by the panel. These include problems of sexual dysfunction (except insofar as these would be improved by measures against coercion and infection or by increased confidence in control over fertility) and cancers of the reproductive organs (except for some consideration of STD prevention and treatment as a cost-effective measure for prevention of cervical cancer). Many diseases and conditions prevalent in developing countries, such as malaria, are

---

[1]The Universal Declaration of Rights, for example, includes "the highest attainable standard of physical and mental health" (United Nations, 1973).

aggravated by pregnancy: we include as reproductive health those programs that help prevent pregnancy but not those that disrupt malaria transmission. The framework we use does not include actions to improve child survival after the first week of life, though many of the interventions we discuss (improved pregnancy and delivery care and child spacing and fertility limitation) would have positive effects on child health.

For practical purposes, the panel concentrated on health problems for which causes, consequences, and effective remedies are linked programmatically. We recognize that in drawing limits around our subject we risk neglecting some useful linkages. The boundaries around our topics should be considered permeable membranes, not rigid walls.

The next four chapters of this report follow the sequence suggested by our organizing framework, dealing with healthy sexuality (Chapter 2), infection-free sex (Chapter 3), intended pregnancies and births (Chapter 4), and healthy pregnancy and delivery (Chapter 5). Each chapter discusses both the magnitude of problems and what is known about the effectiveness of interventions. The next two chapters deal with themes that link the interventions: program design and delivery (Chapter 6) and costs and financing (Chapter 7).

A recurring theme in this report is the need for more research. Although enough is already known to move programs and policies in more effective directions, continued organizational learning and adaptation is still needed. This need spans the spectrum from development of new diagnostic tools, pharmaceuticals, and contraceptives to field trials, survey measurement of reproductive morbidities and risk behaviors, operations research, and cost-effectiveness analysis of interventions. The panel finds good reason to believe that the investment in this research will pay off in terms of improved quality of life, especially for the people who are now the least well served.

2

Healthy Sexuality

We use the term "healthy sexuality" to incorporate a sense of volition in sexual relations and control over one's body. Sexual autonomy is thus part of healthy sexuality, if choices are informed and responsible. Rational adults need to know the potential consequences of their actions, and one person's autonomous decisions cannot be called healthy if they are coercive to another person.

Healthy sexuality is related to reproductive health in three ways. First, it is a determinant of reproductive or sexual health, in physical terms, because its lack can result in higher risk of problems such as unintended pregnancies and sexually transmitted diseases (STDs), including human immunodeficiency virus (HIV) infection. Second, healthy sexuality may be a determinant of future reproductive health, since it affects people's ability to make use of reproductive health services, and coercion and childhood sexual experience may affect adult sexual satisfaction and risky behaviors (Finkelhor, 1995). Third, healthy sexuality can be viewed as an intrinsic aspect of health, defined to include emotional and mental well-being.

Although we concentrate on healthy sexuality in women, many of the arguments made here can be extended to men. In addition, although there is variation in sexual expression, many of our arguments are valid across a range of kinds of sexual expression.[1] Yet, there is significant

---

[1]At the same time, there is also a gradient of social acceptability of these other forms of sexuality, with the greatest agreement across cultures in disapproval of deviant forms of sexual behavior such as commercial sexual exploitation of children, and the least agreement about different kinds of sexual relationships between consenting adults.

cultural variation in sexual norms and practices and in the social *meaning* of healthy sexuality. We identify three different aspects of sexuality over which individual control is possible and on which there would be varying levels of agreement with regard to autonomy:

(1) control in the sense of protection from sexually related violence or coercion, including rape and sexual exploitation of children. This aspect of sexuality is the one most likely to find consensus across cultures.

(2) control over sexual relations within a stable union, in particular the right to *refuse* sexual relations, whether physically safe or "unsafe" (that is, likely to lead to infection or to an unwanted pregnancy). The right of women to refuse sexual relations is now more openly discussed and is also being officially acknowledged, at least in principle; the Fourth World Conference on Women in Beijing in 1995 endorsed this right in its Platform of Action.

(3) control over access to sexual relations, that is, the right to *seek* sexual relationships. This aspect of sexuality has the least agreement across cultures, and we do not make policy recommendations in this area.

Not only do these three kinds of control vary across and, at times, within cultures, they can also vary during a person's life. Norms, behavior, and their implications for reproductive health can also change over time.

In this chapter we first examine sociocultural variations in these three aspects of healthy sexuality. We then look at two special problems in healthy sexuality, sexual violence and female genital mutilation. The role of public policy and interventions to promote reproductive health is discussed in the last section. We emphasize cross-cultural variations in norms and institutions and highlight the major changes in sexual behavior that are occurring.

CULTURAL CONTEXT OF SEXUALITY

Volition in sexual relations can have distinct meanings, defined as conditions under which women would have an acknowledged right to refuse sexual relations:

- when there is the possibility of exposure to an unwanted pregnancy,
- when there is the possibility of exposure to an infection, especially of the reproductive tract, and
- when the sexual relationship in general or at any particular time is unwanted for other reasons (including physical tiredness).

The third condition is a topic of much disagreement. Though the concept of rape of a spouse has been defined under legal codes in some areas, husbands have been considered to have a right to sexual relationships with their wives in most cultures, though in virtually no culture is this right unconditional in principle, even if it is sometimes in practice. Even separation or divorce may not always limit men's right of sexual access. For example, some Latin American studies suggest that once a woman has been "possessed" by a man at one point, she loses her right to refuse sexual relationships with him (Pick, Givaudan, and Aldaz, 1996).

The formal and extreme form of refusal of sexual relationships with a socially sanctioned partner is the seeking of a separation or a divorce. The woman's *real* (as opposed to notional) access to this step is determined by a mixture of legal, social, and economic factors. Not least important is the emotional and physical support that the separated woman can expect from her natal family, friends, or others. All these factors differ widely across cultures and societies: for example, practices such as village exogamy often make it physically difficult for a girl's parents to be even aware of, let alone do anything about, their daughter's marital difficulties. Such practices are related to norms that forbid parental interference in a married daughter's life.

The first act of sexual intercourse can be particularly traumatic in many cultures because it is typically the time that a woman's right of refusal is the weakest, whether such sexual activity occurs in a casual relationship or a formal union. Ignorance, a weak bargaining position, and social pressure (as well as the desire to please) create a situation in which the loss of virginity takes place under conditions similar to those that would conventionally be considered rape (see, e.g., reports of researchers in India and Algeria, in Heise, Moore, and Toubia, 1995). In some cultures in the Middle East, a "deflowering" ceremony to demonstrate the virginity of a new bride is held on the wedding night, and relatives, friends, and neighbors are invited: guests wait outside while the hymen is ruptured by sexual intercourse (or, sometimes, by hand) and a woman relative attending brings out proof of virginity in the form of a handkerchief soaked with blood. This experience is typically traumatic for women (Khattab, 1996).

Norms about abstinence at specified times, such as postpartum abstinence (Caldwell and Caldwell, 1981), may not be gender neutral when sexual activity is allowed for men but denied to women. For example, between 42 and 49 percent of currently married men report a casual sexual relation in the past year in Guinea Bissau, Lesotho, and Côte d'Ivoire, while for women it is less than 20 percent in all the countries studied (Caraël, 1995); see Table 2-1. Nonregular sexual activity is generally greater among single than among currently married women, but formerly

TABLE 2-1 Men and Women Aged 15-49 Reporting One or More Nonregular Sexual Partners in Last 12 Months, by Current Marital Status: in percent

	Men			Women		
Country or City	Currently Married	Formerly Married	Never Married	Currently Married	Formerly Married	Never Married
Africa						
Burundi	8	6	6	3	0	0
Central African Republic	14	12	14	4	11	4
Côte d'Ivoire	49	61	54	10	38	29
Guinea Bissau	42	49	49	19	7	28
Kenya	21	75	44	3	35	32
Lesotho	46	55	36	19	21	14
Lusaka	35	46	35	10	15	8
Tanzania	21	64	49	7	43	28
Togo	21	8	17	2	0	1
Asia						
Manila	8	20	23	1	5	1
Singapore	6	40	13	0	8	0
Sri Lanka	5	11	3	3	18	1
Thailand	17	59	45	1	14	1
South America						
Rio de Janeiro	31	91	69	5	34	17

SOURCE: Adapted from Caraël (1995).

married and even currently married men report higher rates than do single men. Many Africans consider it legitimate for a man to have sexual access to cowives, mistresses, or commercial sex workers during any particular wife's postpartum period. Indeed, the ease of availability of alternative sexual partners is cited by many women as an important reason for reducing the period of postpartum abstinence. In this sense, the right of a wife to refuse sexual relations may be a double-edged weapon. When submission to sexual advances, however unwanted, is the only route to other kinds of economic or domestic security, the right to refuse sex may mean very little in practice.[2]

One reason for refraining from sexual activity in many cultures has been the fear of an unwanted pregnancy in the absence of other fertility control methods. This issue can be separated into two parts. First, can a woman insist on the use of contraception in such cases, and then if her partner is noncompliant, can she refuse sexual intercourse? This question in turn hinges on a woman's ability to practice contraception herself, with or without her partner's consent. If fears of unwanted pregnancy legitimize a woman's refusal of sex, then freer access to contraception can in one sense worsen women's control over their bodies: while contraceptives may free women from the burden of unwanted pregnancies, they may at the same time remove one of the few excuses accepted by men to avoid unwanted intercourse (Folch-Lyon, Macorra, and Shearer, 1981).

The health implications of the lack of a right to refuse sexual intercourse are even more serious when one examines the right to refuse unsafe sex. The current evidence on this matter is scarce, but there is some evidence that in many parts of Africa, the fear of infection is slowly becoming a legitimate ground for refusing sexual relations, most likely due to the increasing prevalence and awareness of HIV infection. For example, Orubuloye, Caldwell, and Caldwell (1993) report that among the Yoruba in Nigeria, women now feel more free to refuse sex with infected partners. Similarly, Awusabo-Asare, Anarfi, and Agyeman (1993) found their female respondents in Ghana relatively free to refuse sexual relations with a partner infected with an STD. However, a refusal based purely on a partner's promiscuity, where an infection was not established, was not believed to be similarly valid.

Healthy sexuality in the more positive sense of access to sexual relations can be thought of under three separate aspects: control over when sexual activity starts, control over the choice of one's sexual partner, and

---

[2]Sexual relationships are as hierarchical as, and often mirror, other kinds of gender inequality and power structures. Increasing women's sexual autonomy may result from improvements to female status in areas that have no obvious connection with their sexuality.

control over the frequency or intensity of sexual activity. But numbers reveal little about motives; one cannot infer women's levels of autonomy from high or low levels of premarital sexual activity.

Asian cultures, on the whole, are characterized by discouragement of premarital sexual behavior, and Middle Eastern cultures are generally even more insistent on premarital chastity. There has reportedly been no "sexual revolution," though political and feminist efforts have been made to encourage greater gender equality and female autonomy in spheres of life other than sexuality (Hathout, 1989). Premarital sexual control is not just an ideal in many societies: institutions and cultural practices support enforcement of this norm, although such institutions and practices are under increasing pressure to change. For example, one frequently stated reason for the traditionally early marriage of girls in South Asia and the Middle East has been the need to ensure their virginity at the time of marriage. The literature of South Asia is replete with real and fictional accounts of the methods used to confirm such virginity, as well as the opprobrium heaped on brides who fail to meet the requirement.

Female seclusion is also a common way of preventing unwanted male-female interactions. Seclusion has obvious implications for the ability of women to use clinical services of all types, particularly when it is their own health needs rather than those of their children for which they seek care. Seclusion of women as a way to control their sexuality operates not just through overt seclusion, but also through norms about matters such as the correct occupations for women (see, e.g., the constraints on working class women in Naples described by Goddard, 1987). Norms about seclusion and work can also operate to limit women's ability to serve as health care and family planning providers (see, e.g., the discussion of Bangladesh by Koenig and Simmons, 1992).

More often, adolescent sexual activity in traditional societies is restricted by less drastic means. For example, in South Asia, norms about female seclusion do not necessarily require young girls to be secluded from all males in the household or even in the village. Instead, premarital chastity is promoted by a cultural proscription on intrakin or intravillage marriage so that all men in a girl's village of birth are in principle her brothers and any relationship that develops is by definition incestuous. In many cultures the importance given to virginity may reflect not so much a concern about premarital sexual activity as about premarital pregnancy. Strategies to preserve the virginity of unmarried girls may therefore emphasize the latter. Whiting, Burbank, and Ratner (1986) record several such strategies, ranging from a ban on all sexual activity to relatively unlimited freedom to experiment with sexual activity that stops short of actual intercourse (see also Du-Toit, 1987).

Prohibitions against male sexual activity before marriage are univer-

TABLE 2-2 Males and Females Who Had Not Had Intercourse at Time of First Marriage/Partnership, Among Ever-Married Men and Women, by Current Age: in percent

Country or City	Age							
	25-29		30-34		35-39		40-49	
	M	F	M	F	M	F	M	F
Africa								
Côte d'Ivoire	35	52	24	56	23	58	29	68
Kenya	15	31	8	25	5	30	6	32
Tanzania	30	66	24	77	28	82	42	83
Lusaka	38	51	26	56	23	68	28	65
Asia								
Manila	36	83	29	88	21	85	24	87
Singapore	57	92	71	95	56	95	68	94
Thailand	28	98	26	96	27	95	37	99
South America								
Rio de Janiero	17	71	14	69	9	75	13	81

SOURCE: Adapted from Caraël (1995).

sally weaker and less strictly enforced than prohibitions against female sexual activity before marriage. Condonement, and even encouragement, of sexual experience by young men affects the reproductive health of both men and women. Table 2-2 shows data from surveys, carried out by the Global Programme on AIDS, on sexual intercourse prior to marriage or partnership among ever-married men and women. Males and females in the Kenya survey and males in the Rio de Janeiro survey were most likely to report sexual activity prior to their first stable union. Thai, Singaporean, and Manila women reported the lowest rates of sexual activity prior to marriage or union.

Quite apart from the gender inequality implied by such differences in sexual norms, in an environment in which adolescent females are denied such activity, adolescent males seeking sexual activity turn to other partners—usually commercial sex workers, as the anthropological and survey evidence from Thailand describes (see, e.g., Thongkrajai et al., 1993) or to older married women, often within the larger extended family (see, e.g., Goparaju, 1994, on India). Because their husbands have often had such sexual contacts, young married women are put at risk of acquiring STDs at a stage in life when they are culturally least able to identify or seek medical or nonmedical help for socially embarrassing conditions such as reproductive tract problems. Many popular magazine or newspaper columns on health-related matters include letters from readers that refer to female reproductive tract problems for which the letter writers are embarrassed to seek medical help (see, e.g., Basnayake, 1985). The anthropological literature also stresses the inability of young women to admit to and seek help for reproductive health problems because this kind of illness, especially if it is feared to result in infertility, can lead to legitimizing a husband's search for a new wife (see, e.g., Bourquia, 1990; Doniger, 1991); this is discussed further in Chapter 3.

Many religious or cultural traditions pay at least lip service to the idea of male fidelity or to the idea of carefully restrained male infidelity. The latter approach includes norms about polygyny and about male access to other women during periods of postpartum abstinence. These social and cultural traditions have implications for the reproductive health of women in two ways: directly, if it means that they lose their sexual access to their husbands when husbands have other alternatives;[3] indirectly, because the wider sexual networks increase their risk of infections. The practices of polygyny, premarital commercial sex, extramarital sex during postpartum abstinence (and during periods that males travel to cities, usually for work) are all at least partly institutionalized in the belief that males need sexual release.

In contrast, very few cultures have similar beliefs or condoned practices for women who do not have access to regular sexual relations. Women who are unmarried, widowed, or separated from their husbands because of migration are usually expected to have a celibate life. The restrictions are particularly severe in Asia and the Middle East and particularly stringent in the case of widow remarriage. In South Asia in particular, universal marriage is generally prescribed, while widow marriage is generally proscribed, though a strong reform movement in India has led to a much greater tolerance of widow remarriage. Restraints on the sexual lives of women are not necessarily the cause of sexual dissatisfaction for most women in traditional cultures. Various norms and institutions serve to legitimize the restraints. Because of social conditioning, as well as women's lack of information about female sexuality, most women may be content with restricted sexual expression.

Beliefs about female sexuality are strongly connected to notions of shame and honor, which seek to determine how women may express their sexuality and how their activities need constant monitoring to prevent an undue expression of such sexuality. For example, folklore refers

---

[3]Polygyny may not always have this connotation, since wives may welcome cowives for a variety of reasons (Bledsoe and Cohen, 1993).

often to women's sexual greed or wantonness that makes them neglect home and family in the search for lovers and to the need to control this tendency (see, e.g., Constantinides, 1985). This image of women's insatiable sexuality can affect their sexual and reproductive health. In the early days of Mexico's family planning programs, men's fear that women who were not pregnant and exhausted from child care would become sexually promiscuous and cheat on their husbands was found to be a potential barrier to the success of the programs (Folch-Lyon, Macorra, and Shearer, 1981).

There are also cultures in which premarital sexual activity by young girls is condoned, even encouraged, and a resulting pregnancy is welcomed; this is a pattern in much of sub-Saharan Africa (see, e.g., Caldwell, Caldwell, and Quiggin, 1989; Meekers, 1990, 1992; van de Walle, 1990). One difficulty in interpreting the meaning of this practice lies in the fluid definition of marriage that prevails in much of Africa and the Caribbean, so that sexual activity is hard to classify as either pre- or postmarital (for a review, see Bledsoe and Cohen, 1993). Marriage is a process in which cohabitation, ceremonies, and childbirth can occur in varying sequence: the issue is not so much whether a birth occurs to parents who have had a marriage ceremony, but whether the birth is considered socially legitimate. That legitimacy involves, among other things, whether the newborn has an acknowledged father, whether the adolescent parents are in a stable union, whether the union has the approval of the larger kin group, and so on.

Even in cultures that have traditionally frowned on premarital female sexual activity, there have recently been strong signs of change. There are reports of increases in premarital sexual activity from all regions. Several surveys of young unmarried women report that they are now under strong social and peer group pressure to engage in premarital sex: in Thailand (see, e.g., Thongkrajai et al., 1993); Nigeria (Renne, 1993; Feyisetan and Pebley, 1989; Oyeneye and Kawonise, 1993); Senegal (Diawara, 1979); Ghana (Anarfi, 1993); Kenya (Ferguson, Gitonga, and Kabira, 1988); Côte d'Ivoire (Meekers, 1990); Liberia (Taylor, 1984); North Africa (Mernissi, 1977); and India (Kapur, 1973; Savara and Sridhar, 1994).

Two major reasons for an apparent rise in premarital sexual activity have been proposed. The first is that ages at first marriage have risen, so that women now have more years "at risk" of premarital sexual activity. This reason has been proposed as the major cause of the rise in premarital adolescent sexual behavior in much of Africa (Bledsoe and Cohen, 1993). Premarital pregnancies can pose an increasing social problem if they disrupt young women's schooling, their chances for desirable marriage, and other preparation for adult roles, even when age-specific fertility rates are decreasing (Bledsoe and Cohen, 1993).

The second reason is the increasing "sexualization" of cultures world-wide (see, e.g., Udry, 1993; Burt, 1990). The hypothesis is that various features of modern life have greatly increased both the desire for sexual activity as well as the possibilities for such activity. Among the factors thought to be responsible for such sexualization are the mass media; increased migration and urbanization with resulting opportunities for social interaction; and increased materialism and relative or absolute impoverishment, which have led to sharp rises in commercial sex. Given the variety of factors, it is impossible to determine whether increased adolescent sexual activity is associated with increased female sexual autonomy.

The term "commercial sex" covers a very wide variety of practices (Gillies and Parker, 1994), and it is difficult to quantify the extent of the behaviors, to generalize about the motivations of those who provide the sexual services, or to estimate adequately the consequences for sexual and reproductive health (Cohen and Trussell, 1996). The United Nations Global Programme on AIDS sponsored a series of household surveys of sexual behavior in developing countries, which included questions on commercial sex, defined as contacts within the last 12 months, with a nonregular partner, for which gifts or money were exchanged. This is a broad definition, and it is likely that interpretations varied among countries, that commercial sex workers were underrepresented among respondents, and that the behaviors were underreported because of social stigma or illegality (Caraël, 1995). The proportions of men reporting such contacts ranged from 1 percent in Sri Lanka to nearly 25 percent in Tanzania: "In some populations, sex in exchange for money and gifts represents an important part of sexual behavior, while in others it plays only a marginal role." (Caraël, 1995:122).

Smaller, more intensive studies of commercial sex work have documented a wide variety of motivations and economic circumstances. Pickering and Wilkins (1993), in a careful study of women sex workers in the Gambia, found many from relatively well-off homes, in contact with their families, for whom commercial sex was an economic choice, an attempt to make a lot of money quickly and possibly become mistresses of rich men. Orubuloye, Caldwell, and Caldwell (1994) found that commercial sex workers in urban Nigeria tended to be better educated than the general population. Other studies have found more evidence that commercial sex is a result of families' economic hardship and very limited alternative opportunities for employment. For example, Ghanaian women migrants to the Cote d'Ivoire who engage in commercial sex are often single mothers from poor families with few alternative sources of income (Anarfi, 1993). Commercial sex workers in Thailand have little education, come from poor families, and send back a large proportion of their incomes as remittances (Archavanitkul and Guest, 1994). Sexual "autonomy" can have little positive meaning for women (or men) who feel forced to sell sexual services. Even if selling sexual services is not invariably defined as the result of coercion, women and men who do so are at high risk of sexual violence (discussed in the next section), as well as high risk of sexually transmitted diseases (see Chapter 3).

SEXUAL VIOLENCE

Sexual violence, both within and outside a formal relationship, occurs in many women's lives (Heise, Pitanguy, and Germain, 1994; Heise, 1994). Data on it are limited, in part because violence has only recently been recognized as a public health issue and an important topic of research and in part because of methodological problems, such as unwillingness to discuss or report the problem and differences among existing studies in definitions, samples, and research methods. Enough is known, however, to justify inclusion of violence against women as a serious reproductive health problem. In population-based surveys in developing countries (using various reference periods), 30 percent of women report being beaten by spouses in two Caribbean islands; between 56 and 67 percent in stratified samples in Papua New Guinea; 20 percent in Colombia; and 60 percent in Santiago, Chile (summarized in Heise, Pitanguy, and Germain, 1994:Table 1). In a recent survey in Uttar Pradesh state, India, more than one-third of men reported that they beat their wives (Martin et al., 1997).

Violence against women resulting in death is seen across a range of economic and cultural conditions.[4] The scope of the problem cannot be deduced from figures for homicide alone. Suicide, whether real or apparent, is often the outcome of predeath violence. The classic example is provided by the phenomenon of "dowry deaths" in parts of northern India, where young married women are often found to have died in accidents or committed suicide and where there is a very fuzzy dividing line between suicide or accidental injury and homicide. A cross-cultural survey drawn from research in Africa, Peru, Papua New Guinea, and other Melanesian islands found that marital violence was a defining feature in female suicide (Counts, 1987).[5]

---

[4]Several anthropological and ethnographic reviews have documented the existence of societies and cultures in which male violence against women is not endemic, showing that current high levels in other societies are hardly inevitable (see, e.g., Gilmore, 1990; Levinson, 1989; Sanday, 1981; Counts, Brown, and Campbell, 1992).

[5]Men are more likely to die from intentional injuries (homicide and suicide combined) than are women. Murray, Yang, and Qiao (1992) show death rates for males ranging from 2.5 to 10 times those for females in populations at different levels of adult mortality. Our focus here is on violence against women, though, because violence and the threat of violence against women are more directly connected to sexual coercion and other reproductive health problems than is the case for men.

Gender-based violence has an obvious impact on women's control over their sexuality and therefore their sexual health. The negative consequences of violence that have a direct bearing on reproductive health include physical injuries, STDs, pelvic inflammatory disease, unwanted pregnancy, and unsafe abortion or miscarriage—as well the mental or psychological aspects of sexuality, such as depression, anxiety, and sexual dysfunction (Jenny et al., 1990; Koss, Heise, and Russo, 1994). The fear of domestic violence can make a woman unable to negotiate condom use or practice contraception, if, for example, she fears accusations of infidelity (Folch-Lyon, Macorra, and Shearer, 1981; Fort, 1989) Rape can change a woman's relationship with her partner and her family or have serious consequences for her social or economic status. The social and psychological consequences are particularly negative because most acts of violence against women, including rape, are committed not by strangers but by persons known to the woman, especially family members (Koss, Heise, and Russo, 1994). Studies in India (Paltiel, 1987), Egypt (Mashaly, Graicer, and Youssef, 1993), Kenya, Bangladesh, and Thailand (United Nations, 1989) report that females are more frequently murdered by family members, especially male partners, than by other aggressors.

Although most societies do not explicitly condone violence against women, they often explicitly or implicitly support the socialization of the male psyche as one based on domination and aggression. Such gendered socialization is related to the expression of domination and aggression through violence against those perceived as weak (Heise, 1994). Even if societies do not explicitly condone violence against women, they may do little to stop it through legal channels. The concept of rape does not exist in many penal codes. In many Latin American countries, rape, even by strangers, is considered a "crime against morality" rather than a crime against the person, like homicide. As a consequence, if the judicial system does not consider rape victims to have impeccable morals, the crime may not be prosecuted (Barricklow, 1993). Domestic violence is also neglected by the police and by the courts in many countries. For example, in Bolivia, aggressors who injure family members can only be punished by the legal system if the injuries incapacitate the victim for at least 30 days (Ford Foundation, 1992). In some Islamic countries, there are stringent requirements for corroboration from eyewitnesses to prove sexual violence against women, and women who fail to prove their complaints leave themselves open to accusations of adultery or fornication. Such laws and practices reflect social norms that condone violence against women, both within the home and outside it. A culture of violence, as well as the individual experience of violence, can breed an atmosphere of fear and tension among women that is detrimental to their sexual health, as well as their full participation in many activities of daily life.

One particular kind of sexual coercion deserves separate mention, the sexual exploitation of young children. The consequences of this form of coercion are likely to be even more traumatic and long-lasting than those of violence against adult women. Child abuse is even more likely than abuse against women to be perpetrated by persons known to the young person. Evidence from the United States indicates that a history of childhood sexual abuse is associated with unhealthy sexual behavior as an adolescent or adult and greater incidence of sexually transmitted diseases (Laumann et al., 1995:Table 9.15; Browne and Finkelhor, 1986). Children in difficult circumstances—street children, orphans, refugees—are especially vulnerable to abuse (Rajani and Kudrati, 1996; Shamim and Chowdhury, 1993).[6]

FEMALE GENITAL MUTILATION

Several authors have argued that maintaining virginity until marriage is a main purpose of the practice of female genital mutilation (El-Saadawi, 1982; Dualeh and Fara-Warsame, 1982; van der Kwaak, 1992). Female genital mutilation is the term now used by the World Health Organization (WHO) to cover a spectrum of procedures for which the older term "female circumcision" has often been used.[7] The practice has been reported in more than 30 countries on the African continent, 7 in the Middle East, and 4 in Asia and in other areas to which certain ethnic groups from these countries have migrated, including Western Europe, the United Kingdom, and the United States (World Health Organization, 1994). It is estimated by the Institute of Medicine that there are currently 114 million women and girls who have been "circumcised," with 2 million new procedures performed each year (Howson et al., 1996).

There are three primary kinds of procedures, with wide variation among and even within groups. The most widely practiced, often called "Sunna" circumcision, from an Arabic word meaning "tradition," consists of the removal of the prepuce or the tip of the clitoris or both. The clitoris is not completely ablated. Clitoridectomy, or excision, consists of

---

[6]In 1996 representatives of 119 governments, and of United Nations agencies and nongovernmental organizations, met in Stockholm, Sweden, for a World Congress Against Commercial Sexual Exploitation of Children. They unanimously adopted an Agenda for Action, which called for a broad range of actions, including criminalization of commercial sexual exploitation of children, education and social mobilization to inform both children and their guardians of children's rights, and programs and counseling for victims.

[7]WHO defines "female genital mutilation" to encompass clitoridectomy, infibulation, and other related practices, which vary in their severity. In 1993 the 46th World Health Assembly passed resolution WHA46.18 using the term FGM.

the removal of the entire clitoris, both prepuce and glans, and may include the removal of the adjacent labia, either minora, majora, or both. Sunna circumcision and excision affect 85 percent of the women who have undergone genital mutilation (World Health Organization, 1994). The most extreme procedure, infibulation, also referred to as pharaonic circumcision, involves the removal of the clitoris, the adjacent labia (minora and majora), and the joining of the sides of the vulva across the vagina, securing them with thorns or with silk or catgut thread. A small opening is left to allow the passage of urine and menstrual blood. The infibulated vagina is forced or cut open to accommodate sexual penetration and childbirth (World Health Organization, 1994).

The immediate health consequences of female genital mutilation can include infection, including tetanus and HIV, septicemia, hemorrhage, injuries to adjacent tissues, urinary retention, shock, and death (World Health Organization, 1994; Howson et al., 1996). Antiseptic techniques and anesthesia are generally not used. The sequelae of infibulation are the most serious (Howson et al., 1996). The sequelae of all procedures may be exacerbated by unsanitary conditions in which women live and give birth and lack of access to routine health care, safe surgery, and antibiotics.

In some countries, nationally representative samples of women have been asked about their experience of female genital mutilation. Circumcision is nearly universal among Egyptian women (El-Zanaty et al., 1996). In the Sudan, "pharaonic circumcision" is the most prevalent type of female genital mutilation, experienced by three-quarters of all women (Department of Statistics, Sudan, 1991). In the Central African Republic, 43 percent of women aged 15-49 reported that they had been circumcised (Nguelebe, 1995).

The long-term effects include loss of sexual sensitivity and sexual frigidity caused by painful intercourse, delayed menarche and crypto-menorrhea or dysmenorrhea, chronic pelvic complications, dysuria, recurrent urinary retention and kidney infection, vaginal stenosis, keloid formation, neuroma, retention cysts, and disfigurement of the external genitalia (Howson et al., 1996). Forcible sexual penetration of an infibulated woman can cause lacerations of the perineum, rectum, and urethra. Obstetric consequences range from sterility due to infection of the uterus and fallopian tubes to exposure of a fetus to infectious diseases, risk of damage to the baby's skull as it passes through the damaged birth canal, and fetal asphyxia or brain damage due to prolonged labor. An infibulated woman must be "opened" to ensure safe delivery of her child, a procedure that poses further risks to the mother and baby (Howson et al., 1996; World Health Organization, 1994).

POLICY AND PROGRAM IMPLICATIONS

Policies and programs to promote healthy sexuality on the dimensions of freedom from violence, the right to refuse unwanted sexual relations, and the ability to seek to express and to enjoy one's sexuality can be divided into three broad types: policies and programs that increase the information and knowledge base needed to promote reproductive health, including the need to *collect* more information, as well as the need to *disseminate* such information to those who need and can use it; policies and programs that provide individuals the means to achieve such healthy sexuality; and policies and programs that provide the social, legal, and community support needed to prevent sexual violence as well as to protect and treat the victims of such violence.

Culturally appropriate interventions are needed at a variety of levels: social and political structures, norms, communities, families, couples, and individuals. For example, a woman's ability to refuse sexual relations with her husband may depend on the possibility of support from several of these levels. If her refusal occasions violence, she will require support from social and political structures in order to defend herself, or from her community to make clear that violence is not acceptable and that her refusal is valid. She and her husband as a couple need support in understanding her needs and the basis for her refusal. A woman's initial impulse to refuse and state her needs comes from individual characteristics such as sufficient information, self-esteem, and communication skills.

The extent to which each of these levels is involved in protecting healthy sexuality is culturally and situation specific. The term "community" may not have real meaning for some people in urban areas. It may be all-important in other situations, in which neighbors and extended families are the guardians of the norms that govern sexuality. Gender also determines the relative importance of intervening at different levels. Men, with more power, have more decision-making capacity. Therefore, interventions concentrating on individual behavior change may be more effective for men than for women, whose behavior is curtailed by family, community, and societal factors.

There is some experience in developing countries with programs of each type. Their effects on reproductive health and costs have rarely been evaluated, however, and the evaluations that do exist typically deal with programs in high-income countries. But each of these program and policy types warrants wider implementation and research.

Research and Dissemination

A high priority for research should be documenting the extent of the problems discussed in this chapter, including violence and sexual coercion, the sexual exploitation of children, and female genital mutilation, and the forms they take in particular societies. Research is also needed on the meaning of female genital mutilation for women and its consequences for health in the communities in which it is practiced.

Since open discussion of sexuality is limited in most societies, information does not circulate about beliefs or behaviors. As a result, people may believe that they are the only ones who feel or behave a certain way. They may not discuss their sexual beliefs and behaviors, even with close friends or family, out of the fear that they are not "normal." Comprehensive dissemination of research to the communities where it was carried out is a powerful tool that allows people to publicly acknowledge their true beliefs and behaviors.

This is the case in much of Latin America with regard to certain beliefs about sexuality. For example, in Mexico, it was assumed that sexuality education in the schools was a radical idea that would disturb the Catholic majority's sensibilities. As a result, the government was hesitant to implement a comprehensive program of sexuality education. The Mexican Institute for Research on Family and Population (IMIFAP), a nongovernmental organization, commissioned a nationwide survey that demonstrated a consensus among Mexicans that their children's formal education needed to include extensive preparation in personal development, including basic aspects of sexuality. Even more surprisingly, the survey showed that parents wanted this education to begin in elementary school (IMIFAP and Gallup Corporation, 1993). IMIFAP gave these study findings extensive dissemination through press conferences, television and radio interviews, and communication with education authorities. In addition, a film that contained the poll results was shown on national television. In meetings with parents' groups at which the film was shown and the poll results discussed, IMIFAP representatives discovered that parents felt liberated by the fact that it was considered "normal" to want assistance in giving their children information about sexuality.

This example illustrates how focused research on opinions and behaviors can, if adequately disseminated, open discussion on previously taboo topics. Research findings can be used effectively to test community assumptions about sexuality and, through accurate information, open discussion that can lead to policy changes.

Sexuality Education Programs

In many regions sexuality education is already an accepted part of the response to high adolescent pregnancy rates and the threat of HIV infection. Approximately one-half of Latin American adolescents receive some type of sexuality education in school, much of it designed and provided by nongovernmental organizations (International Planned Parenthood Federation, 1995). In addition, governments and nongovernmental organizations in several countries have attempted various strategies to reach young people who are outside the formal educational system.

Most programs provide information about reproduction, contraception, and diseases. They may also include psychosocial components related to self-esteem, gender roles, or decision making. Programs that want to address a wider range of issues in healthy sexuality might include components on gender roles, sexual and domestic violence, and rights and obligations within couples, families, and society. Concepts of gender equality would need to be introduced into other areas of education since sexuality education courses will always constitute a very small part of young people's educations. (Evidence on the effect of course duration is equivocal; Kirby, 1994.)

There is also a need to reexamine the selection of target populations for sexuality education. Young people are easier to reach than adults because of their participation in the educational system. However, adults are also misinformed and require orientation on issues related to sexuality. Programs can consider reaching adults through their place of employment, their children's schools, or organizations like unions and community kitchens. A Mexican program to train parents to inform their children about sexuality found that participants had many doubts about their own sexuality that they wanted addressed (Pick et al., 1992). The Women and AIDS Program of the International Center for Research on Women is identifying innovative ways to reach adults through STD and AIDS education, including training for traditional women's groups in Africa and holding group informational sessions at STD treatment clinics. Education programs can also have an impact at the family and community levels by training parents to provide sexuality education directly to their children and by involving community leaders in establishing goals for family life and sexuality education programs.

Published evaluations of sexuality education pertain mostly to the United States (Kirby, 1994; Kirby et al., 1994; Mauldon and Luker, 1996). A recent review concluded that HIV and sexuality education programs did not promote earlier initiation of sexual relations nor lead to more partners or more frequent sex among young people (Kirby, 1994). Some curricula were associated with delayed initiation of sexual intercourse. Results of evaluations of the effects of HIV and sexuality education programs on the use of condoms and other contraceptives are equivocal. The programs that have consistently appeared successful in meeting their goals have a number of common characteristics, including: a theoretical grounding in social influence or social learning theories, focus on specific behaviors, instruction on social influences and pressures, and activities to practice specific skills and to increase young people's confidence in their skills. We have not found evaluations dealing specifically with the influences of sexuality education on attitudes and behavior related to violence and sexual coercion.

Health Services

The concepts behind healthy sexuality need to be integrated into reproductive health service provision. Service providers have access to clients' attention and trust and should receive training that allows them to move beyond providing contraceptive services to explore the factors that might influence clients' misuse of contraceptives or exposure to STDs. In male family planning clinics in Brazil and Colombia, the staff found that men will participate if clinics offer a wide range of services not directly related to family planning, such as sexuality counseling, sexual dysfunction treatment, and infertility treatment (Rogow, 1990). Two Brazilian experiments in incorporating women's concerns about sexuality into reproductive health care demonstrated that this type of model attracts clients and removes obstacles to effective contraceptive use (Bruce, 1990). A more comprehensive approach that integrates concerns about sexuality with reproductive health needs could help women achieve healthy sexuality and improve reproductive health markers, such as consistent contraceptive use (Dixon-Mueller, 1993). (See the description of an information and counseling program at a family planning clinic in Brazil, in Diaz, 1996.)

Access to and enjoyment of sexuality in both men and women is conditioned by their physical reproductive health. Reproductive tract infections, impotence, and the strain of repeated childbearing greatly limit the expression of sexuality. Health and family planning services need to take account of the concerns of their clients on these issues, but they must do so in a culturally sensitive way. Only then will women be able to shed the "culture of silence" (Khattab, 1992) in which they treat reproductive tract problems as part of a normal existence or else are too embarrassed to seek help for such problems even if they are perceived to be abnormal.

Health services need to play a stronger role in detecting domestic violence and sexual abuse of children, counseling and treating victims, and interventions. The health system may be the only public service with which victims come into contact (Belsey, 1996).

Information and Communication

In many different parts of the world, media campaigns have been successfully used to spread information about AIDS, as well as to increase awareness of family planning, which may lead to positive behavior changes. Television and radio are widely accessible and influential, particularly among young people. The commercial media already manipulate sexual images in many ways. It is therefore critical to analyze the media's role in formulating norms and attitudes related to sexuality and to use mass media to promote images of healthy sexuality. Extensive research would be necessary to determine how the mass media could best promote healthy sexuality. Campaigns could focus on such previously neglected issues as domestic violence and, where relevant, female genital mutilation. Collaboration with entertainers who are interested in promoting healthy messages about sexuality should be an important part of interventions directed at young people.

All interventions have to be designed with respect for religious beliefs and local culture. This is particularly important in designing reproductive health strategies in places where female genital mutilation is common; work should include research on its meaning to local women and measures to educate the public and formal and informal health care providers about its harmful effects on women's health. Some countries have implemented education programs and media campaigns to discourage female genital mutilation. These programs may be directed at the general population, specifically at mothers of young daughters, or to medical practitioners, including midwives who traditionally perform the procedure (Kiragu, 1995).

Increased Educational, Economic, and Organizational Opportunities for Women

A principal barrier to women's control over their sexuality is their dependence on men (or on their children) for economic survival. If women have no alternative, they will enter into unions in which they exchange sexual availability for support on their partners' terms. They will have few options for escaping such unions if their partner is abusive or unfaithful. Therefore, one key to women's achieving control over their sexuality is more economic participation and control in their households and in the larger community. In addition, it has to be socially acceptable both for women to delay marriage and to leave abusive unions. A comprehensive reproductive health strategy should include development efforts that assist women in gaining access to education and finding employment. This type of intervention will need to work through social and political structures and societal norms that restrict or facilitate women's economic autonomy.

Legal and Policy Changes

Legal and policy changes to promote healthy sexuality can include reform of laws related to sexual and domestic violence, policies that include sexuality education in public schools, reform of family laws to increase the rights of women to property and inheritance, and enforcement of laws against cultural practices harmful to reproductive health (such as female genital mutilation). Legal changes promoting healthy sexuality can help foster changes in public attitudes, and changing attitudes in turn make enforcement of the laws more likely and more effective.

Governments around the world have already taken some important steps toward policies favorable to healthy sexuality. For example, Mexico, Colombia, and Chile passed laws in 1994 making sexuality education obligatory. In India, a recent law stipulates that if a woman dies within 7 years of marriage from "unnatural" causes (including accidents and suicide), the police are obliged to investigate the possibility of a dowry- or marriage-related death. The police departments in many parts of the country also have special units to deal with complaints about domestic violence, although there has been much criticism about how they really operate. In Brazil, there are now 200 police stations staffed entirely by women to deal with domestic violence (Ford Foundation, 1992).

Female genital mutilation is now outlawed in some African countries (Kenya, Senegal, and the Central African Republic). However, even where it is outlawed, the practice may continue in secrecy, with those suffering complications inhibited from seeking help (World Health Organization, 1994). In 1994 the United Nations 47th World Health Assembly adopted a resolution to encourage all countries to "establish national policies and programs that will effectively, and with legal instruments, abolish female genital mutilation. . . . and other harmful practices affecting the health of women and children."

Nongovernmental organizations have contributed in vital ways to improve health services and health policies and laws in most parts of the world. In Africa, a network of organizations is working to change public attitudes about female genital mutilation and to encourage government leaders to speak out against the practice and to enforce laws against it where they exist. Other organizations have focused on the issue of violence against women, providing counseling and support and practical help to victims and working to change public attitudes and law enforcement. In Zimbabwe, for example, a group called Musasa has conducted training sessions for the police and other government agencies (Stewart, 1996). There is a need for improved communication both among nongovernmental organizations and with governments on issues affecting women's health and sexuality. Such dialogue will enable them to be more effective agents for policy change.

3

Infection-Free Sex and Reproduction

Sexual relations and reproductive events should be free of infection. Reproductive tract infection (RTI) is a generic term we use to cover three types of infection: sexually transmitted diseases (and infections) (STDs), endogenous vaginal infections, and infections related to reproductive tract procedures.

RTIs are caused by a variety of bacterial, viral, parasitic, and fungal microorganisms, and they have major consequences that include infertility, ectopic pregnancy, chronic pelvic pain, genital neoplasia, and enhanced transmission of the human immunodeficiency virus (HIV). The sexually transmitted infections are associated with a spectrum of acute, chronic, and pregnancy-related conditions (Brunham and Ronald, 1991); see Table 3-1. Endogenous vaginal infections include bacterial vaginosis and candidiasis, both the result of overgrowth of organisms normally present in the vagina. Endogenous infections have also been associated with prematurity and low birth weight (Gravett et al., 1986). Procedure-related infections can involve the lower or upper reproductive tract and can result in both acute sepsis and such long-term complications as infertility.

RTIs are a persistent global health problem: as syphilis preoccupied clinicians at the beginning of the twentieth century, RTIs are a major international public health problem as it ends (Holmes et al., 1990; Wasserheit, 1994; Piot and Islam, 1994). Trends in STDs have become increasingly important indicators of unsafe sexual behavior in both developed and developing countries, and changes in trends monitor the effec-

TABLE 3-1 Major Sexually Transmitted Infection Microbial Agents and Their Effects

Sexually Transmitted Infection	Acute Disease	Chronic Disease	Pregnancy-Associated Disease
Bacterial			
Neisseria gonorrhoeae	Urethritis Cervicitis Salpingitis	Infertility Ectopic pregnancy Chronic pelvic pain	Prematurity Septic abortion Ophthalmia neonatorum Postpartum endometritis
Chlamydia trachomatis	Urethritis Cervicitis Salpingitis	Infertility Ectopic pregnancy Chronic pelvic pain	Ophthalmia neonatorum Pneumonia Postpartum endometritis Prematurity (?)
Treponema pallidum	Primary and secondary syphilis	Neurosyphilis Cardiovascular syphilis Gumma	Spontaneous abortion Stillbirth Congenital syphilis
Haemophilus ducreyi	Genital ulcer	None known	None known
Viral			
Human immunode-ficiency virus (HIV)	Mononucleosis-like syndrome	AIDS	Prematurity Stillbirth Perinatal HIV infection
Human papilloma virus (HPV)	Genital warts	Genital cancer	Laryngeal papillomatosis
Herpes simplex virus type 2 (HSV-2)	Genital ulcer	Recurrent genital herpes	Congenital and neonatal HSV Prematurity
Hepatitis B virus (HBV)	Acute hepatitis	Chronic hepatitis Cirrhosis Hepatoma Vasculitis	Perinatal HBV
Parasitic			
Trichomonas vaginalis	Vaginitis Urethritis		Prematurity Low birthweight

(?), Evidence is weaker than for other effects.

SOURCE: Adapted from Brunham and Ronald (1991:62).

tiveness of STD prevention programs, including those aimed at controlling the spread of the HIV.

In this chapter we examine RTIs in both the developed and developing world: their magnitude and dimensions, their determinants and
consequences, the available means to prevent and treat them, and the
strengths and limitations of possible intervention strategies. Unfortunately, the goal of infection-free reproductive health appears as far away
today as it did 100 years ago, and we conclude that a multifaceted public
health approach is necessary to get us closer to the goal of infection-free
sex.

REPRODUCTIVE TRACT INFECTIONS

Measures

Estimates of the incidence and prevalence of RTIs vary according to
the source of data and the methods used to detect them (Rothenberg,
1990). In most developed countries, sources generally include reportable
infections (e.g., gonorrhea and syphilis), visits to office-based practices,
national surveys of representative populations, and data on patients at
specialized health facilities (e.g., STD clinics, family planning clinics).
Unfortunately, each of these sources has limitations. Data on reported
infections are affected by differences in the completeness of reporting
among different health care sources. Infections diagnosed in public facilities are reported more frequently, so these data are susceptible to biases
related to the characteristics of individuals who tend to use public clinics.
Data from private clinicians' practices are often affected by the absence of
diagnostic validation. National surveys are limited by their sporadicity
and the superficial nature of the analytic variables. Data from specific
health facilities suffer from the problem of patient selection bias, as well
as geographic variation.

In developing countries, data sources are even less representative
(Meheus, Schulz, and Cates, 1990; Wasserheit, 1989; Over and Piot, 1993;
World Health Organization, 1995b). Few nations have even rudimentary
surveillance systems, so RTI incidence is usually derived from patient
visits to health care facilities. RTI prevalence is typically extrapolated
from studies of selected high-risk populations. Although these data provide useful estimates, they must be viewed with even more caution than
reports from the developed world. Studies have shown wide discrepancy
between women's self-reported symptoms and medical diagnoses of
prevalent conditions (Younis et al., 1993; Zurayk et al., 1995). This discrepancy could be due to two factors: RTIs are sometimes asymptomatic,
and even when symptomatic, women's perceptions of the symptoms may

not prompt help-seeking behavior. For example, women may consider vaginal discharge a "normal" occurrence, even when accompanied by color or odor, because it is so widespread in the community (Zurayk et al., 1995). Alternatively, women may recognize the symptom but may not want to report it because of stigmatization. In developing countries, research is needed on women's perceptions of reproductive health conditions in order to design better instruments to measure RTIs at the community level.

Finally, data on specific RTIs also vary by the type of infection (Centers for Disease Control and Prevention, 1994; Laga, 1994; World Health Organization, 1995b), depending on whether current or cumulative infection is being measured. In both developed and developing countries, symptomatic viral infections (measured by physician visits) occur less frequently than serologic or cytologic indicators of the cumulative number of infected persons. Thus, care must be used in making comparisons among different measures of RTIs.

Prevalence in Developed Countries

In North America and Europe, the incidence of genital chlamydial infections and viral STDs steadily increased during the 1970s and 1980s, while the incidence of gonorrhea generally declined (Gershman and Rolfs, 1991); levels of syphilis varied among different population subgroups (Wasserheit, 1994; Over and Piot, 1993). Endogenous infections such as bacterial vaginosis and candidiasis remained high, accounting for up to 5 percent of all primary care visits (Berg, 1990).

Overall, syphilis incidence rose during World War II, but fell thereafter, coinciding with the introduction of penicillin. The lowest levels were observed at the end of the 1950s, increasing from the 1960s on. A rapidly rising male-to-female ratio coincided with the spread of syphilis among men having sex with men throughout the 1970s. In the 1980s, however, probably as a result of the safer sexual behaviors stimulated by HIV prevention messages, syphilis rates in gay males declined dramatically (Rolfs and Nakashima, 1990; Webster and Rolfs, 1993). At the same time, in the United States and other developed countries with heterogeneous populations, syphilis rates climbed during the late 1980s among heterosexuals of minority races. By the mid-1990s, syphilis levels were again falling in most developed countries.

The trends for gonorrhea have been more consistent. Gonorrhea incidence generally increased in the 1960s, and then, depending on the country, declined at different points in the 1970s. In the United States, most of the decline occurred among older, white populations, with gonorrhea rates remaining high among minority races and adolescents (Webster,

Berman, and Greenspan, 1993). Overall, gonorrhea is associated with a younger mean age than syphilis among all gender and race categories.

Chlamydia infections became the most prevalent bacterial STD in the developed world during the 1970s, when gonorrhea levels began declining. Chlamydia is not a universally reported infection; therefore, syndromes have been used as proxies to monitor trends. In England and the United States, nongonococcal urethritis diagnoses exceeded those of gonorrhea in the early 1970s, with the gap widening in recent years (Centers for Disease Control and Prevention, 1994). In one rural Canadian province, active surveillance showed rates of chlamydia nearly three times higher than those of gonorrhea (Alary, Joly, and Poulin, 1989). In all developed countries, chlamydial infections in women exceed those in men, and chlamydial prevalence is strongly correlated with younger age and heterosexual behaviors.

Sexually transmitted viral infections are widespread. In the United Kingdom and the United States, the numbers of symptomatic genital herpes and genital warts cases increased 5- to 15-fold during the 1970s and 1980s (Centers for Disease Control and Prevention, 1994). In the developed world, symptomatic genital herpes causes over 10 times more genital ulcer cases than does syphilis. Moreover, recent investigations have shown that symptomatic infections with herpes simplex viruses (HSV) are only a small fraction of the total prevalence (Johnson et al., 1994): for example, HSV-2 has occurred among an estimated 30 million Americans, even though less than one-quarter perceive themselves ever to have had genital herpes. Similarly, diagnoses of both symptomatic genital warts caused by the human papilloma virus (HPV) and of asymptomatic infection have increased enormously during the last two decades (Centers for Disease Control and Prevention, 1994). HPV infections of the cervix and vagina have emerged as the most common STD among sexually active adolescent populations. Since no serologic test is available to determine previous infections and HPV cannot be recovered through tissue culture, determining the full extent of these infections is extremely difficult.

The epidemiologic pattern of HIV infection in the developed world is different from that in the developing world (Over and Piot, 1993). Beginning in the mid-1970s, HIV was transmitted among homosexual and bisexual men and resulted in acquired immune deficiency syndrome (AIDS) by the early to mid-1980s. The virus entered the injection drug-using populations in the early 1980s and rapidly spread in Western Europe and North America during the decade. Limited heterosexual transmission occurred in these regions until the late 1980s; since 1989, however, the greatest proportionate increase of reported AIDS cases has been among heterosexuals and this trend is expected to continue (Centers for Disease Control and Prevention, 1995). By the end of 1996, an estimated 1.3 million persons in North America, Western Europe, Australia, and New Zealand were living with HIV/AIDS (UNAIDS and World Health Organization, 1996) Among all AIDS cases reported to the World Health Organization (WHO) by 1993, more than one-half came from the United States and Europe (40% and 13%, respectively) (Way and Stanecki, 1994). However, because reports from the developing world are less complete than those from the developed world, WHO estimates that cases reported by the United States actually represent less than one-sixth of the world total of AIDS cases (World Health Organization, 1995a).

Overall, in most developed countries, the incidence of classical RTIs such as gonorrhea and syphilis declined rapidly during the 1980s among middle and upper socioeconomic strata; in North America, however, the incidence of these same RTIs remained stable or actually increased within young, low-income, minority populations. HIV infection has also become entrenched in these same disenfranchised groups, and the proportion that is spread through heterosexual behaviors is increasing.

Prevalence in Developing Countries

The epidemiology of RTIs in developing countries differs greatly from that in developed countries (Wasserheit, 1989; Brunham and Embree, 1992; Over and Piot, 1993; Piot and Islam, 1994; World Health Organization, 1995b). Overall, RTIs are a more frequent health problem in developing countries. WHO estimates at least 333 million new cases of curable STDs occurred globally in 1995 (World Health Organization, 1995b), mostly in developing countries. RTIs are among the top five causes of consultation at health services in Cameroon, representative of many African countries; and among adults, RTI is the leading diagnosis (Meheus, Schulz, and Cates, 1990). In Zimbabwe, up to 10 percent of the population had a documentable RTI (Laga, 1994). Intensive studies of women in India, Bangladesh, and Egypt have found RTI rates ranging from 52 percent to 92 percent, less than one-half of which were recognized by the women as abnormal (Bang et al., 1989; Wasserheit et al., 1989; Younis et al., 1993; Singh et al., 1995). Among RTI syndromes, the etiology of genital ulcer infection differs significantly from that in the developed world: syphilis and chancroid are the major causes of genital ulcers in tropical countries, with genital herpes accounting for a smaller proportion (Brunham and Ronald, 1991). Table 3-2 shows the prevalence of RTIs among pregnant women in some developing countries for which there are data.

Syphilis in developing countries remains at levels that were seen in developed countries a century ago. One must be cautious in looking at the data, however, because a seropositive serological test for syphilis

TABLE 3-2 Prevalence of Selected Reproductive Tract Infections Among Pregnant Women, Selected Developing Countries, 1980s: in percent

Country	Syphilis[a]	Gonorrhea[b]	Chlamydia[b]
Cameroon	—	14.5	—
Central Africa Republic	9.5	9.5	—
Ethiopia	16.9	—	—
Gabon	—	5.5	9.9
Gambia	11.0	6.7	6.9
Ghana	—	3.1	—
Kenya	—	6.6	29.0
Malawi	13.7	—	—
Malaysia	2.0	0.5	—
Mozambique	6.3	—	—
Nigeria	2.1	5.2	6.5
Saudi Arabia	0.9	—	—
Somalia	3.0	—	—
South Africa	20.8	11.7	12.5
Swaziland	33.3	3.9	—
Tanzania	16.4	6.0	—
Uganda	40.0	—	—
Zaire	2.0	—	—
Zambia	12.5	11.3	—
Zimbabwe	—	7.0	9.9

[a]Diagnosis is based on Treponema Pallidum Haemagglutination test (TPHA) and Fluorescent Treponemal Antibody test (FTA-Abs).
[b]Diagnosis is based on culture of vaginal secretion.

SOURCE: Data from World Health Organization (1986), Wasserheit (1989), and Over and Piot (1993).

could be due to sexually transmitted infection or to previous infection with nonvenereal treponematoses (Larsen, Hunter, and Creighton, 1990). WHO estimates that in 1995, approximately 12 million new cases of adult syphilis will occur worldwide, with the greatest number in South Asia and sub-Saharan Africa (World Health Organization, 1995b). With this limitation in mind, past syphilis infections among pregnant women have ranged from less than 1 percent in Saudi Arabia to more than 33 percent in Swaziland (see Table 3-2). In one population of rural Somalia, nearly one-quarter of men and women in the general population had past evidence of syphilis (Over and Piot, 1993). Overall, syphilis is highly prevalent in developing countries, and considerable risk for congenital syphilis exists in many areas (Brunham and Embree, 1992).

Gonorrhea, like syphilis, is more prevalent in developing countries than in developed countries. Estimates for large cities in Africa suggest an annual gonorrhea rate of between 3,000 and 10,000 cases per 100,000 inhabitants (Laga, 1994). These frequencies have been extrapolated mainly from attendance at general health care centers or from special surveys of prevalence in population groups that may not be representative. Surveys of gonorrhea in pregnant women have ranged from one-half of 1 percent in Malaysia to 40 percent in Uganda (see Table 3-2). Among women visiting family planning clinics, rates have ranged from 2 percent in Swaziland to 17 percent in Kenya (Wasserheit, 1989). WHO estimates that approximately 62 million new cases of gonorrhea will have occurred in 1995 among adults worldwide; the largest number will be in South Asia and sub-Saharan Africa (World Health Organization, 1995b).

Genital chlamydial infections in the developing world have a prevalence similar to those in the developed world, both occurring at high levels. Among pregnant women, chlamydial infections are more frequent than gonococcal, with rates ranging from 6 percent in Nigeria to 29 percent in Kenya (see Table 3-2). Among men with symptoms of urethritis, rates of chlamydial infection (as measured by nongonococcal urethritis) appear to be lower than in the developed world. However, because chlamydia causes less symptomatic infections, patients may not be motivated to seek treatment in resource-poor areas where health care is difficult to obtain (Laga, 1994). WHO estimates that approximately 89 million new cases of chlamydia will have occurred in 1995 among adults worldwide; again, as with syphilis and gonorrhea, the greatest number will be in South Asia and sub-Saharan Africa (World Health Organization, 1995b).

Chancroid is highly endemic in many tropical countries, in particular Southeast Asia and eastern and southern Africa (Piot and Islam, 1994). The global incidence of chancroid is probably equivalent to that of syphilis. (There is a resurgence of interest in this infection due to the availability of new methods for detecting the causative organism, *Haemophilus ducreyi*.) In both developed and developing countries, commercial sex workers and their clients play a crucial role in the spread of chancroid.

On the basis of extrapolations from selected local studies, WHO estimates trichomoniasis is the most common curable STD (World Health Organization, 1995b). Trichomonal infection is frequently asymptomatic in men. Prevalence rates among women attending antenatal clinics range from 12 percent in Kenya to 47 percent in Botswana (World Health Organization, 1995b). Cross-sectional screening has found this infection in 11 percent of Nigerian adolescent women (Brabin et al., 1995). WHO estimates that 170 million new cases of trichomoniasis will have occurred in 1995 among adults worldwide, especially in developing countries (World Health Organization, 1995b).

The level of sexually transmitted viral infections appears to be quite high. Serologic studies have found that asymptomatic herpes simplex type 2 infections are frequently more common than evidence of past syphilis (Corey, 1994). Likewise, HPV has been the most prevalent RTI found in selected studies, even in comparison with vaginal bacterial infections (Singh et al., 1995). In Asia and elsewhere, hepatitis B virus (HBV) is widespread (Lemon and Newbold, 1990); this virus is transmitted not only among sexual partners, but also from mothers to their newborns.

HIV infection in the developing world has been predominantly transmitted through heterosexual behaviors (Way and Stanecki, 1994). By the end of 1996, more than 22 million persons were infected worldwide, of whom 14 million were in sub-Saharan Africa (UNAIDS and World Health Organization, 1996). The HIV epidemic emerged later in Asia; however, rapid increases have occurred in both South and Southeast Asia. A striking increase in the percentage of HIV-infected commercial sex workers in Thailand and India, for example, provides a harbinger of future levels of HIV infection among the general population in these countries.

The level of endogenous RTIs among women in developing countries is typically even higher than that of the traditional STDs. In rural India, with careful physical examination and laboratory investigation, 92 percent of women were found to have genital infections (Bang et al., 1989). Less than one-half of these women had reported any RTI symptoms when interviewed prior to being examined. Similar situations were found both in Egypt (Younis et al., 1993) and in another region in India (Singh et al., 1995). The type of dominant endogenous infection varied among the populations, although bacterial vaginosis and candidiasis were both common. Until recently, the inability to mount a coordinated prevention response, even in the face of the pervasive HIV epidemic, has led to continued high levels of all RTIs in developing countries.

DETERMINANTS OF RTIs

Many factors affect the current high level of RTIs in both developed and developing countries (Wasserheit, 1994; Holmes, 1994; Cates and Holmes, 1992), and the factors differ not only from nation to nation, but also from community to community. Three interrelated environmental levels affect RTI patterns: physiological microenvironment, personal behavioral environment, and sociocultural macroenvironment. These levels can be further stratified according to specific effects related to the organism, the host, or the situation under which transmission occurs.

At the microenvironmental level, microbiologic, hormonal, and immunologic variables most directly influence individual susceptibility, infectiousness, and the development of RTI sequelae. These microenvironments are shaped, in part, by the personal environments created by an individual's sexual and health-related behaviors (Wasserheit, 1994).

Substance use behaviors also affect reproductive health. Most direct and dramatic is the role of intravenous drug use in HIV transmission, which has been prominent in the developed countries and in parts of Asia and Latin America. Use of alcohol and other drugs is associated with casual sex (Ferry, 1995), sexual violence and coercion, resulting in unwanted exposure to infection. Besides affecting acquisition of infection and the development of sequelae, personal behaviors mediate risk of exposure to infection. They are, therefore, the determinants that most directly affect changing infection patterns characterized by the emergence, maintenance, or reemergence of RTIs at a community level.

Individual behaviors and risk are, in turn, molded by powerful macroenvironmental forces that include socioeconomic, demographic, geographic, political, epidemiologic, and technological factors. Over the past 20 years, the profound changes that have occurred in the macroenvironment of both the developed and developing worlds have largely shaped patterns of RTI prevalence.

Physiological Microenvironments

Trend data are not available for most of the biological indices of the microenvironments that affect RTI patterns. For example, although it is known that the vaginal flora and acidity (pH) of the microbiological microenvironment influence susceptibility to RTIs (Hillier et al., 1992), it is not known how these factors have changed over time in either developed or developing countries. Similarly, manifestations of the hormonal microenvironment—such as the size of the zone of cervical ectopy, the penetrability of the cervical mucus, the patency of the cervical canal, the phase of the menstrual cycle, and possibly even the composition of seminal and prostatic fluids—may contribute to susceptibility to RTIs or their sequelae (Ehrhardt and Wasserheit, 1991).

Trend data are obtainable, however, for a few of the microenvironmental parameters. By altering cervicovaginal ecology, modulating vaginal pH, or other mechanisms, one RTI may increase susceptibility to other RTIs and their complications (Wasserheit, 1992). Thus, recent increases in RTIs may have fueled some of the changing disease patterns biologically, as well as epidemiologically. Moreover, high levels of RTIs have been implicated in the rapid spread of HIV—particularly among homosexual men in the developed countries and heterosexual men and women in Africa and Asia (Over and Piot, 1993). Decreases in the age of menarche, a manifestation of the nutritional and hormonal microenvironment, have been documented in both developed and developing countries (Rees,

1993). Competing factors that influence the immunological microenvironment, such as nutrition, pregnancy, HIV infection, and prior exposure to STDs, can also be traced over time in some populations.

Personal Behavioral Environments

Both sexual and health-related behaviors affect the prevalence of RTIs; see Figure 3-1.

Sexual Behaviors

Risky sexual behaviors have been one of the primary determinants of changing patterns of RTIs, including HIV infection. Early sexual debut appears to be associated with subsequent patterns of multiple sexual partners and sex with risky partners in both developed and developing countries (Kost and Forrest, 1992; Caraël et al., 1995). Furthermore, the hormonal microenvironment is age dependent: for young adolescents, behavioral risk factors such as multiple, risky partners combine with biological risk factors such as large zones of cervical ectopy to cause high RTI rates.

Both commercial sex (exchange of sex for money or drugs) and specific sexual practices (such as anal intercourse, intercourse during menses, or "dry sex") have also been linked to increased risk of RTIs or their sequelae (Caraël et al., 1995). Occupations that require long intervals away from home (e.g., truck drivers, migrant workers, military personnel) also place persons in higher risk personal environments. In developing countries, marked variability exists among different nations in the reported level of risky sexual behaviors (Cleland and Ferry, 1995). For

FIGURE 3-1 Behavioral Personal Environments that Affect RTI Patterns

Sexual Behavior	Health Behavior
Age at coital debut	Barrier contraceptive use
Number of sex partners	Hormonal contraceptive use
Commercial sex	Use of intrauterine device (IUD)
Sexual practices	Vaginal douching
	Circumcision
	Early health care utilization
	Compliance with therapy
	Provider screening

SOURCE: Wasserheit (1994)

example, in 18 countries participating in a standardized WHO survey, the proportion of men reporting five or more sex partners in the past year ranged from 0 percent in Sri Lanka to 11 percent in Thailand (Caraël et al., 1995); for women, the level never exceeded 3 percent.

Health-Related Behaviors

Health-related behaviors are also a crucial component of the personal environments affecting RTI patterns (see Figure 3-1). Several of these behaviors, such as early health care utilization, compliance with therapy, and provider screening, primarily affect the distribution of the curable bacterial RTIs by reducing the duration of infectiousness and by preventing the occurrence of long-term complications.

Other health-related behaviors, such as contraceptive use, vaginal douching, and circumcision, may influence RTI patterns more broadly. Correct and consistent condom use decreases the risk of STDs, including HIV infection (Roper, Peterson, and Curran, 1993; Cates and Stone, 1992). The new polyurethane vaginal sheath (the "female condom") has also been shown to decrease the risk of some STDs (Soper et al., 1993). Chemical barrier methods (spermicides) apparently decrease rates of bacterial cervical infection, although their influence on viral RTIs remains unclear (Feldblum and Joanis, 1994). Hormonal contraceptive use, in contrast, may increase the risk of chlamydial cervicitis, but it seems to decrease risk of symptomatic pelvic inflammatory disease (PID). Both of these effects are probably mediated by hormonally induced changes in the microenvironment, such as expanded zones of ectopy and decreased penetrability of cervical mucus. Use of both hormonal methods and the intrauterine device (IUD) may increase RTI risk by reducing the likelihood of using condoms (Wasserheit, 1994).

Male circumcision is associated with lower levels of both bacterial and viral STDs (Moses et al., 1994). Moreover, close correlation exists between areas in Africa with high percentages of circumcision and low STD and HIV rates. Douching has been associated with higher rates of upper genital tract infection (Wolner-Hansen et al., 1990), although whether this effect is confounded by a self-treatment response to vaginal symptoms remains unclear.

Data on health care utilization, compliance with therapy, and provider screening behaviors are also quite limited. Clearly, financial and social barriers to early and effective care disproportionately affect adolescents and people in poor communities, both of whom are particularly common in developing countries.

The Sociocultural Environment

The most difficult task in addressing infection-free reproductive health lies in affecting the macroenvironmental forces, both in developed and developing countries; see Figure 3-2. Such factors as poverty, the low status of women, racism, social upheaval, and migration promote high-risk sexual behaviors, primarily because they increase economic marginalization (Aral and Holmes, 1990). These social and economic factors also result in fragile or nonexistent public health infrastructures, thus presenting barriers to health-related behaviors among the populations most in need of services. Communities of high RTI prevalence result. Extreme social upheaval may ultimately precipitate extensive outmigration and the spread of infection (Wallace, 1988).

The demographic characteristics of the populations frequently compound the problem. Young age composition and sex ratio imbalance are linked with many of those factors, as well as with RTI risk behaviors. In developing countries, relatively large and growing segments of populations are sexually active adolescents and young adults. Moreover, the gender imbalance in sexual relationships contributes to community situa-

FIGURE 3-2 Macroenvironments that Affect RTI Patterns

Socioeconomic
  Poverty
  Status of Women
Political
  Public health infrastructure
  Social upheaval imbalance
Demographic
  Young age structures
  Sex ratio
Geographic
  Urbanization
  Domestic and international travel
  Migrant labor
Technological
  RTI tests
  RTI therapies
  Prevention technologies (e.g., microbicides)
Epidemiologic
  RTI prevalence
  Sociosexual networks

SOURCE: Wasserheit (1994).

tions in which males have multiple sex partners and females are unable to control their exposure to sexually transmitted infections.

Poverty has been a particularly important force in shaping RTI patterns (Toomey et al., 1993). In developed countries, poverty is associated with other factors that are correlated with infection, including substance abuse, commercial sex, poor access to health services, and young age at first intercourse. In developing countries, the absence of preventive and curative services among poor and poorly served populations perpetuates high RTI prevalence.

These socioeconomic trends have been accompanied in many places by changes in the political environment that further limit access to public-sector RTI care: at the same time that RTI levels are rising, the public health infrastructure in many countries is deteriorating (Mosley, Bobadilla, and Jamison, 1993). Ironically, these trends have occurred despite advances in diagnostic and therapeutic technologies that could improve RTI prevention efforts.

CONSEQUENCES OF RTIs

RTIs have serious implications for reproductive health. For example, chlamydia and gonorrhea significantly reduce a woman's chances of becoming pregnant. Moreover, virtually every organism that is sexually transmitted can be passed to the fetus or infant—often with tragic consequences.

Pelvic Inflammatory Disease

"Pelvic inflammatory disease" (PID) has come to represent clinically suspected endometritis or salpingitis that has not been objectively confirmed pathologically or visually (i.e., by laparoscopy) (Kahn et al., 1991). Investigations over the past decade have emphasized the polymicrobial nature of PID. In general, three major groups of microorganisms play an etiologic role in PID: *Neisseria gonorrhoeae*, *Chlamydia trachomatis*, and a wide variety of anaerobic and aerobic bacteria. A leading hypothesis is that *N. gonorrhoeae* and *C. trachomatis* initiate tubal infection and that anaerobic and aerobic bacteria from the cervix or vagina are secondary invaders (Cates and Wasserheit, 1991).

In some European locations, *N. gonorrhoeae* has been cultured in fewer than 10 percent of samples taken from women diagnosed with PID (Cates et al., 1990), while in some developing world populations, *N. gonorrhoeae* has been cultured in up to 80 percent of women diagnosed with PID (Cates, Rolfs, and Aral, 1990). This variation is probably due to true differences among the populations studied and variations in the severity of infection, as well as differences in laboratory standards. In general, gonococcal PID is associated with more clinically severe symptoms than chlamydial upper genital tract infections, although the latter are more insidious.

Teenagers have a particularly high rate of PID, especially when the data are corrected for level of sexual activity (Shafer and Sweet, 1989). In the United States, for example, sexually active 15- to 19-year-old females have a one in eight estimated lifetime risk of suffering PID (Shafer and Sweet, 1989). Rates are probably higher in developing countries, given the higher prevalence of infection and more limited access to care. As described above, biological, behavioral, and social determinants raise the risk of RTIs among teenagers, so creative interventions are needed to reach this high-risk age group.

The role of atypical (also called "subclinical" or "silent") PID in causing adverse reproductive sequelae is becoming increasingly apparent (Cates and Wasserheit, 1991). Atypical salpingitis accounts for a sizable proportion of tubal infertility. Many investigations have found that more than one-half of women with documented tubal occlusion reported no history of previous PID, despite serologic evidence of past chlamydial or gonococcal infection (Cates and Wasserheit, 1991). Moreover, morphologic and physical analysis of tubal epithelium from women with distal tubal obstruction found extensive ultrastructural damage, even among women who had no knowledge of previous PID (Patton et al., 1989). Women with atypical salpingitis had levels of tubal abnormalities similar to those with overt salpingitis. No demographic or clinical determinants have been found that differentiate women with atypical salpingitis from those with symptomatic PID (Cates, Joesoef, and Goldman, 1993). Thus, clinical evidence of symptomatic PID is not a necessary precursor for the eventual development of tubal dysfunction or obstruction.

Infertility

Women with a self-reported history of PID are more likely to be infertile than those without. A WHO multicenter study of infertile couples showed the proportion of infectious causes of infertility in different parts of the world: in Africa, nearly four-fifths of couples had an infectious etiology, compared with about two-fifths of infertile couples in other developing countries and one-fifth of couples seeking infertility services in developed countries (Cates et al., 1985).

Infertility as a consequence of RTI occurs primarily through the damage caused by salpingitis, which in turn leads to tubal dysfunction and occlusion. Usually this damage involves antecedent lower genital tract infections with either *N. gonorrhoeae* or *C. trachomatis*.

The etiologic role of previous chlamydial infection in causing tubal infertility has been exhaustively studied. Multiple retrospective investigations have examined the relationship between serologic evidence of past chlamydial infection and tubal infertility. Despite wide variations in study design, results uniformly document that tubal infertility is significantly associated with previous chlamydial infections (Cates and Wasserheit, 1991). The majority of women with tubal infertility have no prior history of clinical PID; thus, the role of subclinical (or chronic) tubal inflammation in the pathogenesis of tubal infertility is quite important.

Ectopic Pregnancies

After fertilization, postinfectious tubal occlusion can still influence pregnancy outcome through its effect on potentially fatal ectopic implantation. In developed countries, the public health effects of ectopic pregnancies have been well documented: both increased incidence and decreased death-to-case rate (Centers for Disease Control and Prevention, 1994). Several factors have contributed to these trends, but the most powerful etiologic correlate is PID (Chow et al., 1987). Moreover, many of the other conditions frequently associated with ectopic pregnancy—lower genital tract infection, past IUD use, postabortal infection, and pelvic surgery—have a primary link with PID. However, few studies have examined the pathogenesis of ectopic pregnancy. The roles of such possible cofactors as douching, previous abdominal or pelvic surgery, and cigarette smoking are not known. Finally, as with tubal infertility, the preventive impact of antibiotic treatment for PID has not been firmly established.

Pregnancy Outcomes and RTIs

Nearly all RTIs can significantly influence pregnancy outcomes for both mothers and neonates (Cates, 1995). Vertical transmission, resulting in congenital infection, is a particularly serious outcome of perinatal RTIs; see Table 3-3. Fetal wastage, low birth weight, and prematurity are also adverse pregnancy outcomes commonly associated with RTIs.

Gonorrhea

Among pregnant women, the incidence of gonorrhea has ranged from less than 1 percent to 7.5 percent in developed countries and from 2 percent to 30 percent in developing countries. The majority of pregnant women with gonococcal infection are asymptomatic. Preterm delivery, premature rupture of membranes, and histologic evidence of chorio-

TABLE 3-3 Neonatal Effects of Reproductive Tract Infections

Organism	Maternal Infection Rate (%)	Infant Effects	Transmission Risk from Infected Mother	Treatment of Neonate	Prevention
Neisseria gonorrhoeae	1-30	Conjunctivitis, sepsis, meningitis	Approximately 30%	Screening: maternal culture; ocular prophylaxis	Penicillin, Ceftriaxone
Chlamydia trachomatis	2-25	Conjunctivitis, pneumonia, bronchiolitis, otitis media	25-50% conjunctivitis 5-15% pneumonia	Screening: maternal culture; ocular prophylaxis	Erythromycin
Treponema pallidum	0.01-15	Congenital syphilis, neonatal death	50%	Serologic screening in early and late pregnancy	Penicillin
Herpes simplex virus	1-30	Disseminated, central nervous system, localized lesions	3% recurrent at delivery, 30% primary at delivery	Cesarean delivery if lesions present at delivery	Vidarabine, Acyclovir
Human papilloma virus	10-35	Laryngeal papillomatosis	Rare	None	Surgery
Human immunodeficiency virus	0.01-20	Pediatric AIDS	22-39%	Pregnancy prevention Zidovudine prophylaxis	Zidovudine

SOURCE: Adapted from Cates (1995).

amnionitis are more frequent in mothers with gonorrhea than in comparison groups. Clinical symptoms of sepsis in newborns, as well as maternal puerperal fever, have been associated with positive *N. gonorrhoeae* cultures of the orogastric contents of newborns. Prevention of neonatal gonococcal ophthalmia, which can lead to blindness, relies on ocular prophylaxis with silver nitrate or antibiotics at birth.

Chlamydia

The prevalence of cervical infection with *C. trachomatis* among pregnant women ranges from 2 percent to 25 percent in both developed and developing countries, but in most samples it is 8 percent to 12 percent. Untreated, cervical chlamydial infections in pregnancy cause approximately 20 percent higher rates of preterm delivery and low birth weight (Cohen, Veille, and Calkins, 1990). The consequences for infants of maternal infection at term include conjunctivitis and pneumonia. Ideally, prevention of chlamydial infection in pregnancy and among infants relies on detecting and treating prenatal infections. However, a tertiary prevention strategy is neonatal ocular prophylaxis with erythromycin ophthalmic ointment.

Syphilis

Syphilis can be transmitted transplacentally throughout the course of untreated maternal disease at every stage, from incubation to tertiary syphilis. The early stages, however, when spirochetemia is highest, pose the greatest risk to the fetus. Untreated syphilis in pregnant women results in adverse pregnancy outcomes, including abortion, prematurity, stillbirth, or neonatal death. Prevention depends on prenatal diagnosis and maternal treatment (Hira, Bhat, and Chikamata, 1990). Effective treatment of the mother, even late in pregnancy, generally results in cure of the fetus.

Most congenital syphilis occurs because the health care system fails either to detect maternal infection or to pursue it to adequate treatment. Current prevention recommendations for developed countries emphasize extending prenatal care where possible. In developing countries, where adequate prenatal care is largely unaccessible, screening and treatment for syphilis whenever a pregnant woman contacts a health system is crucial.

Herpes

The prevalence of symptomatic genital herpes infection among pregnant women is less than 1 percent at the time of delivery (Randolph, Washington, and Prober, 1993). Intermittent asymptomatic shedding occurs from either the cervix or vulva, and the majority of neonatal herpes is transmitted from asymptomatic mothers. The role of screening in pregnancy for herpes infection is currently being evaluated. In developed countries, acyclovir may have a role in prophylaxis of infants born to mothers who demonstrate cervical infection at delivery.

Human Papilloma Virus

HPV infection is transmitted from an infected mother to her newborn during delivery by direct contact with infected cervical and vaginal tissue. Little is known about what factors may predispose the infant to symptomatic infection. No effect of maternal HPV infection on infant birth weight or gestational age has been reported; however, vaginal delivery is sometimes complicated by large warts. Although infants delivered to women with genital HPV infection occasionally have oral and anogenital warts, the most serious complication for the infant is laryngeal papillomatosis—fortunately, a rare outcome of this highly prevalent infection.

Human Immunodeficiency Virus

HIV can be transmitted from infected women to their offspring during pregnancy or soon after. Perinatal transmission rates vary from 22 percent to 39 percent, but they can be markedly reduced with zidovudine prophylaxis (Centers for Disease Control and Prevention, 1994); however, zidovudine is not generally available in developing countries. Breastfeeding has been demonstrated to be a mode of postpartum infection, particularly for infants whose mothers are infected after delivery. Clinical symptoms of HIV infection occur earlier in the course of illness among children infected perinatally than among adults. Moreover, the overall mortality rate after diagnosis of HIV infection is relatively high for those infected perinatally: one-half die before they reach 36 months of age (Brown et al., 1991).

RTI-Related Neoplasia

At least five squamous cell neoplasms—carcinomas involving the cervix, vagina, vulva, anus, and penis—have been strongly associated with HPV infection, particularly with HPV types 16, 18, 31, and 45 (Bosch et al., 1995). Squamous cell carcinoma of the cervix has also been strongly correlated with both the number of sexual partners (Buckley et al., 1981;

Harris et al., 1980) and (in some but not all studies) with smoking (Harris et al., 1980; Brinton et al., 1986) and HSV-2 infection (Hulka, 1982). Hepatocellular carcinoma is often caused by HBV, another sexually transmitted virus. Finally, some of the tumors associated with AIDS, namely, Kaposi's sarcoma and non-Hodgkin's lymphomas, although related to the profound immunosuppression caused by HIV, may themselves have an underlying viral etiology (Moore and Chang, 1995).

INTERVENTIONS TO PREVENT AND TREAT RTIs

The design and implementation of interventions to prevent and treat reproductive tract infections requires the effective coordination of a multifaceted public health response. Comprehensive programs must respond at both the individual and societal level, promote private and public investments in infection-free sexual and reproductive health, and encourage intersectoral coordination. Given local differences in available technological, human, and financial resources, the specific elements of programs can be expected to vary considerably in different settings, but common themes should be addressed in every program. Although many unanswered questions remain regarding the design of optimal approaches to RTI prevention and treatment, the most immediate challenge lies in the implementation of strategies already shown to be both feasible and cost-effective.

A tension often exists among the objectives of programmatic interventions, particularly for sexually transmitted infection. One objective is to relieve individual suffering and the serious personal sequelae of RTI. Another is to minimize the community impact of infections by reducing transmission. Although many interventions address these two objectives in concert, meeting these objectives may require different, complementary strategies if resources are limited.

An example of this tension often arises in regard to the traditional STD control approach that targets interventions to high-risk "core transmitters" (Moses et al., 1991). Studies show a tight cluster of some STDs, such as gonorrhea, in specific geographic areas (Rothenberg, 1983; Wasserheit, 1989). From a community perspective, the efficacy of a targeted approach is supported by cost-effectiveness modeling that demonstrates a greater benefit than other approaches, as measured by disability-adjusted life-years saved per dollar invested (Over and Piot, 1993). Others have questioned the wisdom of relying exclusively on a highly targeted approach, however, noting that such an approach fails to address the needs of individuals outside the identified core groups (Elias, 1991). Although these individuals are "less important" at a community level and may be more costly to reach, they certainly have real personal needs for the prevention and treatment of RTIs. Consider the monogamous woman who faces the risk of sexually transmitted infection solely as a result of the extramarital sexual activity of her husband (McGrath et al., 1993). Once infected, she is unlikely to further spread infection in the community (except through reinfection of her husband or perinatally). Interventions exclusively targeted to core transmitters will not directly meet her needs for either prevention or treatment.

The trade-offs involved in choosing a particular set of intervention strategies in any given locale should be made explicit so that the various options can be the subject of discussion in the community. Where available, such choices should be guided by data concerning the relative cost-effectiveness of different intervention strategies. A mixture of responses will most often be warranted.

Different settings call for different intervention approaches. The manager of a busy family planning clinic serving women in the general population may not have a key role in controlling STDs at a community level. Clinic clients in most parts of the world are probably not responsible for transmitting infections widely within the community. In a family planning clinic, counseling to guide appropriate contraceptive choice, standardized case management of symptomatic infections, patient-initiated partner notification, prevention of iatrogenic infections, and selected screening efforts are appropriate (and feasible) programmatic interventions (Elias and Leonard, 1995). In contrast, aggressive condom promotion, regular STD screening and treatment, and clinic-assisted partner notification focused on commercial sex workers and their clients may be important intervention choices for the manager of a community's STD control program.

A cost-effectiveness analysis of options for STD control that used as an outcome measure only the reduction of STD prevalence in the community might show that scarce resources should be directed exclusively to the intense efforts aimed at core transmitters. However, as we argue further in Chapter 7, reproductive health programs have multiple related goals. For family planning programs, these include helping clients achieve their reproductive intentions in a healthful manner (Jain and Bruce, 1993). Preventing infertility by managing syndromes related to RTIs is thus part of their mission and may be important for credibility as health providers (among staff as well as clients). The type and intensity of STD prevention, detection, and treatment efforts aimed at general populations should vary, as we argue below, according to such factors as the prevalence of STDs and the effectiveness of local interventions and treatment algorithms.

Unfortunately, a failure to consider relevant intervention options in context has too often resulted in inaction. Consequently, family planning and maternal-child health services have often missed important opportunities to meet the needs of their individual clients, while STD control programs have focused almost exclusively on high-risk core transmitters. What is needed is a more coordinated approach in which all health programs serving those at risk of RTIs recognize the scope of the problem and design the most appropriately balanced local response. Recognizing the important role played by family members, traditional practitioners, pharmacists, and the private sector in preventing and treating RTIs and their consequences is an important element of such a coordinated response.

Limitations in the Data on RTI Interventions

One of the major limitations in developing recommendations for RTI intervention programs is the paucity of data available concerning the effectiveness and cost of various intervention strategies. Few interventions have been thoroughly evaluated (Aral and Peterman, 1993; Oakley, Fullerton, and Holland, 1995). Even when evaluations have been attempted, too often study designs have been weak, and the results have consequently been inconclusive (O'Reilly and Islam, 1995). For example, evaluations of primary prevention efforts have rarely contained adequate controls. Programs with partial success have not often been refined and retested or replicated in other settings. Many studies accept changes in attitudes and knowledge as proxies for behavior change, a conclusion not justified by the available knowledge (DiClemente et al., 1992; Temmerman et al., 1990). At the same time, expectations of the effectiveness of behavioral interventions have often been too high, with the result that partially successful interventions have been undervalued (O'Reilly and Islam, 1995).

A further limitation relates to large degrees of variability in the quality of intervention efforts. The same intervention strategy can have diverse effects in different settings, reflecting both differences in the populations served and in local program implementation. For example, with HIV discordant couples in Europe, fewer than 50 percent of couples regularly used condoms despite repeated counseling (de Vincenzi, 1994); in California, however, there was more condom use, perhaps due to greater intensity of the intervention program, as well as an emphasis on counseling couples together (O'Reilly and Islam, 1995; Padian, Vittinghoff, and Shiboski, 1994). Generally, little information exists about "which" interventions work, and even less addresses "how" or "why" any given intervention works in a particular setting. As a consequence, there is little guidance available on how to design effective program packages, especially for individuals in the general population.

This lack of information has long been a concern in the field of interventions research (Chen and Rossi, 1983; Stoeckel, 1992). Many intervention efforts may have limited effects not because they lack a causal influence on the phenomenon of interest, but because they have been poorly implemented at a local level. At the extreme, program efforts may fail primarily because of unsuccessful implementation, causing program planners to abandon an otherwise promising intervention. In the health education literature, this is sometimes referred to as a "type III error"—something does not work simply because it does not actually "happen" with sufficient intensity or in the way in which it was intended (Basch et al., 1985). The discrepancy between program plans and program realities, as well as weak program effects, is well known in the area of family planning service delivery (Simmons and Elias, 1993). Much more attention must be directed to understanding the "how to" of intervention design, as well as the relative merits of different intervention strategies.

Defining the Content of RTI Interventions

A comprehensive RTI intervention strategy requires three levels of action:

- primary prevention—preventing the acquisition of infection: prevention of sexually transmitted infections, prevention of endogenous infections, and prevention of iatrogenic infections;
- secondary prevention—identifying and treating established infection: management of symptomatic infections, screening for asymptomatic infections, and mass treatment approaches; and
- tertiary prevention—minimizing the adverse consequences of such infection.

Obviously, primary prevention of infection has tremendous intuitive appeal because it diminishes the subsequent need for the other interventions. Identification and treatment of established infection is also crucial, however, as it has important effects at both the individual and community level, particularly for sexually transmitted infections. Indeed, STD case-finding efforts (a secondary prevention strategy) also prevent a large number of primary infections (or reinfections) when they are combined with appropriate clinical management, client counseling, and partner notification, referral and treatment (Cates and Holmes, 1992). Finally, concerted attempts to minimize the adverse sequelae of RTIs (e.g., tubal infertility, ectopic pregnancy, or congenital infection) are also important given the large personal, social, and economic costs of these outcomes.

Primary Prevention

Strategies for the primary prevention of RTIs vary according to the type of infection; see Table 3-4. Primary prevention of sexually transmitted infections predominately involves personal behavioral change, with an emphasis on sexual behaviors and practices (Choi and Coates, 1994; Over and Piot, 1993). Prevention of endogenous infections also requires personal behavioral change, but with an emphasis on a range of hygienic and health-related behaviors. In contrast, prevention of iatrogenic infections requires attention to issues of service quality, with an emphasis on

TABLE 3-4 Strategies for Primary Prevention of Reproductive Tract Infections

Type of Infection	Prevention Strategy
Sexually Transmitted	Delaying sexual initiation (coital debut)
	Reducing number of sexual partners or rate of partner change
	Changing the dynamics of partner selection
	Reducing nonconsensual sexual exposure
	Encouraging safer sexual practices
	Promoting condom use
	Providing voluntary counseling and testing
	Promoting use of other barrier methods
	Encouraging male circumcision (?)
Endogenous	Improving knowledge of reproductive physiology and menstrual and personal hygiene
	Promoting appropriate help-seeking behavior
	Reducing the use of harmful intravaginal substances (i.e., douches and desiccants)
	Reducing the inappropriate use of systemic antibiotics
Iatrogenic	Improving access to safe delivery and abortion services
	Improving infection control practices
	Improving provider technical competence
	Enhancing the management of service delivery (quality of care)
	Providing antibiotics prophylactically (?)

(?), Evidence of effectiveness or cost-effectiveness is weaker than for other strategies.

the technical competence of providers and adherence to infection control practices.

Primary Prevention of Sexually Transmitted Infections

Various behaviors determine a person's risk of acquiring a sexually transmitted infection, thereby providing several opportunities for intervention. Primary prevention interventions stress either reducing an individual's risk of sexual contact with an infected person or decreasing the per-exposure probability of acquiring an infection. Secondary prevention efforts (discussed below) seek to decrease the duration of infectiousness for those STDs (primarily bacterial) that are amenable to treatment. Three factors in combination—the likelihood of contact with an infected person, the efficacy of per-exposure transmission, and the duration of infectiousness—are the principal determinants of the spread of sexually transmitted infection within a population (Anderson and May, 1988).

Strategies to reduce exposure to infections include encouraging a delay in the initiation of sexual activity, a reduction in the number of concurrent sexual partners, a reduction in the rate of sexual partner change, more careful selection of sexual partners, and efforts to reduce the incidence of nonconsensual sex. Strategies to reduce the per-exposure risk of infection include avoiding certain sexual practices, treatment of other RTIs, and the promotion of condoms and other vaginal barrier methods (see Table 3-4).

Delay of Initiation of Sexual Activity   Delaying the initiation of sexual activity is especially important because of the enhanced biological susceptibility of adolescents to sexually transmitted infections and their consequences (Gotardi et al., 1984). Behavioral research findings also suggest that early coital debut is associated with a subsequent higher prevalence of high-risk sexual practices (Kost and Forrest, 1992). A recognition of the difficulties adolescents often face in obtaining reproductive health services (Karim et al., 1992; Flisher, Roberts, and Blignaut, 1992) is another reason to encourage this approach.

Several successful programs have been described (Coates and Makadon, 1995; Kirby et al., 1991; Howard and McCabe, 1990; Walter and Vaugh, 1993). The essential elements of success seem to be peer intervention approaches that stress autonomy and healthy decision making, and the provision of accurate information concerning sexuality, the consequences of unprotected sexual activity, and the available options for avoiding infection and unwanted pregnancy. Providing accurate information on sexuality to adolescents has not been shown to increase early sexual activity; indeed, when an effect has been documented, these interventions have been associated with a significant delay in the initiation of sexual activity (Kirby et al., 1994; Holtzman et al., 1994; Kirby et al., 1991).

Reduction of Number of Partners Encouraging a reduction in the number of sexual partners is an important means of reducing the spread of STDs. As some people, particularly young and unmarried individuals, may have only one partner at a time but high rates of partner change ("serial monogamy"), reducing the rate of new partner acquisition is also important (Anderson, 1989). It should be emphasized, however, that many currently monogamous individuals may still be at some risk of sexually transmitted infection—either through the multiple sexual partnerships of their sole sexual partner or as a consequence of infections acquired prior to a committed, mutually monogamous, relationship. This risk exists particularly for chronic viral infections, such as HPV, hepatitis B, and HIV infection, but also to those pathogens that may have long periods of asymptomatic carriage (e.g., trichomonas or chlamydia).

The risk that any particular sex partner has an STD is determined by a complex set of factors, including the overall prevalence of infection in the community, the variance in the rates of sexual partner change within that community, and characteristics of the particular sexual networks from which partners are selected (Caldwell, Orubuloye, and Caldwell, 1991; Anderson, 1989). Many of the macroenvironmental determinants discussed above serve to highly structure both the local epidemiology of infection as well as the social interactions that comprise any particular individual's network of sexual contacts. As a consequence, the same sexual behaviors can have different consequences depending on where and with whom they are practiced.

Awareness and Education Large investments have been made in mass communication efforts aimed at encouraging AIDS awareness, providing accurate information regarding the routes of HIV transmission and the available means of STD/HIV prevention, and minimizing discriminatory responses against those with HIV or perceived to be at risk of infection (Choi and Coates, 1994; Kelly et al., 1992). In general, the more successful campaigns have used a range of media, have been designed with appropriate attention to local cultural norms, and have employed audience segmentation and professional production and pretesting. Efforts to evaluate these approaches have focused primarily on their ability to improve knowledge and influence attitudes and, in this regard, have been fairly successful. However, convincing data that these approaches have, in themselves, resulted in significant behavior change are generally lacking. Indeed, a number of studies show a relatively poor correlation between improved knowledge and reduced risk behaviors (DiClemente et al., 1992; Aral and Peterman, 1993). Yet public awareness and knowledge of AIDS and other infectious diseases are necessary conditions for control of diseases, even if they are not sufficient by themselves. Continued provision of information is useful even while work continues on ways to affect behavior.

Within family planning programs, HIV/AIDS information and prevention messages have been successfully incorporated into existing information, education, and communication efforts. When such efforts have been evaluated, they have accomplished their purposes without any adverse effects on contraceptive service provision. For example, in Colombia, community-based family planning field workers were randomized into two groups (Vernon, Ojeda, and Murad, 1990): the providers in the experimental group were requested to dedicate 20 percent of their time to AIDS prevention activities and encouraged to establish outreach to groups of potentially high-risk clients; the control group was to simply respond to clients' requests for AIDS information. The authors found community-based field workers could successfully incorporate AIDS prevention activities into their responsibilities without harming their contraceptive sales. A variety of other less rigorously evaluated efforts have also demonstrated the feasibility of incorporating STD and AIDS awareness efforts into existing family planning programs (Stover, 1988; Apao and Darden, 1993; Finger, 1994). Such efforts require resources, however, particularly for training and materials development. Resource limitations have limited service integration in many settings.

A broad variety of peer interventions have also been developed as primary prevention programs. These typically focus on both promoting condom use and reducing the number of partners. In one well-designed and -evaluated peer intervention among gay men in the United States, popular opinion leaders were trained to deliver HIV prevention messages to men in gay bars. The intervention was successful, producing significant reductions in unprotected anal intercourse of 15-29 percent from baseline levels (Kelly et al., 1992). The peer interventions literature is characterized by sizable variability in observed program effects, arising from broad variability in specific program approach and design, the intensity of intervention, and the outcome measures. Even more than other types of primary prevention efforts, peer interventions require further exploration, documentation, and description of the tenets for success.

Change in the Dynamics of Partner Selection Changing the dynamics of partner selection, while addressing a potentially important determinant of infection risk, is difficult. First, sexual behaviors are private. Second, the probability that a potential partner has an active infection cannot be readily discerned. Indeed, attempts to do so based on sociodemographic characteristics often invite stigmatization, with its attendant social discrimination. Consequently, opportunities for intervention in this area are somewhat limited. One approach is to encourage men to refrain from the purchase of commercial sexual services. For example, it has been suggested that large industries employing sizable migrant labor forces should consider providing for the relocation of workers' spouses as a means of reducing the demand for commercial sex (Sweat and Denison, 1995). Another approach is to encourage more open communication between all sex partners concerning the risk of sexually transmitted infection and the available means of protection. This latter approach may be most important in facilitating condom or other barrier method use among intimate partners, but it may also discourage partnership with individuals unwilling to discuss and negotiate these issues. Intervention in this area will require an emphasis on skills building, not just didactic information. Other structural approaches that promote women's economic independence (e.g., changing wife inheritance laws) or aim to change harmful cultural practices (e.g., those forms of ritual cleansing that involve sexual intercourse) may also be an important means for changing the dynamics of partner selection (O'Reilly and Islam, 1995; Lamptey et al., 1995; Sweat and Denison, 1995).

Reduction of Nonconsensual Sexual Exposure   Program efforts to reduce the incidence of nonconsensual sex are an important—and often overlooked—means of reducing the risk of exposure to sexually transmitted infections (Heise and Elias, 1995). In these situations, by definition, sexual partners are not selected, but some structural attempts can be made to reduce exposure to those settings where unwanted sexual activity may be encountered. Efforts to encourage more responsible sexuality among men are the most important in this regard. For example, a number of approaches—mostly involving peer interventions and the reduction of substance use—have recently been described as means for reducing the occurrence of "date rape" (Holcomb et al., 1993; Baylis and Myers, 1990; Hanson and Gidycz, 1993; Miller, 1988; Funk, 1993; Dating Violence Intervention Project, 1988).

Encouragement of Safer Sexual Practices   Information concerning the higher relative risk of infection associated with certain specific sexual practices—such as receptive anal intercourse—can be included in health promotion messages, along with accurate information concerning the effectiveness of barrier methods of contraception. Some programs have also encouraged alternatives to penetrative sexual intercourse, sometimes referred to as "outercourse." These messages encourage couples to explore alternative expressions of sexual intimacy that do not carry a risk of sexually transmitted infection. The messages, as well as attempts to eroticize safer sex, have been effective at changing behavior on a short-term basis in peer interventions among gay men (Kelly et al., 1992; Kegeles, Hayes, and Coates, 1995). Few intervention efforts have singled out specific sexual practices, however; consequently, it is not possible to discern the relative contribution of safer sexual practices and increased use of barrier methods of contraception to the observed outcomes.

Condom Promotion   When properly and consistently used, latex condoms are highly effective in reducing the spread of sexually transmitted infections (Centers for Disease Control and Prevention, 1988a; Feldblum and Joanis, 1994). Some recent data are also available concerning the effectiveness of the polyurethane vaginal sheath (female condom), and this device has been approved by the U.S. Food and Drug Administration (FDA) for marketing as a means of STD prevention (Feldblum and Joanis, 1994; Centers for Disease Control and Prevention, 1993b). Approval for several new nonlatex "plastic" male condoms is also being sought.

Efforts to promote the consistent use of good quality latex condoms, like reducing the number of partners, have been one of the principal AIDS prevention strategies for the past decade. Not surprisingly, condom promotion efforts have used many of the same approaches—and have most often been combined with—efforts to encourage partner reduction. The biggest challenge for condom promotion is encouraging use with steady partners. In many settings where men have become willing to use condoms with casual, commercial, or new partners, there is still little use within steady relationships (Van Landingham et al., 1995). Similarly, even among commercial sex workers who routinely use condoms with clients, there is a much lower rate of condom use with boyfriends (Dorfman, Derish, and Cohen, 1992).

Condom promotion efforts have included mass communication, peer interventions, and a number of innovative approaches, such as the use of street theater and commercial social marketing (see below). Condom promotion poses an additional challenge when compared with partner reduction strategies, however: not only must programs achieve the goals of accurate information provision and motivation for behavioral change, but they must also ensure that condom commodities of sufficient quality are readily available to those motivated to use them. Periodic failures in condom procurement, distribution logistics, and supply have sometimes been a major impediment to the successful implementation of condom promotion efforts.

One of the most successful strategies has been condom social marketing (Population Services International, 1994). Using the full range of techniques of commercial marketing, condom social marketing programs have used a wide range of print and broadcast media, widespread outlet distribution, and point-of-purchase advertising to greatly increase the volume of condom sales (which can plausibly be taken as an indicator of use), even in some of the world's poorest countries (Population Services International, 1994).

Successful condom promotion among vulnerable groups of women, such as sex workers, has posed a number of challenges and spawned a number of innovative community approaches. Several intervention trials among sex workers in Africa using community organizing techniques and training peer educators to conduct outreach among sex workers and clients have shown consistent improvements in reported condom use (Lamptey et al., 1995; Williams et al., 1992; Wilson, Myathi, and Whariwa, 1992; Asamoah-Adu et al., 1994). More recently, some programs have begun to explore structural or "enabling" approaches to promoting condom use, which are explicitly targeted to the broader determinants of infection risk (Tawil, O'Reilly, and Verster, 1995). In these approaches, public policies that facilitate safer sexual behaviors are promoted. The most successful of these efforts has been the 100 percent condom use policy established in brothels in Thailand (Rojanapithayakorn, 1992). In this program, the Thai government made condom use mandatory: local health officials use STD rates from monthly screening of registered sex workers to assess compliance and hold brothel owners and clients responsible. Recent surveillance data suggest a dramatic decline in STD incidence in recent years (Hanenberg et al., 1994). Other structural approaches focus on changing inheritance laws and funereal customs that involve sexual exchange between the bereaved spouse and other family members (O'Reilly and Islam, 1995).

Voluntary Counseling and Testing Another tactic for primary prevention has been voluntary counseling and testing for HIV antibodies. This approach has been a cornerstone of the HIV prevention effort in the United States since the mid-1980s (O'Reilly and Islam, 1995). The effect of these interventions have been mixed, however, with considerable variability between sites (Higgins et al., 1991; Choi and Coates, 1994). As with other intervention strategies, the various effects probably reflect underlying variation in the content and intensity of the counseling and support services provided.

In general, better results have been found when both partners are counseled and in settings in which clients actively seek out the services in comparison with those in which they encounter counseling and testing in the course of seeking other services (i.e., in an STD clinic). In the only randomized, controlled trial of counseling and testing that has been published (Wenger et al., 1991), subjects were randomized to receive "AIDS education alone" versus "AIDS education plus voluntary counseling and testing." Twice as many people in the second group were using condoms 8 weeks after the intervention, but that was still less than one-half of those who participated in the intervention. Given the costs of counseling and testing, mostly for adequate pre- and post-test counseling, this strategy may not be cost-effective as a way to promote condom use in developing countries. Several further evaluations are planned (O'Reilly and Islam, 1995). The most important unanswered questions concern issues of consent and the need for counseling. One study in Kenya found that, even after giving informed consent, many women did not actively request their test results, suggesting that other factors beside interest in their HIV serostatus influenced their decision to accept testing as part of a study protocol (Temmerman et al., 1995). Some researchers have suggested that the requirement for extensive counseling be abandoned; they propose instead the widespread availability of home testing for HIV, using saliva diagnostic kits (Frerichs et al., 1994). The pros and cons of the home testing debate have recently been summarized by Krieger and Stryker (1995).

Promotion of the Use of Other Barrier Methods   Data concerning the use of chemical barrier methods—such as spermicides containing nonoxynol-9 and other biodetergents—for primary prevention of STDs are mixed. Similarly, published data concerning the effectiveness of other physical barriers (such as the diaphragm and cervical cap) for infection prevention are limited. Based on a review of 10 observational studies, Rosenberg and Gollub (1992) estimate that use of existing female barrier methods reduces the transmission of gonorrhea and chlamydia by roughly 50 to 75 percent. Some data also suggest that regular use of spermicides is associated with a lower risk of cervical cancer, an event known to be associated with HPV infection of the reproductive tract (Hildesheim et al., 1990). Spermicidal products are not currently approved by the U.S. FDA for use as microbicidal agents, and data concerning the efficacy of these products for prevention of HIV remain inconclusive (Cates and Stone, 1992; Feldblum and Joanis, 1994). One study of sex workers in the Cameroon demonstrated substantial protection from HIV infection among women using the vaginal contraceptive film (Zekeng et al., 1993). Another study among sex workers in Kenya, however, showed no protection and raised the concern that, in high doses, spermicides might enhance infection by causing vaginal inflammation or ulceration (Kreiss et al., 1992).

The public policy question of whether to include a broad recommendation to use chemical barrier methods as a means of infection prevention when condom use cannot be successfully negotiated is still a matter of considerable debate (Stein, 1992; Rosenberg and Gollub, 1992; Niruthisard, Roddy, and Chutivongse, 1992). The New York State Health Department has produced materials outlining a "hierarchy of prevention options" that recommends using other woman-controlled barrier methods in the event that a woman is unsuccessful in negotiating condom use with her male partner (Cleary, 1994). Obviously, the availability of safe and effective vaginal microbicidal products would be an important addition to the prevention armamentarium (Elias and Heise, 1994).

Male Circumcision   Given the known association between male circumcision and a lower incidence of both genital ulcer disease and HIV infection (Moses et al., 1994), some public health officials have suggested the strategy of recommending male circumcision as a means of primary infection prevention. Such an approach would require extensive community consultation, sensitivity to cultural norms, and an understanding of its potential acceptability. No published evaluations of this type of intervention are available.

Prevention of Endogenous Infection

The prevention of endogenous RTIs, such as bacterial vaginosis and candidiasis, requires efforts to improve women's and men's knowledge of reproductive physiology, menstrual and personal hygiene, health-seeking behavior, and adherence with prescribed therapy. It also requires reducing the use of harmful intravaginal substances (i.e., douches and desiccants), as well as curtailing the inappropriate use of broad-spectrum, systemic antibiotics (Wölner-Hansen et al., 1990). These latter approaches will require changing the recommendations and prescriptive practices of both traditional and allopathic health care providers, pharmacists, and family members, as well as individuals. To date, no intervention programs explicitly aiming to reduce the incidence of endogenous infections have been reported in the literature.

Prevention of Iatrogenic Infection

In contrast to preventing sexually transmitted and endogenous infections—which primarily requires personal behavioral change strategies—preventing iatrogenic infections requires intervention to improve the overall quality of reproductive health services and, in particular, transcervical medical procedures. Preventing such infections will require careful consideration of the current inadequacies of the medical care system, especially for provider training, infection control, and accessibility of services.

The greatest opportunity to prevent unnecessary morbidity and significant mortality associated with iatrogenic RTIs is to eliminate the need for unsafe abortion procedures. This goal is likely to be promoted by improving the supply of contraceptive services to those who desire them, widely promoting the use of emergency contraception, and decriminalizing abortion services (Alan Guttmacher Institute, 1994; Ellertson et al., 1995). Chapter 4 discusses some of the training and quality assurance efforts that could lead to lower rates of iatrogenic infection from abortion procedures. Given that a large number of septic procedures still occur in some areas, even where abortion has been legalized, successful intervention will also require ensuring an adequate number of trained abortion providers and, ultimately, the availability of safe alternatives to surgical abortion in the form of medical abortifacients that do not require transcervical procedures. Better training of providers to ensure the optimal treatment of abortion complications before infection develops will also be necessary.

Reducing the number of infections associated with other transcervical procedures, such as IUD insertion, will require more attention to adherence with infection control guidelines, improved provider technical competence, strengthening client counseling to help guide optimal contraceptive choice and proper use, and enhancing the overall management of service delivery programs. Given that some number of procedure-related infections occur even with optimal technique, the utility of antibiotic prophylaxis administered at the time of these procedures has also been investigated (Ladipo et al., 1991; Sinei et al., 1990). These results have been mixed, largely because of the unexpectedly low incidence of PID observed even among those IUD users who have received placebo regimens. Further studies, particularly studies involving new single-dose therapeutic regimens, may be necessary to fully understand the benefits and costs of use of antibiotics.

Secondary Prevention

Secondary prevention—the identification and treatment of established infections of the reproductive tract—is also an important element of a comprehensive intervention strategy; see Table 3-5. Appropriate treatment relieves symptomatic morbidity, prevents the more serious complications of infection that result in additional morbidity and occasional mortality, and serves to limit the duration of infectiousness—a critical determinant in the sustained spread of sexually transmitted infection. Unfortunately, a large proportion of RTIs are asymptomatic, especially in women. This characteristic of RTIs limits the utility of approaches that only treat symptomatic infection. Thus, while clinical management of symptomatic infections is essential, it is not adequate in itself. There

TABLE 3-5 Strategies for Secondary Prevention (Identification and Treatment) of Reproductive Tract Infections

Kind of Identification or Treatment	Strategy
Management of symptomatic infections	Standardized case management Encouraging prompt care seeking Improving treatment adherence Encouraging abstinence during treatment Clinic-based counselling for prevention
Screening for asymptomatic infections	Serologic screening Urine, pelvic exam(?) Case finding, especially for cervical infections (e.g., gonorrhea and chlamydia) Partner notification and referral
Mass treatment	Prophylaxis for neonatal gonococcal ophthalmia "Epidemiologic" treatment of core transmitters and communities with high rates of RTI prevalence

(?), Evidence of effectiveness is weaker than for other strategies.

are two general strategies for addressing asymptomatic RTIs: case finding or screening, an effective approach although limited by the cost of diagnosis, follow-up, and treatment; and selective mass treatment. In the latter approach, there is no attempt to identify specific infections; rather, all members of a target population believed to be at risk are empirically treated with effective therapy. This approach has had limited application to date, but some interesting studies are under way.

Management of Symptomatic Infections

While a sizable proportion of RTIs are asymptomatic, many infections are symptomatic. Symptomatic men and women with RTIs can be classified with a number of clinical syndromes, including urethral discharge, vaginal discharge, genital ulcer, lower abdominal pain, and inguinal swelling. The World Health Organization (1991, 1994) has developed a set of standardized flowcharts or algorithms to help guide the clinical management of these syndromes in a variety of service settings, including those with and without microscopy facilities. Appendix A reproduces the most recent revision of WHO guidelines for the management of STD-associated syndromes.

Unfortunately, the performance of these algorithms in practice has been variable: the algorithms work well for genital ulcer disease and symptomatic urethral discharge in men; however, in the case of those syndromes most common among women—vaginal discharge and lower abdominal pain—their performance is less than optimal (Vuylsteke et al., 1993). A number of studies have shown a poor correlation between women's symptoms, clinical observations made during vaginal and pelvic examination, and the presence of infection as detected by laboratory testing (Bang et al., 1989; Wasserheit et al., 1989; Grosskurth et al., 1994; Younis et al., 1993; Zurayk et al., 1995). For example, in one study conducted in Zaire to assess the diagnostic validity of the WHO flowcharts, the hierarchical algorithms for vaginal discharge and lower abdominal pain had only 48 percent sensitivity and 75.2 percent specificity when applied to pregnant women and 54.9 percent sensitivity and 52.2 percent specificity when applied to female sex workers (Vuylsteke et al., 1993). A poor correlation with the actual presence of infection means that a large proportion of women are unnecessarily treated, while others who have infections remain undetected.

This situation is further compounded by the complexities of health-seeking behavior among men and women who experience symptoms of infection. Many people with RTI symptoms follow a sequence of therapeutic practices, beginning with self-treatment in the home and progressing through remedies provided by family members, pharmacists, and a variety of traditional healers before seeking health services from allopathic providers (Olukoya and Elias, 1994). Whether the development of health education efforts that encourage more prompt health-seeking behavior among symptomatic individuals will improve the utility of clinical algorithms remains to be tested. More timely health-seeking behavior will change the characteristics of the population presenting for syndromic management, which may influence the performance characteristics of the therapeutic algorithms. Consequently, it is important to validate standardized clinical management tools among the populations in which they will actually be used.

Although the current WHO algorithms are not ideal, standardized case management must be considered a mandatory intervention for the responsible delivery of contraceptive and other reproductive health services. Many men and women currently come to services complaining of symptoms related to RTIs. Unfortunately, providers are often poorly informed about women's perceptions of reproductive tract symptoms and the cultural idioms of symptom presentation (Zurayk et al., 1995). Failure to address a client's concern undermines the credibility of the service delivery system. Too often individuals in need of care are sent away without any attention given to their presenting complaint, or they are given a vague referral to an STD treatment facility to which they cannot or will not go.

The challenge is to refine current guidelines for clinical management of symptomatic RTIs within existing reproductive health facilities. Ideally, this would be done in the light of data concerning the local epidemiology of infection and antibiotic resistance patterns. One benefit of such an approach would be to minimize the costly and unnecessary overtreatment of clients and potentially improve clinical outcomes through standardizing therapy, thereby allowing program managers to select the most cost-effective therapeutic regimens (again, ideally based on local data) and streamline drug procurement processes.

In refining the algorithms, one important issue that urgently requires clarification is the utility of linking syndromic management to behavioral risk screening. WHO flowcharts have included a number of screening questions regarding sexual behavior (World Health Organization, 1991). Risk assessment is positive only if patient answers yes to: Does your sexual partner have a discharge from his penis or open sores anywhere in his genital area? Or if she answers yes to two or more of the following: Are you younger than 21 years? Are you unmarried or not in union? Have you been with your husband or sexual partner for less than 3 months? Have you had more than one sexual partner in the last 4 weeks?

The purpose of these questions is to help distinguish between cervical infections (which have more serious complications and require more intensive treatment) and vaginal infections (which are more common). Given the generally poor predictive performance of the vaginal discharge algorithm, treating all women with a discharge syndrome for cervical infection has the potential to result in high levels of overtreatment with broad spectrum antibiotics, an outcome that has significant costs both in terms of resources and the possible emergence of antibiotic resistance. Unfortunately, there are few data to determine whether these questions significantly improve the diagnostic performance of the algorithms in the majority of settings in developing countries where they will be applied. As discussed further below, risk screening approaches have sometimes had paradoxical results (e.g., when applied to interventions to reduce maternal morbidity and mortality; Rooks and Winikoff, 1990). Therefore, caution must be used in recommending the combination of an essential, potentially highly cost-effective intervention strategy (standardized case management) with a behavioral risk screening approach that has had limited testing.

The combined approach may be helped by local definition of the risk screening criteria. One recent study conducted in a Jamaican STD clinic, for example, evaluated the sensitivity of diagnosing cervical infection with an algorithm designed to combine a woman's symptomatology with an assessment of her risk status. In that population, the WHO flowchart, including risk assessment, was 84 percent sensitive and 40 percent specific for cervicitis diagnosis (Behets et al., 1995). Adaptation of the algorithm on the basis of local data was found to be slightly more specific, though somewhat less sensitive, and a modification of the WHO algorithm was defined for local use. Behets et al. (1995:15) concluded that "the generation of regional data enhanced local acceptability of algorithm approaches."

Ultimately, the predictive performance of standardized algorithms may be further improved by the development of newer and simpler diagnostic tests for RTIs. Recently, a number of initiatives to promote the development of STD diagnostic technology applicable in resource-poor settings have been launched (Berkely, 1994), and there has been some early success. For example, the use of a simple dipstick test for the presence of leukocyte esterase may greatly improve screening efforts among men who either have asymptomatic urethritis or experience mild symptoms without gross discharge (Shafer et al., 1989; Mayaud et al., 1992). Rapid advances in gene amplification and the use of urine as a specimen source for antigen detection (Quinn, 1994) are also promising approaches, but they are still experimental and prohibitively expensive.

Developing an acceptable flowchart for standardizing the management of symptomatic individuals is only the first step in treatment. Experience in primary care settings routinely using flowcharts to manage other clinical conditions (e.g., acute respiratory infections in children) suggests that more operational research is needed to successfully introduce such strategies to a variety of providers in a range of clinical practice settings (Pan American Health Organization, 1983). At a minimum, the widespread use of standardized case management strategies will require a sizable investment in provider training and retraining.

Efforts to upgrade diagnostic facilities and ensure adequate antibiotic supplies are also needed. One randomized community trial in Mwanza, Tanzania, has recently shown that improved STD case management had a significant impact on HIV incidence (Grosskurth et al., 1995). Primary health care clinics in six rural intervention communities received STD health education, staff training on the use of syndromic treatment algorithms, a regular supply of antibiotics, supervisory visits, and access to an STD reference clinic. The HIV incidence was reduced by more than 40 percent in this population after the integration of this package of STD services within the primary health care system. (In comparison with randomly matched communities, the prevalence of other STDs was also consistently lower in the intervention communities, but these results were not statistically significant.)

In addition to using standardized case management to choose therapeutic interventions, efforts are also needed to improve treatment adherence (compliance) and encourage sexual abstinence for the duration of therapy among those diagnosed with STDs. Clinics also have to allow sufficient time for providers to conduct appropriate counseling regarding the primary prevention of RTIs, condom use, and the importance of partner notification and treatment. Some public health researchers have suggested that the opportunity to provide such directed prevention advice may be as important as the treatment itself in reducing the spread of RTIs (O'Reilly and Islam, 1995).

Screening for Asymptomatic Infections

Interventions aimed at screening for asymptomatic infections (case finding) have historically been an important strategy for STD control. For example, serologic screening for syphilis infection is a standard component of routine antenatal care in many settings (Centers for Disease Control and Prevention, 1988b, 1993a). Providing prompt treatment for mothers has proven to be an extremely cost-effective strategy for preventing congenital syphilis, even in extremely resource poor settings (Hira, Bhat, and Chikamata, 1990; Stray-Pederson, 1983). Syphilis screening requires minimal diagnostic facility, is relatively inexpensive, requires therapy with antibiotics that could be readily available and affordable in most settings, and requires a modest level of client follow-up and treatment adherence. Therefore, the widespread implementation of screening for asymptomatic syphilis infections in antenatal clinics can be seen as a "sentinel" intervention. Yet although the necessary steps to ensure antenatal syphilis screening, maternal follow-up, and appropriate treatment are all relatively simple, they are rarely successfully coordinated in most developing country settings (Temmerman, Mohamedali, and Fransen, 1993). Successful establishment of antenatal syphilis screening could, therefore, serve as a benchmark of the programmatic capacity to design and effectively achieve more complicated interventions, such as case finding for other infections (Schulz, Schulte, and Berman, 1992).

In considering screening for other asymptomatic infections, cervical infections in women (primarily caused by gonorrhea and chlamydia) are an important priority, given the high costs associated with PID and its complications. Diagnostic screening for these infections with currently available technology is neither simple nor inexpensive, however, so such screening must be rationed. A number of studies are available to suggest that screening for asymptomatic cervical gonococcal and chlamydial infections is cost-effective in family planning settings in industrialized countries (Trachtenberg, Washington, and Halldorson, 1988; Handsfield et al., 1986; Begley, McGill, and Smith, 1989). Selective screening is most cost-effective when prevalence is generally low (i.e., 2-3%); in high prevalence settings (> 5%), universal screening is the more cost-effective approach, if affordable (Marrazzo et al., 1997). Hence, in selecting those for screening, sub-populations known to have a higher prevalence of infection are sought (Over and Piot, 1993; Aral and Peterman, 1993). Again, the relative cost-effectiveness of this screening may improve as simpler and less expensive diagnostic tests become available.

Another potentially important method for identifying people with asymptomatic sexually transmitted infections is through partner notification and referral efforts (formerly known as contact tracing). Identification and treatment of infected partners could also help lower the risk of reinfection for women who have been treated for STDs. Partner notification may be either passive—infected people are expected to personally notify their partners concerning the possibility of infection and the need for treatment ("patient referral")—or active—clinic staff solicit names of sexual contacts and attempt to contact them ("provider referral"). The second approach is obviously more costly, but it is also more effective (Judson and Wolf, 1978). However, studies of the effectiveness of partner notification efforts in both developed and developing country settings have had mixed results (O'Reilly and Islam, 1995; Andrus et al., 1990; Winifield and Latif, 1985; Asuzu, Rotowa, and Ajayi, 1990). More research concerning the optimal design of partner notification efforts is needed to refine this set of interventions.

Mass Treatment Approaches

Treatment of an entire group of individuals at risk of infection (without diagnosing individual infections in the population) requires that the therapy administered be safe, highly effective, inexpensive, and associated with minimal side effects. A mass treatment approach requires that the intervention be acceptable to the community concerned and that the number of infections prevented be sufficient to justify the expense and any possible risks (World Health Organization, 1986). For many years, putting silver nitrate or antibacterial eyedrops in the eyes of newborn infants as a prophylaxis against ophthalmia neonatorum caused by gonorrhea has met these criteria (Brunham, Holmes, and Embree, 1990). This intervention ranks among the most cost-effective in terms of preventing serious morbidity (preventable blindness) at exceptionally low cost (Laga, Meheus, and Piot, 1989).

Another mass treatment strategy involves the treatment of populations with high STD prevalence with antibiotics known to be effective against pathogens prevalent in those communities. To be effective at the population level, mass treatment interventions require high treatment compliance and coverage and need to take into account local migration patterns and sexual networks. After considering these factors, STD mass treatment interventions have generally focused on treating either specific subpopulations known to have high STD rates (such as sex workers and migrant laborers) or entire communities with high STD rates. A "selective mass treatment" program among female sex workers (introduced as an addition to a long-established screening program) in the Philippines had a strong initial effect on the prevalence of gonorrhea, but this effect dissipated after a few months because of high rates of reinfection (Holmes et al., 1996).

Recently, several authors have suggested that "epidemiologic" STD control may also be a worthwhile HIV intervention strategy (Wawer et al., 1995; Cates, Rothenberg, and Blount, 1996). The potential for bacterial and parasitic infections of the reproductive tract to augment the transmission of HIV (Wasserheit, 1992; Clottey and Dallabetta, 1993) makes this an attractive strategy in areas where HIV is highly endemic.

One STD mass treatment trial is currently being conducted among communities in Rakai, Uganda. Twenty-six villages have been randomly selected to receive the intervention: mass treatment of all consenting individuals aged 15-59 every 9 to 10 months with antibiotics, in addition to an intensive health education and condom distribution campaign. In 26 control villages, the population receives the health education and condom distribution campaign, but not mass treatment for STDs; people will be referred for STD treatment based on their symptoms or positive serologic test results for syphilis (Wawer, 1995). The sustainability of this type of mass treatment intervention has been questioned, however, given the high costs of the treatment regimens involved (*Science*, 1995). The trial may also provide further information concerning the nature of STD/HIV synergy in both asymptomatic and symptomatic populations.

When comparing a mass treatment approach with other STD treatment strategies, one should consider the estimated rates of reinfection and the feasibility of providing adequate clinic-based STD services within a population. In practice, a mass treatment approach may be best used as an initial, one-time intervention to lower overall STD prevalence, in conjunction with the establishment of adequate STD diagnostic and treatment services to sustain the reduction in STD prevalence over time.

Tertiary Prevention

The third set of interventions is tertiary prevention, minimizing the impact of complications of infection. The main components of tertiary prevention are clinical management of septic abortion, alarm and transport for ectopic pregnancies, the management of infertility, and cervical cancer screening. As noted above, these complications are a major source of reproductive morbidity and mortality. For many of these conditions, the associated disability costs are fairly high, but so are the perceived costs of intervention. Consequently, the threshold to intervene is often quite high and a vicious cycle has developed. Because interventions have rarely been attempted, proven models for successful program development in resource-poor settings are lacking, and inexperience fuels programmatic complacency.

Strengthening the clinical management of women who go to health facilities with complications of septic abortion is a priority area for intervention. Effective programs have the potential to avert many of the deaths that occur each year as a result of unsafe abortion (McLaurin, Hord, and Wolf, 1990). A number of programs for training providers in the use of appropriate technology, such as manual vacuum aspiration, have been developed and implemented. Of course, efforts to manage the complications of septic abortion must be accompanied by concerted efforts to prevent septic abortion in the first place. Strengthening postabortion contraceptive services is an important strategy.

Another life-threatening complication of some RTIs is ectopic pregnancy. When this occurs, it typically presents as a medical emergency requiring urgent surgical intervention. Successful clinical management of this uncommon, but serious, condition will depend largely on the availability of appropriate diagnostic and transport systems to ensure safe maternity (see Chapter 4). This is particularly important for women in rural areas who must travel considerable distances to surgical facilities.

The management of infertility and the development of screening programs to detect and manage cervical neoplasms are examples of other areas where interventions are needed to manage the complications of reproductive tract infection. Recently, the WHO Special Programme on Human Reproduction has developed a manual on "simplified infertility management" for developing countries (Rowe et al., 1993). A number of pilot projects for cervical cancer screening have also been recently started (Blumenthal et al., 1994; AVSC International and Program for Appropriate Technology in Health, 1994). To date, however, little data are available concerning cost-effective interventions to reduce the impact of these complications.

RECOMMENDATIONS

We present first our general recommendations for the promotion of infection-free reproductive health. Specific recommendations are then discussed in three areas: immediate priorities for existing reproductive health programs, including those programs initially established either primarily or exclusively to provide family planning services; program gaps, highlighting the need to expand services to those groups currently not reached by any reproductive health services, especially men and young adults; and research priorities.

As noted above, data concerning the cost and effectiveness of the many interventions for preventing and treating RTIs and their consequences are extremely limited. With finite resources, difficult choices will need to be made. These choices will be shaped by existing facility infrastructures, health personnel, research capacity, among other factors, and should be the outcome of considered debate in local communities.

General Recommendations

1. Policy makers and program managers should design locally relevant and culturally sensitive RTI prevention and treatment programs.

2. The actual content of intervention programs and the challenges posed by their implementation should be accurately monitored and evaluated.

3. The cost and effectiveness of the various intervention strategies to prevent RTIs should be evaluated and compared.

Immediate Priorities

Much can be done right now by family planning programs to respond to the concerns of their clients and staff about RTIs, STDs, and HIV/AIDS. All clinic staff need to be well-informed about HIV/AIDS so that they can answer their clients' basic questions. In this respect, it is important that staff learn to work through any fears they may have about AIDS or any judgmental attitudes they may harbor toward people with STDs. This will enable them to respond accurately and with sensitivity to those who may be infected or at risk of becoming infected.

Clinic staff also should be aware of the symptoms of RTIs so that even if diagnosis and treatment are not available on site, their knowledge can be taken into account when considering the method of family planning most appropriate for each client. Family planning programs should also consider clients' risk of exposure to RTIs in determining protocols for providing various contraceptive methods. Barrier methods, particularly condoms, could be a better option for some clients despite being considered "less effective" contraceptive methods. For some clients, the secondary benefits of RTI prevention may be as important as the primary benefit of contraception. Programs should have well-designed informational materials dealing with RTIs, STDs, and AIDS available for staff and clients. For example, simple, pictorial instructions on how to correctly use and dispose of condoms are essential. All clinicians cannot assume that people know how to use condoms. Many do not, and embarrassment about such ineptitude has been shown in some studies to be a major reason why some people at risk still do not use condoms (Richters, 1994).

Program managers should encourage provision of basic RTI treatment services in clinics whenever possible. If services cannot be offered on site, providers should make the effort to learn which testing and treatment services for RTIs, STDs, and AIDS are available in their area and refer clients to these services as appropriate. Clinics and community-based distribution programs should have ample condom supplies for distribution to clients. Moreover, clients should be resupplied as quickly, efficiently, and as unobtrusively as possible.

Program Gaps

Health systems, particularly those in resource poor settings, often fail in their attempts to recognize or coordinate an effective response to RTI prevention or treatment. This failure occurs for a number of reasons, including weak management information systems, poor logistics and commodity distribution, inadequate provider training, and a narrow policy focus. Periodic disruptions of the supply of condoms and antibiotics are a particularly unfortunate example of this type of programmatic deficiency. Lapses in infection control practices are another common program failure.

The overall management of reproductive health services should be strengthened as a means to ensure implementation of interventions known to be effective. The establishment and monitoring of infection prevention standards for clinical services could be seen as a "sentinel" intervention. Infection prevention, consisting of simple measures such as hand washing, appropriate use of gloves, and adequate sterilization of instruments should be a minimum standard for all service delivery. Monitoring services for lapses in infection prevention practices will allow program managers to identify gaps in provider training and motivation, interruptions in supply and logistics systems, and difficulties in coordination between different service elements. If basic infection prevention practices cannot be ensured, it is unlikely that other, more complicated interventions for RTI prevention or treatment will succeed. This overall monitoring may best be accomplished by an explicit attempt to build an alliance with service providers as a means of promoting a general climate of organizational development within service programs. The COPE (client-oriented, provider-efficient) method of self-assessment developed by AVSC International is an excellent example of such an approach (Dwyer and Jezowski, 1995).

One of the problems facing program managers in large service delivery systems is the lack of well-defined mechanism for "going to scale" with successful small-scale pilot projects. This is especially a problem in the government sector in developing countries. Larger scale demonstration projects that are developed with the input of all relevant community groups (including government, nongovernmental service organizations, advocacy groups) and attempt to implement a broad range of RTI interventions within the constraints of a typical community's budget would be helpful in gaining experience in this area. The participation of community decision makers is an essential element for the sustainability of these intervention efforts.

Another urgent need is to expand the range of clients served by reproductive health programs. Adolescents, men, and the current users of traditional and informal sector services are examples of groups not reached through current programs. There is also a need to work with private sector services to improve the quality of their efforts to prevent and treat RTIs. Expanding services may require relaxing some of the current restrictions on nonphysician providers and changing some cultural assumptions regarding the presumed sexual abstinence of certain groups of women (i.e., adolescent, postpartum, or postmenopausal women). Correcting the current deficiency of trained female service providers through augmented training and support is also needed.

Research Priorities

Many unanswered questions concerning the optimal approach to achieving infection-free reproductive health would benefit considerably from both basic and applied research.

Seven topics should be the main priority areas for future research:

1. local characterization of RTI epidemiology and antibiotic sensitivity—and a low-cost methodology for making such assessments;
2. the relationships between perceptions of reproductive morbidity, syndromic presentation, and biomedical definitions of infection (including documentation of the current patterns of help-seeking behavior and the perceptions of men);
3. sexual behavior and factors influencing decision making concerning the use of prevention technologies, such as condoms and spermicides;
4. development and validation of case management strategies, as well as operations research on all aspects of service organization and delivery;
5. demonstration and pilot projects, focusing on models of integrated services;

6. product development research on low-cost RTI diagnostics, therapeutics, vaccines, and woman-controlled prevention technologies, such as vaginal microbicides; and

7. documentation of the interactions of RTIs and existing contraceptive technology.

4

Intended Births

The nations that signed the Programme of Action of the International Conference on Population and Development (ICPD) committed to try "... by the year 2015, ... to provide universal access to a full range of safe and reliable family-planning methods and to related reproductive health services which are not against the law" (United Nations, 1994:sect 9.1). Family planning programs contribute to reproductive health in two main ways: by allowing women and men to exercise the "freedom to decide if, when and how often" to have children (as included in the ICPD definition of reproductive health) and by reducing the number of times that a woman is exposed to the risks of unsafe pregnancy and delivery. In addition to these direct effects, there is evidence for a long-term impact as well: families that are not burdened by excess fertility can and do invest more in the nutrition, schooling, and health care of their wanted children. This investment, in turn, can be expected to improve the reproductive health of the next generation, among other benefits.

In this chapter we first discuss the evidence that unintended pregnancies and births are common. We next summarize the evidence that unintended pregnancies are harmful for the health and well-being women and their families. The bulk of this chapter then deals with some of the main problems confronting family planning programs and provision of safe abortions, which are the primary means through which public policy facilitates achievement of the goal of intended births. The final section deals with the broader policy environment.

DEFINING AND MEASURING INTENDED FERTILITY

There is no unambiguous definition of "intended birth" that would apply to the different societies covered by this report, nor to all families within any society. "Intentions" fit actual decisions and behavior only imperfectly: the answers to standardized questions used in household surveys cannot fully capture the complexity of the process by which intentions are formed or their intensity. However, some measures, even imprecise ones, are needed to gauge the extent of the problem of unintended pregnancy, and survey data on fertility intentions have been found to predict subsequent fertility behavior well, at least at a population level (Westoff, 1990).[1]

The best recent source of comparable data for large populations in developing countries is the Demographic and Health Surveys (DHS). Using different items in the standard DHS questionnaires, there are two broad approaches to measuring intentions. One approach relies on answers to direct questions about the last birth or current pregnancy. In most DHS surveys, women are asked, for each live birth that occurred less than 5 years before the interview: "At the time you became pregnant with [Name], did you want to become pregnant then, did you want to wait until later, or did you want no more children at all?" Women who are pregnant at the time of the interview are asked analogous questions about their current pregnancy.

We use the term "unwanted" to refer to a pregnancy or birth to a woman who reports that she did not want any more children; "mistimed" for a pregnancy or birth to woman who wants more children, but not in the near future, and "unintended" to cover both.[2]

The second approach relies on hypothetical questions about all children. Most DHS surveys include this question: "If you could go back to the time when you did not have any children and could choose exactly the number of children to have in your whole life, how many would that be?" The answers can be averaged for a population, or a desired total

---

[1]The Technical Note at the end of this chapter discusses some of the problems of existing measures of the prevalence of unintended pregnancies and abortions.

[2]Other researchers use different terms. Some use "unplanned" to describe pregnancies that were not wanted at the time of conception or recognition of pregnancy, distinct from "unwanted," referring to the woman's wishes at the time of birth or interview. Asif and his colleagues (1994), analyzing data collected from pregnant women in Uttar Pradesh, India, distinguish between "unwanted," "unwanted but accepted," and "wanted" pregnancies; nearly half the pregnancies in his sample were classified unwanted but accepted. Brown and Eisenberg (1995) discuss the implications of various definitions of intention and wantedness.

fertility rate can be estimated by deleting recent births to women who report an ideal family size lower than their actual number of living children (Cochrane and Sai, 1993; Bongaarts, 1990). An alternative is to construct a "synthetic estimate" of desired total fertility rates, summarizing estimates of proportions of women at each parity who report that they want no more children. These indirect methods do not allow estimation of mistimed (as opposed to entirely unwanted) pregnancies, and they require a hypothetical recasting of respondents' lives that may not be especially meaningful. But they avoid one weakness of the direct questions about specific pregnancies: "[U]nderreporting is apparently common and is presumably caused by a reluctance of women to classify their offspring as unwanted" (Bongaarts, 1991:223).

Since desired family size has fallen in almost all developing countries for which it has been measured, it has been conventional to focus on only one aspect of failure to achieve reproductive goals, namely, unwanted childbearing. Yet as Kingsley Davis (1967) noted three decades ago, "family planning" literally construed should include the notion of couples planning to have a family. Infertility can lead to loss of social status, divorce, and other negative consequences, as well as being a cause of tremendous unhappiness.

Larsen and Menken (1989) provide useful evidence on the prevalence of infertility from a combination of demographic surveys and microsimulation of populations with varying amounts of deliberate fertility control. Larsen (1994) estimates that the proportion of women sterile by age 34 in 17 sub-Saharan African countries varied from a low of 11 percent in Burundi to a high of 31 percent in Cameroon. She concluded that "the true prevalence of sterility in sub-Saharan Africa is so substantial that it ceases to be a merely individual problem and has become a public health issue" (Larsen, 1994:469). As in previous reviews, Larsen found great geographic variation in apparent infertility, which she plausibly ascribes to geographic variation in the incidence of reproductive tract infections. In Chapter 3 we discuss the needs for programs to control sexually transmitted diseases (STDs), which is the most effective way to prevent infertility in the countries most affected.

Whose Intentions?

A crucial question in all societies is whose fertility intentions count in deciding if a birth is "intended." The potential mother is obviously most directly affected, and any definition of intention that did not include her wishes and interests would be unacceptable. Potential fathers also have, or are expected to have, a lot at stake in fertility decisions. A widely shared ideal would call for good spousal communication and socially approved methods of reconciling disagreements that respect the rights of all involved.

A recent review of published studies, based on both surveys and qualitative research, showed (Mason and Taj, 1987:632;631) "more often than not . . . women's and men's fertility goals are very similar. When gender differences do occur . . . they usually are small and are of both types (men more pronatalist than women and vice versa)." These are population averages, which could be consistent with some degree of offsetting disagreement between spouses. More importantly, general agreement on preferences for the number of children does not imply agreement among spouses about the desirability of particular behaviors (modern contraception, periodic abstinence, or induced abortion) to implement those goals. Husbands' disapproval is one of the most common reasons for women's not using contraception reported in surveys by women at risk of an unwanted pregnancy. As Bongaarts and Bruce (1995) point out, more than one-half of such women in most African countries also report that they have never discussed contraception with their husbands, suggesting that they may feel powerless to influence the decision or even raise the topic. Casterline, Perez, and Biddlecom (1996) report similar results from more intensive interviews in the Philippines.

Intergenerational differences in family size goals may be more pronounced than interspousal differences. It is commonly believed by family planning program managers in South Asia, for example, that the chief opponents of small families are domineering mothers-in-law. Caldwell (1986) has argued that the patriarchs in West African lineage systems have a strong interest in seeing their sons have many children who can perform economic and religious services and generate prestige for their grandfathers. We know of no studies directly comparing the stated preferences of older people for grandchildren with the fertility goals of their adult children. The notion of a couple as the only decision makers whose preferences should count is probably a minority view in the world as a whole, and a recent development even where it is now the dominant view. Marriage and fertility decisions are widely regarded as too important to leave solely to prospective spouses and parents, particularly young ones. In practice, methods for estimating the extent of unwanted fertility and unmet needs for family planning implicitly take the woman's (potential mother's) stated intentions as paramount. The justification is that a woman is the person whose physical health is directly at risk in pregnancy and delivery; in all societies women, on average, bear the major share of responsibilities for child care.

Unwanted Pregnancies and Births

Direct Measures

Figure 4-1 shows the proportions of recent births and current pregnancies reported as unwanted in the most recent DHS survey in 34 countries, grouped by region.[3] The proportion varies widely among countries within regions, but it is clearly lowest in sub-Saharan Africa, where large desired family sizes are still reported, and generally highest in Latin America, the Middle East, and North Africa. Outside Africa, the proportion of births unwanted ranges in most countries from 12 to 34 percent.

Figure 4-2 shows the proportion of unwanted births in the same countries, grouped by the percentages of married women aged 15-49 currently using any form of contraception (the contraceptive prevalence rate). The countries with the lowest contraceptive prevalence (most of which are in sub-Saharan Africa) have low proportions of unwanted births. The median is 18 percent among the nine countries with contraceptive prevalence of more than 50 percent, considerably higher than the median of 5 percent among the ten countries with contraceptive prevalence of less than 20 percent. This difference does not necessarily mean that women in the highest contraceptive prevalence countries are more likely to have an unwanted birth in a particular year. Precisely because they use contraception more, they are less likely to have a baby than are women in countries where contraceptive use is uncommon. This can be seen in Figure 4-3, showing the range of values for the unwanted birth *rate* (unwanted births per 1,000 women per year) for countries in the same contraceptive prevalence categories as in Figure 4-2.[4] Countries with contraceptive prevalence above 50 percent tend to have lower unwanted birth rates than countries with contraceptive prevalence between 20 and 30 percent, despite having higher proportions of unwanted births, because they have much lower overall birth rates. Women are most at risk of unwanted births in countries where contraceptive use is in the range 20-40 percent, presumably because contraceptive behavior and fertility are lagging behind the more rapid change in fertility preferences.

The proportion of unwanted births is the appropriate measure for discussing the consequences of unwantedness for children. It highlights

---

[3]Countries chosen for DHS do not represent a random sample of all countries in a region, but they do cover a wide variety of conditions in developing countries outside China.

[4]The unwanted birth rate was calculated as the product of the proportion of most recent births or current pregnancies reported as unwanted multiplied by the general fertility rate (births per 1,000 women aged 15-49 per year) as estimated by the United Nations.

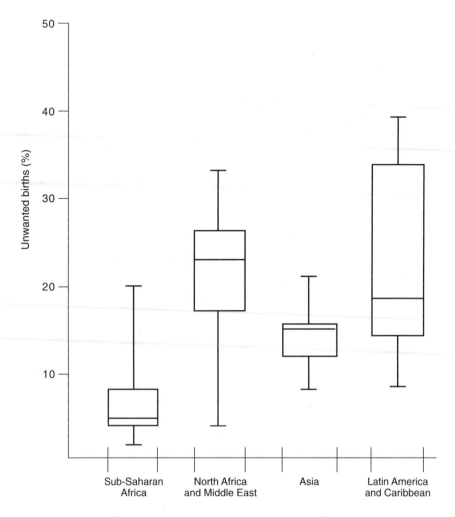

FIGURE 4-1 Percentage of most recent births or current pregnancies unwanted in countries with recent DHS surveys, by region. Wide bars show 25th centile, median, and 75th centile for countries in each category; narrow bars show lowest and highest values. SOURCE: Demographic and Health Surveys.

the situation in many low-fertility societies where contraception and safe abortions are already widely available and well known. The second measure, the unwanted birth rate, is appropriate for gauging the effects of unwanted fertility on women's lives. It shows that women in low-fertility societies are less likely than those in societies with higher fertility rates to be affected by the consequences of unintended pregnancies and births.

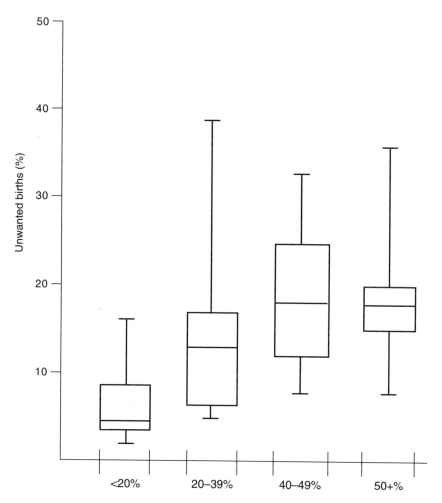

FIGURE 4-2 Percentage of most recent births or current pregnancies unwanted in countries with recent DHS surveys, by contraceptive prevalence. Data are for married women aged 15-49. Wide bars show 25th centile, median, and 75th centile for countries in each category; narrow bars show lowest and highest values. SOURCE: Demographic and Health Surveys.

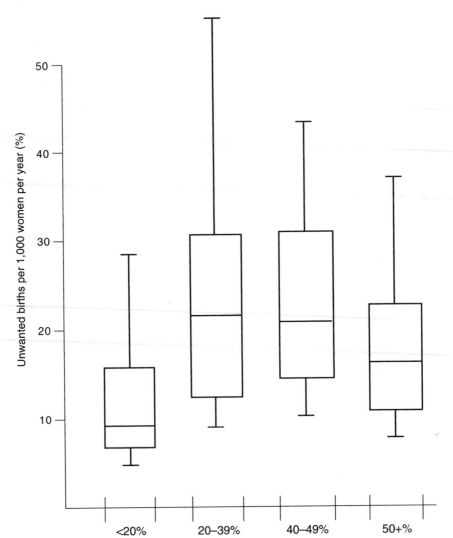

FIGURE 4-3 Unwanted births per 1,000 women aged 15-49 per year in countries with recent DHS surveys, by contraceptive prevalence. Wide bars show 25th centile, median, and 75th centile for countries in each category; narrow bars show lowest and highest values. SOURCE: Demographic and Health Surveys.

Indirect Measures

The indirect approaches to measurement also produces high aggregate estimates of the extent of unwanted fertility. Cochrane and Sai (1993) estimate that in developing countries outside China, 30 percent of fertility is unwanted. Bongaarts' aggregate estimates (also based on comparison of ideal with actual family size) show that in countries with high fertility (total fertility rates [TFR] above six births per women), only 16 percent of births appear unwanted. The highest percentages of unwanted births are found in countries in the middle range of fertility rates (between four and six births per woman), where nearly one-third of births are inferred to be unwanted. In low-fertility countries (TFRs below four births per woman), 25 percent of births appear unwanted.

Figure 4-4 shows the proportion of recent births or current pregnancies reported as mistimed in DHS surveys, with countries grouped according to contraceptive prevalence rates.[5] These data show no consistent association: the median proportion of mistimed births is just above one-fifth for all countries, across the range of contraceptive prevalence rates. This evidence suggests that the potential demand for family planning for purposes of spacing births can be high even when desired fertility is high. Country-level analyses of DHS data by Westoff and Bankole (1995) confirm that much of the unmet need for contraception inferred from women's replies, especially in sub-Saharan Africa, is motivated by the desire to delay first pregnancies or to space pregnancies, rather than by a desire to stop childbearing.

Determinants

The determinants of unintended fertility are complex, not easily reduced to factors such as lack of education, unfamiliarity with contraception and abortion, or unavailability of services. In Indonesia, for example, Weller et al. (1991) found no significant association between women's education and the wantedness of their most recent child born within the last 5 years. The researchers ascribed this lack of an association to the offsetting effects of education on preferences for lower fertility and on ability to control fertility.

Data for the United States—a country where nearly all adults are literate, publicly funded family planning clinics have existed across the

---

[5]The percentages shown in Figure 4-4 do not include the births and current pregnancies reported as unwanted (shown in Figure 4-2).

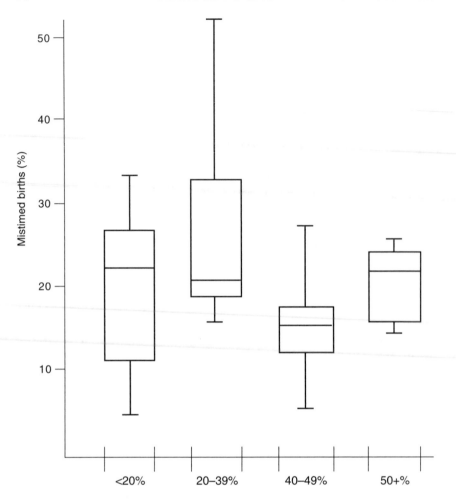

FIGURE 4-4 Percentage of most recent births or current pregnancies mistimed in countries with recent DHS surveys, by contraceptive prevalence. Wide bars show 25th centile, median, and 75th centile for countries in each category; narrow bars show lowest and highest values. SOURCE: Demographic and Health Surveys.

country since the late 1960s, private outlets for contraceptive supplies and advice are widespread and costs of contraception are very low in relation to incomes (by international standards), and abortion is safe and common (about 30 percent of all pregnancies not ending in miscarriage are terminated by induced abortion)—are revealing. In the United States, nearly one-half of all births in 1988 were unintended (Kost and Forrest, 1995): more than one-quarter of births to women with 16 or more years of schooling were unintended, and births to women with three or more previous births were more likely to be unintended than were first births. The evidence demonstrates that making contraception and abortion safe and widely available and ensuring that women have high levels of education do not, by themselves, reduce the proportions of unintended pregnancies and births.

Thus, despite the increased use of effective contraception, the proportion of births that are unwanted or mistimed may rise in the early stages of the fertility transition before leveling off or falling. Changes in fertility preferences that accompany the fertility transition make the goal of eliminating unintended births a moving target. There is good evidence that fertility intentions change during the course of the transition to low fertility. Desired family size has fallen in almost every country where trend data are available from DHS and the World Fertility Survey, and the decline has sometimes been dramatic: in Kenya, the average fell by more than three children per woman in 20 years (Rutstein, 1995). Desired family size has fallen quite consistently for almost all birth cohorts of women, and for both educated and uneducated women, in 28 countries for which two or three comparable surveys are available (Rutstein, 1995).

Lloyd (1994:191) argues that "the emergence of 'unwanted fertility' is symptomatic of parents' rising aspirations and their increasing awareness of alternatives to their own and their children's current condition." This gap between intentions and experience appears to grow in the early stages of the demographic transition, when declining mortality, particularly for infants and children, results in larger numbers of children growing up for given numbers of live births. As actual fertility declines, wanted fertility may decline even faster, so that the proportion of births that are unintended may actually grow even while fertility control is becoming more prevalent.

Induced Abortions

The evidence about the prevalence of unintended pregnancy discussed so far is based on women's reports about their intentions and contraceptive behavior. Further evidence that large proportions of pregnancies are unintended comes from the limited available data on the prevalence of induced abortion. The most authoritative estimates are that in 1987, worldwide, there were between 26 and 31 million legal abortions and 10 to 22 million illegal abortions (Henshaw and Morrow, 1990).

By combining direct reports with incomplete data on treatment of abortion complications, Henshaw estimated that in 1990, there were total of 20 million "unsafe abortions," that is, those "not provided through approved facilities and/or persons" (World Health Organization, 1994:2).

These 20 million unsafe abortions are estimated to have resulted in 70,000 deaths of women, of which 69,000 are in developing countries, one-third of them in Africa (World Health Organization, 1994:Table 3). Although some abortions result from pregnancies that were desired at the time of conception, the great majority are likely to have been unintended from the outset.

Abortion complications are not uniquely problems of the young and the unmarried, whose sexual activity may not be considered legitimate. For example, in low-income urban communities in Kenya, women who had recently had abortions were typically in their 20s and had previously given birth (Baker and Khasiani, 1991). "While not denying that induced abortion is a growing problem among young, educated women [in Africa], evidence suggests that the problem is not limited to them" (Coeytaux, 1988:187).

CONSEQUENCES OF UNWANTED PREGNANCIES AND BIRTHS

Unwanted pregnancies and births can have a variety of negative consequences, for the children themselves, their siblings, their parents, and society as a whole. Unwanted births impose psychological and financial costs to the family, and high fertility, much of it unintended, imposes costs on society as well.

Unwanted pregnancies expose women, especially poor women, to health risks simply by increasing the number of pregnancies and deliveries in their lifetimes. The lifetime risk of complications is determined in great part by the number of pregnancies a woman has. The lifetime risk of maternal mortality is a function of the number of pregnancies and the quality and likelihood of utilization of available health care. For a given level of access and utilization of effective health care, a reduction in the number of pregnancies will bring about lower maternal mortality rates (Koenig et al., 1988).

In adequate medical settings, abortions are not dangerous procedures, yet most abortions in developing countries are carried out in inadequate settings, and the procedure can be dangerous (World Health Organization, 1994; Mashalaba, 1989). Incomplete and septic abortions are one of the four leading causes of pregnancy-related mortality and also account for a huge number of nonfatal injuries (see Chapter 5). Since most induced abortions result from unwanted pregnancies, and safe and effective methods of preventing pregnancies exist and are acceptable in most societies, the morbidity and mortality caused by unsafe abortion are preventable. Contraception can be regarded as primary prevention of complications of abortion; ensuring medically adequate abortions and post-abortion care are secondary and tertiary prevention.

Unintended births are disproportionately risky for the infant. Tables 4-1, 4-2, and 4-3 show, respectively, the proportions of most recent births (or current pregnancies) reported as unintended in six recent DHS surveys, by age of mother; by birth order, and (for second or subsequent pregnancies) by the time since previous (most recent) birth. In every country, births to women over age 35 and fifth- or higher order births are most likely to be reported as unintended.

Similar results have been found in analyses using the ideal family size questions. In 27 countries covered by the DHS surveys in the late 1980s, the majority of women who had given birth to more than five children reported an ideal of fewer children than the number they actually had in every country outside sub-Saharan Africa (except Guatemala). For the African countries, the cutoff for excess fertility was usually eight children—although in all countries, substantial numbers of women with five children (four, in much of Latin America) also reported that they had more children than their ideal number.

Births or pregnancies coming after intervals of 24 months or less are more likely to be reported as unintended, although the differences are less stark than are those associated with high parity and older maternal age.

Since older maternal age, high parity, and short pregnancy intervals are all associated with the risk of infant mortality (Working Group on the Health Consequences of Contraceptive Use and Controlled Fertility, 1989), delaying mistimed pregnancies or eliminating unwanted ones could im-

TABLE 4-1 Most Recent Birth or Current Pregnancy Unintended in Selected Countries, by Mother's Age: in percent

Country (Year)	Mother's Age		
	<20	20-34	35+
Bolivia (1993)	41.5	53.9	74.0
Colombia (1986)	34.9	48.3	60.5
Egypt (1988)	13.9	41.3	75.0
Kenya (1993)	61.2	55.3	65.4
Nigeria (1990)	13.7	12.5	21.6
Philippines (1993)	37.6	46.4	58.2
Tanzania (1991)	22.7	26.1	31.7
Thailand (1987)	28.3	38.4	47.2

SOURCE: Data from Demographic and Health Surveys, unpublished tabulations.

TABLE 4-2 Most Recent Birth or Current Pregnancy Unintended in Selected Countries, by Birth Order: in percent

	Birth Order		
Country (Year)	1	2-4	5+
Bolivia (1993)	32.7	50.1	78.6
Colombia (1986)	25.0	50.7	68.8
Egypt (1988)	3.8	39.5	67.2
Kenya (1993)	52.1	52.1	66.2
Nigeria (1990)	11.2	9.9	22.7
Philippines (1993)	22.3	47.4	63.6
Tanzania (1991)	18.7	25.0	39.5
Thailand (1987)	20.7	36.3	64.4

SOURCE: Data from Demographic and Health Surveys, unpublished tabulations.

TABLE 4-3 Recent Higher Order Birth or Current Pregnancy Unintended in Selected Countries, by Interval from Prior Birth to Conception: in percent

	Interval	
Country (Year)	Less than 24 months	24 or more months
Bolivia (1993)	68.4	60.1
Colombia (1986)	67.6	49.2
Egypt (1988)	54.0	50.2
Kenya (1993)	67.2	56.1
Nigeria (1990)	21.1	13.0
Philippines (1993)	62.1	49.3
Tanzania (1991)	33.5	27.5
Thailand (1987)	53.4	36.7

SOURCE: Data from Demographic and Health Surveys, unpublished tabulations.

prove infant and child health simply by reducing disproportionately the number of pregnancies defined as high risk.[6]

A few studies have shown higher mortality risks for unwanted chil-

---

[6]Zimicki (1989) discusses the degree to which associations of maternal age, parity, and birth spacing with maternal morbidity and mortality are directly causal through biomedical mechanisms, and the degree to which they are markers for risk factors of other types (e.g., poverty and low social efficacy, lack of access to health services and information). Haaga (1989) summarizes similar evidence for associations with infant health. Both conclude that

dren (e.g., Frenzen and Hogan, 1982, for Thailand), especially for un-wanted girls (Muhuri and Preston, 1991, for Bangladesh). It would be a mistake to limit consideration of the consequences of unintended fertility to the relatively easily measured effects of morbidity and mortality. Par-ticularly as increasing numbers of young women remain unmarried into their 20s and seek more formal schooling to prepare for new roles, unin-tended fertility can become more burdensome. In West Africa, for ex-ample, it has been argued that adolescent fertility, once expected and welcomed, is increasingly a problem since unmarried girls have to quit school and have diminished chances of good jobs and marriages if they become pregnant (Bledsoe and Cohen, 1993).

The threat as well as the actuality of unintended pregnancy can cause considerable suffering. Dixon-Mueller (1989:145) argues:

> An unwanted pregnancy or birth can drive women to attempt a danger-ous self-induced abortion; to infanticide; or to prolonged hostility, de-pression, and despair. [We] must include under women's health not only reported rates of maternal mortality and morbidity associated with contraceptive use and childbirth but also—and perhaps more impor-tantly—women's fears of such conditions or events; the fear of getting pregnant accidentally, for example, or of not getting pregnant at all; the fear of potentially debilitating contraceptive side effects; and the fear of trauma or death in abortion or childbirth.

Deleterious impacts of unintended births on siblings result from the dilution of parental resources, including time and attention as well as material resources. Numerous studies have shown that children in large families receive less schooling and less health care and have poorer nutri-tional status than children from small families (Lloyd, 1994; Desai, 1995). In Ghana, Lloyd and Gage-Brandon (1994) found that girls are at a par-ticular disadvantage: the more younger siblings they have, the less likely to enroll in secondary school and the more likely to drop out. Cross-sectional associations are insufficient evidence of causation, of course, since there is also abundant evidence that parents make conscious deci-sions to balance the number of children they have with the costs of such investments in child "quality" (e.g., Knodel, Chamratrithirong, and Debavalya, 1987). But there is also some evidence—for example, from an intensive family planning program with a quasi-experimental design (Fos-

---

the associations are partly causal, and health would be improved if pregnancies could be delayed or unwanted high parity pregnancies were prevented. Miller's analyses of data from Bangladesh and the Philippines shows that the association of short intervals with high risk of infant mortality persists even when prematurity, prior child death within the family, and other factors are controlled, strengthening the inference that the association is causal.

ter and Roy, 1996)—showing that the associations are partly causal. Helping people implement their preference for fewer children should result in better schooling and health care for the wanted children. The ICPD Programme of Action emphasized the contribution that increased education of girls could make to lowering fertility rates, and, thus, population growth rates. A similar program of action with increased education of girls as its goal could reciprocally emphasize the contribution that family planning programs could make toward that end.

The effects of unintended births on siblings and parents can be mitigated by institutions and customs that share the economic burden with a wide circle of kin or fellow citizens. Child fosterage in West Africa, for example, "breaks down household economic boundaries and spreads the impact of additional children on family resources across a wider kin network" (Lloyd, 1994:188). However, when social institutions, whether traditional or modern, mitigate the impact of an unwanted birth on the immediate family, however, they are spreading costs of unintended pregnancy more widely within society, not eliminating them.

ROLE OF FAMILY PLANNING AND ABORTION SERVICES

There is a large literature on the design, management, financing, and evaluation of family planning programs, and there have been some very useful recent reviews (Simmons and Lapham, 1987; Phillips and Ross, 1992; Buckner et al., 1995), so this report does not attempt to cover the field in a comprehensive fashion. Rather, we focus on some of the major challenges that face family planning programs in the next decade or two, with an emphasis on those that are shared with other aspects of comprehensive reproductive health services.

Unmet Need for Contraception

A measure of "unmet need" for contraception in developing countries can be formed by cross-classification of responses to survey items on the wantedness of current pregnancies, intentions for childbearing in the near future, and current contraceptive use. Westoff and Bankole (1995), using data from 1990-1994 DHS surveys in 27 countries, calculate unmet need as the sum of currently pregnant women who report that their pregnancy is unintended and nonpregnant currently married women who believe themselves fecund and want no more children (or none within the next 2 years), but are not currently practicing any contraceptive method. The proportions of unmet need vary greatly, from between 10 and 15 percent of women in Turkey, Colombia, and Indonesia (countries with high contraceptive prevalence) to more than 35 percent of women in 4 of 14 sub-Saharan African countries (Westoff and Bankole, 1995).

Such estimates have taken on new importance for policy makers since they provide a way to reconcile an emphasis on reproductive rights and client needs with the aggregate goals of fertility reduction that nearly all developing countries have officially adopted. Sinding, Ross, and Rosenfield (1994) note that meeting existing unmet need would by itself fulfill for most countries their official targets for contraceptive prevalence or lowered fertility rates. In this report, we consider individual intentions as paramount in defining reproductive health: "Every birth wanted and safe" means wanted by the parents, not wanted by the state. Helping individuals achieve their reproductive goals should also result in lower fertility rates in the aggregate if desired fertility rates continue to fall in most places. This congruence provides an additional rationale for family planning programs to help women achieve their fertility goals.

Definitions of unmet need have been criticized on several grounds (Pritchett, 1994; Germain and Dixon-Mueller, 1992; Bongaarts, 1991). One is that the surveys on which they are based typically do not include sexually active nonmarried women or women currently using some method of contraception they should not be using for health reasons, using it ineffectively, or suffering needless side effects. Thus, "unmet need" as conventionally measured might be very low, despite the existence of many sexually active women who do not use contraceptives and so are at risk of unintended pregnancies and many dissatisfied users. The available survey indices also do not measure the intensity of women's preferences or why nonusers are not practicing contraception even though they do not want pregnancies. Despite the importance of these questions for scientists trying to explain and predict fertility behavior and to policy makers trying to achieve reproductive health goals, there is surprisingly little in-depth research on these issues.

Casterline, Perez, and Biddlecom (1996) used a combination of survey, in-depth, and focus group interviews in the Philippines to examine the reasons for high rates of unmet need. Their findings confirm the conclusions of Bongaarts and Bruce (1995), who argue that lack of access to services and cost are relatively unimportant barriers. There was a tendency for women in the unmet need category in the Philippines study to believe themselves less likely to conceive. More important, however, were the women's perceptions of their husbands' fertility preferences (though communications among spouses were typically poor), concerns about the acceptability of contraception, and concerns about the health risks thought to be posed by contraceptive methods. (Health risks were important to contraceptive users as well.) These results, which need to be replicated in other countries, tend to reinforce the view that unmet need will not be met solely by an expansion of services. Rather, they point to a need for better counseling, informed choice, and higher quality services that will build trust and create effective demand for family planning.

Need for New Contraceptive Methods

In the early 1960s, the "contraceptive revolution, ushered in by the pill, was thought to be just beginning, and it was widely predicted that a host of new methods would soon be available—a pregnancy vaccine, a pill for men, a menses inducer and a reversible sterilant for men and women" (Lincoln and Kaeser, 1988:20). But the major advances in the last three decades have been in new ways to deliver synthetic hormonal contraceptives for women (injectable and implantable contraceptives and the Levonorgestrel intrauterine device [IUD]). A recent estimate is that it will take at least a decade for injectable hormonal contraception for men to be available in the United States, and 20 years for the availability of contraceptive vaccines for men and women (Alexander, 1995).

New versions of synthetic hormone-releasing IUDs and new plastic condoms are likely to become more widely available in the near future. The experience with contraceptive introduction in the past has shown a need for evaluation of the capabilities of the delivery system as a whole, not just use-effectiveness trials among small numbers of users. Research and development of new contraceptives are not currently receiving funding commensurate with the needs for new methods of low-cost, safe, and effective contraception and control over STD transmission (Harrison and Rosenfield, 1996).

Emergency Contraception

Emergency contraception—prevention of pregnancy through use of contraceptive methods after unprotected sex—could prove a simple and effective back-up to regular contraceptive use, and it may be particularly important for women who are victims of coercive sex. Emergency contraceptives include combinations of regular oral contraceptive pills (containing estrogen and progestin), progestin-only pills, and the copper-T IUD (Trussell, Ellertson, and Stewart, 1996; Trussell and Ellertson, 1995). Combined oral contraceptives that are available in most countries have been shown to be safe and effective for use as emergency contraceptives, with fewer and less severe side effects than older high-estrogen regimens (Trussell, Ellertson, and Stewart, 1996).

Affiliates of the International Planned Parenthood Federation provided emergency contraceptive information and services to some 40,000 women in 1993, mostly in a few developed countries (Senanayake, 1996).

The main reason that emergency contraception is not more widely used in developing countries is a lack of knowledge on the part of both health care providers and women at risk of unwanted pregnancies (International Planned Parenthood Federation, 1995). More operational research, better education of family planning caregivers, and communication to the public are all needed before emergency contraception can become a significant option for women in developing countries.

Quality Issues in Family Planning Services

The promotion of higher quality services in family planning has been pervasive in the last decade. The need for quality improvements has been revealed by studies of services in a wide variety of settings.

The framework proposed by Bruce (1990) has proved useful both for conceptualizing quality of care in assessments and as a checklist for efforts to improve quality. She found six aspects of services that clients view as critical: choice of methods, information given to clients, technical competence, interpersonal relations, mechanisms to encourage continuity of care, and an appropriate constellation of services (Bruce, 1990). We deal here with the first four of these; we do not consider continuity of care, and the appropriate constellation of services is discussed in Chapter 6.

Modern contraceptive methods are now widely available in developing countries; about one-third of married couples in developing countries outside China use some form of effective contraception (Robey, Rutstein, and Morris, 1992). But this availability does not mean that most women and men have safe access to a variety of contraceptive methods so that they can choose one appropriate to their needs at a particular time of their lives. It is difficult to measure access independent of use, but Ross and Mauldin (1996) have used the pooled judgment of experts in a large number of countries to quantify several dimensions of family planning program effort, including safe availability of multiple methods and services. Their study is one of a series of comparable studies dating back to 1972, so it is particularly useful in showing trends over time. In every region of the developing world except East Asia (where scores were already high in 1982), the safe availability of methods and services was greater in 1994 than it had been 12 years earlier. But sub-Saharan Africa still lagged well behind the rest of the world in availability of methods, and little progress had been made there, or in other parts of the developing world, in improving availability between 1989 and 1994. The rapid progress of the 1970s and 1980s in expanding choices in the developing countries appears to have stalled. At the same time that many people are calling for a "second contraceptive revolution" to better meet the needs for safe and reversible contraception and protection from STDs, large parts of the world have not fully profited from the "first contraceptive revolution" (Harrison and Rosenfield, 1996).

Situation analyses conducted by the Population Council in family planning service delivery points in several African countries showed that counseling dealt far more often with information about resupply than with information on how to use contraceptives effectively. Clinic-based providers did not typically ask whether potential clients were breast-feeding, which should affect the choice and sequence of methods (Winikoff, Elias, and Beattie, 1994). Observations at clinics have shown a widespread tendency for providers neither to elicit information about clients' needs nor to listen carefully when it is offered. This lack greatly reduces the value of the interaction (Winikoff, Elias, and Beattie, 1994; Huntington and Schuler, 1993).

Efforts to improve quality have often been regarded by senior managers as inappropriate demands for luxury services. For decades, the ministries of health in developing countries were criticized for spending most of their resources on tertiary care of relatively high quality for urban elites while short-changing basic services for the much larger poor population. For international agencies and women's health advocates to demand greater attention to quality may seem now like a retrograde step. Yet the analogy with curative health services and the quantity-quality tradeoff could be misleading.

First, many of the problems with technical quality of care revealed by the situation analyses and similar studies could as well be seen as barriers to an adequate *quantity* of services: missing equipment and supplies, clinics left shut or clients turned away because poorly supervised providers do not work when they are supposed to; untrained or poorly supervised workers turning clients away (or never seeing any) because they themselves are unfamiliar with procedures. The steps that are needed to improve quality—attention to logistics, adequate supervision, motivation for workers at every level, real feedback to supervisors and managers, accountability for supplies and money—are the same that would be needed to increase service quantity. The advantage of dealing with these problems under the rubric of quality assurance is that emphasis on quality could focus the attention of managers on factors over which they have some control, rather than dissipating their attention onto the external factors for which they cannot be held accountable.

Second, the service that family planning provides is inseparable from provision of information. For resupply methods (e.g., pills), the continuous active participation of individual clients is required. High discontinuation rates are likely to indicate a poor quality program. There are always some clients who wish to conceive after spacing, or whose needs have changed, and who therefore should be discontinuing a particular contraceptive method. But if large numbers of contraceptive users are discontinuing use of any method, rather than switching to one that better meets their needs, it probably indicates that the program is not meeting their needs (Jain and Bruce, 1994).

Lastly, the measures taken to improve quality of services provided by existing providers in existing facilities may result in great efficiency— more output for a given level of resources—than would the deployment of new workers or building of new facilities. The argument that improved quality will lead to greater demand for services and operation at more efficient scales is still largely untested. In a situation analyses of clinics and other family planning service sites in the same clusters included in the 1991-1992 DHS in Peru, Mensch, Arends-Kuenning, and Jain (1994) found that the quality of local services affected the likelihood of contraceptive use more in the rural than in the urban areas (because, the authors suggest, urban residents had access to a choice of clinics). Extreme differences in the quality index they constructed were associated with a predicted increase in contraceptive use from 33 percent to 38 percent of women; in this sample, that difference is comparable to the differences between uneducated women and women with postsecondary education (although less than the estimated effects of exposure to mass media).

Quality control in health care in most developing countries is typically achieved through routine monitoring or periodic assessments. There is a great need for simple and replicable monitoring techniques, including self-assessments and peer review. The client-oriented program evaluation devised by the Association for Voluntary Surgical Contraception is a form of self-assessment that has proved useful in several countries. Peer review has been tried with some success, for example, by midwives in Indonesia (MacDonald et al., 1995). Quality assurance should be considered primarily as a management responsibility in current programs, rather than simply as a topic for research and pilot programs. But there is a need for more operations research and dissemination of experience on replicable methods of quality improvement.

The type of programmatic linkages between family planning and other reproductive health services, especially infectious disease control and antenatal and delivery care, will vary among settings depending on such factors as whether free-standing services are already developed and patterns of utilization. Family planning programs in many countries reach large numbers of young women and thus are particularly well suited as sources of information about sources of prenatal care and emergency care for obstetric complications (see Chapter 5).

As discussed in Chapter 3, family planning programs have an important role in controlling reproductive tract infections (RTIs). At a minimum, clinical contraceptive services, like other clinical services, should be included in measures to prevent iatrogenic infections. Both clinical and community-based programs need to incorporate into guidelines for counseling some realistic assessment, and discussion, of clients' exposure to STDs, including HIV. Latex condoms and nonoxnynol-9 reduce the risk of STD transmission as well as unwanted pregnancy. As we argue in Chapter 3, family planning clinics providing insertion of IUDs should be able to supply standardized case management of symptomatic infections (using the World Health Organization algorithms) and selected screening efforts.

Information, Education, and Communication

The diffusion of information about modern contraception throughout the world in the last three decades has been a remarkable achievement. In 13 of the 22 countries where DHS surveys were conducted in 1990-1993, more than 90 percent of women said they had heard of one or more modern contraceptive methods. In all countries except Nigeria, more than one-half of the women had heard of one or more modern methods (Curtis and Neitzel, 1996). In every country except 4 of the 11 sub-Saharan African countries, more than one-half of the women had heard of the contraceptive pill, the best-known method worldwide. These survey questions have sometimes been criticized on the grounds that respondents claim knowledge out of politeness or so as not to appear ignorant (e.g., by Bongaarts and Bruce, 1995), but even without prompting, the majority of women in all but five countries could name at least one modern contraceptive method (Curtis and Neitzel, 1996). Men are even more likely than women to know at least one contraceptive method: in 15 countries where men were interviewed in DHS surveys, more than one-half of the men reported that they had heard of at least one modern contraceptive method (Ezeh, Seroussi, and Raggers, 1996).

Of course, knowledge that an option exists is not enough. Informed choice and effective use of contraceptives require basic knowledge of how a method works, what noncontraceptive effects it might have, and how to use it. There is evidence both from standardized survey questions and from more intensive interviews and observations that many women and men do not know such things, even in countries where family planning programs are well established. For example, in the DHS in Egypt in 1992, women who reported using the contraceptive pill were asked to show their packet of pills. Interviewers inspected the packets for evidence that the pills had been taken out of sequence, and they asked the women whether they had missed days and what they would do if they did miss a day. Thirty-seven percent of the women had missed taking at least one pill during the month preceding the interview. Only one-third of those who missed a day knew that they should take two pills on the following day or switch methods temporarily. The lack of information may well be due to inadequate services. Findings from multivariate analysis indicate that women whose source of supply was the government clinics were four times as likely as those with other sources to have taken pills out of sequence or missed days (Trottier et al., 1994).

Bongaarts and Bruce (1995) created an index of contraceptive knowledge using data from 12 DHS surveys. It shows that the percentage of women who could name a contraceptive method spontaneously, knew where to get supplies or services, and had an opinion (either positive or negative) about side effects of the method was less than 50 percent, often well below, in 6 of the 12 countries. To explore reasons for not using contraception, Bongaarts and Bruce (1995) used the DHS data, supplemented by results from intensive studies from women respondents who reported that they did not want to get pregnant but were not currently using contraception. The researchers argue that most unmet need is associated with women's lack of knowledge, concerns about health, side effects, the behavior required to use contraception, and objections from their husbands. Bongaarts and Bruce (1995:64) conclude:

> As a combined consequence of poor community information levels, inadequate services, and low literacy, a large proportion of women may not be sufficiently knowledgeable about the health effects of methods to make an informed and comfortable decision about contraception. In such an environment, the impact of unknowns, unfounded rumors, or negative perceptions . . . will depend largely on the adequacy of the program communication strategies and client-provider exchanges.

Such results show a continuing, important role for information, education, and communication campaigns and face-to-face counseling by providers, especially where nonprogram channels of information about contraception are weak. High rates of method failure likely indicate insufficient knowledge about contraceptive use (though the fact that failure rates are higher for couples who want more children some time in the future indicates that motivation also plays a part). Concerns for health effects can be based either on an accurate appraisal of the risks and benefits of a method, in which case the availability of alternatives is particularly important, or on inaccurate information, in which case family planning programs can be considered to have failed in their most fundamental role. Improving knowledge about the side effects of contraception can make an important contribution to women's health. As Casterline, Perez, and Biddlecom (1996) show, both contraceptive users and women with unmet need (as conventionally defined) in their Philippine samples reported a great deal of worry about health effects in in-depth interviews.

Mass communication, social marketing[7], and community-based distribution of contraceptive information and supplies are all strategies that have proved successful in spreading two basic messages—the existence of safe and effective contraceptive methods and the small family norm—even in countries like Bangladesh where the weight of tradition worked against them (Cleland et al., 1994; Lissance and Schellstede, 1993; Piotrow et al., 1994). Now, family planning programs face a new challenge in trying to convey subtler messages about the advantages and disadvantages of different methods and about effective use. There have been some successes in using proven strategies to convey information beyond the basic messages: for example, experiments with adapting the "training and visit" system of agricultural extension to health and family planning in several Indian states.

Abortions

Access to Safe Abortion

In the past three decades, more than 70 countries have changed their laws to remove criminal prohibitions of abortions or to expand the scope of provisions under which abortion had previously been legalized (Cook, 1989). More than 50 percent of all women in developing countries live in countries where induced abortion is legal under most circumstances, 27 percent live in countries where abortions are legal under various medical or social criteria, and 15 percent live in countries where induced abortion is either always illegal or legal only when a woman's life is threatened if she carries the pregnancy to term. These figures are heavily affected by China and India, however: excluding these countries, the figures are 19 percent (almost always legal), 52 percent (legal under specified criteria), and 28 percent (almost always illegal) (Population Reference Bureau, 1995; Henshaw and Morrow, 1990). The current legal status of induced abortion varies widely across regions: 174 million women live in developing countries where abortion is usually illegal, most of them in Central and West Africa, South Asia apart from India, the Middle East, and South America.

The legal status of abortion is without doubt important in determining whether women have access to safe abortions, but it is not the only

---

[7]Sheon, Schellstede, and Derr (1987: 367) define contraceptive social marketing as the distribution of contraceptives through existing commercial and retail channels, and their sale at low prices, with subsidies from national governments or donors, with the primary aim of achieving high distribution among low-income groups. (See also Sherris, Ravenholt, and Blackburn, 1985, for a review of social marketing.)

determinant. In many countries where abortions are legal, large numbers of women have little access to safe services. In some countries where abortions are meant to be legal under specified criteria, there are in fact few provisions for referring women who meet those criteria to abortion providers, and abortions are treated by the health services as though they were illegal under most circumstances. Conversely, there are countries where most abortions are illegal, but where women can find clinics that provide services with relative impunity, as in Colombia.

The problems of access, interpersonal relations, and technical quality of care may well be linked for abortion and emergency treatment of the sequelae of abortion. Even legal and mandated services can be abusive and accusatory (McLaurin, Hord, and Wolf, 1990). Studies in Brazil show poor technical quality of care—the wrong intravenous fluids used and wrong decisions about procedures (Costa and Vessey, 1993). In many countries, including India, induced abortion is legal under various circumstances, but many hospitals have no provisions for referrals or for performing the procedure: For many women in many countries, the right to a safe abortion exists only de jure, not de facto.

In many developing countries, the most common technique used for abortions in hospitals is still uterine evacuation through dilatation and curettage, although the World Health Organization recommends vacuum aspiration in most cases (World Health Organization, 1986). Dilatation and curettage needlessly exposes women to risks of uterine perforation and the risks associated with general anesthesia. Manual vacuum aspiration can be safely delivered in nonhospital settings (McLaurin, Hord, and Wolf, 1990).

Abortions will likely become more common in developing countries in the next few decades. There is very little information about how the necessary medical or paramedical supervision for medical abortions can be assured in practice, and how these services would best be linked with family planning. When providers are properly trained, manual vacuum aspiration should make early abortion safer and less expensive than the dilation and curettage procedure. For both provision of abortions where legal and treatment of incomplete abortions, the equipment and training for manual vacuum aspiration should be made widely available.

Sex-Selective Abortions

Prenatal diagnostic techniques, even those using sophisticated equipment, have spread to some developing countries, so that deformed or unhealthy—or female—fetuses can be identified. There has been a good deal of speculation about the use of such techniques to identify and abort female fetuses. There are three ways of determining the sex of a fetus:

chorionic villi sampling, amnioscentesis, and ultrasound imaging. Ultrasound imaging is very unreliable before the second trimester of a pregnancy, but it is the safest and cheapest of the methods and the most widely available in Asia, so there is some concern that the number of difficult late abortions may increase as a result of increased use of ultrasound imaging. Ultrasound equipment is available in hundreds of clinics and hospitals in India, no longer confined to the large, modern cities where the problem was first described.

Much of the evidence for widespread prenatal screening followed by sex-selective abortion is indirect, based on sex ratios of reported births. In South Korea, China, and Taiwan, the ratio of male births to female births has been steadily increasing since about 1980. In China, the ratio of male births to female births increases steeply with parity, up to parity four, and this difference increased over time during the 1980s (Westley, 1995). Sex-selective abortion illustrates the problems entailed in adopting a simple policy of goal maximization of individual reproductive choice. The definitions agreed at the ICPD lead to a salutary presumption that individual choices are paramount, but they do not solve all potential disputes about exactly which services are part of "reproductive health." India, Korea, and China have all adopted measures prohibiting fetal screening for sex and sex-selective abortion, but enforcement is likely to be difficult.

The Policy Environment

Fulfilling the goal of "every child wanted" will require changes of behavior on the part of public-sector bureaucracies (national and international), private-sector service providers, and current and potential users of services. In studying family planning programs it has sometimes proven useful to classify the needed changes as supply-side or demand-side factors, but the distinction between the two is artificial (Koenig and Simmons, 1992). New services are provided, or their quality and accessibility increased, or policies made more supportive, in part because political leaders and bureaucratic officials decide that these changes are beneficial for the country and conducive to their own continued rule, and in part because an educated and informed public pressures for changes. Organizations in both public and private sectors create their microenvironment, but are also creatures of the larger policy environment.

As we discuss in Chapters 6 and 7, family planning programs in developing countries are typically subsidized: contraceptive supplies, counseling, and clinical services are distributed either free of charge or at prices well below full cost recovery by government agencies and nongovernmental organizations (NGOs). Because of the large numbers of couples now entering peak ages for childbearing and the increasing reliance on modern contraception for fertility control, the demand for subsidized services could rise rapidly.

Countries with subsidized services that face increasing demand have a limited number of options: they can devote more public funds to subsidizing family planning; they can ration services; or they can reduce the average level of subsidy per contraceptive user. The latter can be done either by making services more efficient or by mobilizing private funds, for example, through user fees. In Chapter 7 we discuss the rationale for public-sector financing and some of the experience with user fees.

Recent discussions of population policy have returned to an issue that dominated much of the debate during the early years of international assistance to family planning in developing countries: whether the provision of contraceptive supplies and information suffice or a wide range of other incentives for fertility control and disincentives for large families (measures "beyond family planning") would be required to create effective demand for contraception. In large measure, this debate was overtaken by events in the 1970s and 1980s as individual demand for contraception proved strong in most countries even without incentives and disincentives. Once fertility declines began in Asian and Latin American countries, they proceeded with such rapidity that they seemed to have their own momentum; few stalled because of a lack of continued efforts to stimulate demand (Cleland and Wilson, 1987; Knodel, Chamratrithirong, and Debavalya, 1987; for a counter example, see Hirschman, 1986).

There is little information on which to base estimates of the likely effects on fertility intentions and behavior of policies in other sectors, such as education and social policies to improve women's status. Most current proposals are based on observations of associations (e.g., of women's education and fertility) rather than evaluations of actual interventions. Increasing girls' schooling is likely to produce a range of benefits for women, their families, and society at large.

In the discussions surrounding the ICPD in 1994, the demand-side proponents were not arguing for top-down incentives and disincentives aimed solely at fertility reduction, but for measures to improve education and literacy of women and to raise women's economic and legal status more generally. The argument is that when women have more decision-making power in their households, communities, and society, they will use it in ways that promote reproductive health in the largest sense. Conversely, where women are powerless, efforts to introduce reproductive health programs as isolated interventions will not achieve much.

When the client environment is supportive, programs are effective. Programs are forced to achieve more by a demanding public, as Nag (1983) has shown with useful comparisons of South Asian health services and Caldwell (1986) has argued with historical examples concerning child health. But there are also examples of family planning programs serving (as opposed to coercing) large numbers of women even in unpropitious circumstances, as in Bangladesh (Cleland et al., 1994). Where women are illiterate, poor, and powerless, an ability to limit fertility may be an important (though not in itself sufficient) precondition for change in their status. This argument can be made not only with examples from what are now poor countries, but with historical examples from what are now rich countries, where improvements in the legal and political status of women typically followed by decades the onset of fertility declines.

The education of girls and the improvement of the legal, economic, and political status of women have much broader effects on society than just their impact on fertility and reproductive health. But in the narrow sectoral perspective of a report on reproductive health, they might be seen as the long-term measures that would ensure the sustainability of all short-term programs targeted directly at improving reproductive health. These are complementary investments working on different time scales and through different organizations in society, rather than substitutes.

In the short run, there are several relatively low-cost ways in which policy reforms can support the goal of intended births. Kenney (1993) provides a convenient "checklist" of laws and administrative regulations that limit the availability of safe contraception: health and safety regulations that restrict the choice of methods or of providers; taxes and barriers to trade; regulation of advertising; and restrictions affecting the private sector (both commercial and nonprofit institutions).

Though it is likely that improved access and quality of family planning services would reduce high rates of abortion in many countries, even widespread and high-quality family planning services will not eliminate the demand for abortions. In practice, the effectiveness of reversible contraception is always well short of 100 percent, and coerced or simply unplanned sexual relations remain common.

It is beyond the scope of this report to assess the arguments about whether abortion is morally justified, and under what circumstances, or whether public financing and provision of abortions is justified in a society where a significant minority believe induced abortion to be immoral. But there are many countries where early abortions, in particular, are completely legal, yet unsafe abortions are common, and complications are a major health problem (World Health Organization, 1994). Even where abortions are largely or entirely illegal, medical care for complications is still provided. Thus, regardless of the legal status of induced abortion, improved care for incomplete abortions and complications must be seen as a part of reproductive health services.

TECHNICAL NOTE

Problems with Measurement of Fertility Intentions and Abortion

Much of the available evidence about fertility intentions comes from verbal reports of respondents' mental states at some time in the past or about hypothetical chances to make decisions all over again in response to standardized questions. It is imprecise, at best, to summarize intentions formed more or less unclearly and desires felt more or less intensely into simple dichotomies (wanted or unwanted; correctly timed or mistimed). Verbal reports can be inconsistent over time or with the subsequent behavior, or they may be too consistent, as when people rationalize whatever they did or come to terms with whatever happened to them by claiming that what happened is what was intended.

Estimates based on survey items like those used in the Demographic and Health Surveys (DHS) have been criticized by Pritchett (1994) and others on several grounds: preferences are unstable (though unstable individual preferences would not invalidate conclusions based on population averages; they are analogous to any type of measurement error in this respect), too hypothetical to be used as definitions of unmet need for contraception, and too much influenced by respondents' knowledge of what the interviewers would consider the "correct" answer. This last concern might diminish the usefulness of these survey items for predicting individual fertility without diminishing their usefulness for examining changes in norms or predicting fertility in a population.

Westoff (1990) has argued that data on fertility intentions are meaningful because in the aggregate they predict behavior: the proportion of women who reported in early surveys of the World Fertility Survey (WFS) or DHS that they want no more children was a good predictor of subsequent contraceptive use. However, this work tests only one of the survey items needed to construct measures of unwanted fertility. It could be that the *forward-looking* survey item ("Do you now want more children?") is an accurate predictor of behavior, at least in the aggregate, but the *recall* items ("Did you want your last pregnancy?") or explicitly *hypothetical* items ("If you could start over, how many children would you have?") are not valid or reliable. For example, we know of no direct attempts to validate the recall data by comparing prospective data gathered around the time of conceptions with data gathered later in pregnancies or after the outcomes. Answers to different questions in the same DHS interview can appear inconsistent, as for example, when women report that their last pregnancy was entirely unwanted (rather than mistimed) yet that they now want another child. (However, Westoff and Bankole [1995] report that removing such women does not much change aggregate estimates of unmet need for contraception.)

For this report, we rely most on the direct measure, for two reasons: the direct items allow consideration of mistiming as well as a desire for complete cessation of childbearing; and the major objection to the direct measure of wantedness is that it produces underreporting. But if significant percentages of pregnancies appear unwanted using a measure that is probably biased then the argument that unwantedness is a big problem is strengthened.

We need to distinguish between the wantedness of conceptions and of births. It is likely that many women change their minds about the impending birth during the course of the pregnancy, either becoming reconciled to the birth or regretting an initially wanted conception. Rosenzweig and Wolpin (1993), using data from a survey in the United States for which women were interviewed by random assignment either before or after a birth, found an 8 percent *decrease* in wantedness after the birth, which suggests that at least in this population regret may be more common than rationalization. In an extreme case, a woman may not have intended the sexual intercourse that produced the conception, or the conception, but report as pregnancy goes on that she wants the birth, perhaps not seeing any acceptable alternative. Such an "intended birth" would not be regarded as an indicator of good reproductive health. Conversely, a change of intentions about an initially wanted pregnancy could come about because of a change in circumstances during a pregnancy—abandonment or abuse by the father, for example. It has been argued that conceptions are intended even when births are not; this may be the case, for example, in cultures where a new or potential wife's proof of fecundity is highly valued.

Data on abortions provide evidence both of the extent of unintended pregnancy and of one of its major potentially harmful consequences in developing countries. But existing data are very incomplete. Direct estimates based on household surveys produce implausibly low estimates of the prevalence of induced abortion. In the United States, for example, where most states had liberalized abortion laws even before laws against first-trimester abortions were ruled unconstitutional in 1973, confidential surveys of providers suggest that induced abortions are more than twice as common as is reported in household surveys (Jones and Forrest, 1992). There has been some recent experimentation with survey methods in both developed and developing countries, and survey researchers may have given up too easily on the prospect of measuring abortion with direct questions (see Huntington, Mensch, and Miller, 1996; Laumann et al., 1994:457). The estimates produced by the Alan Guttmacher Institute and the World Health Organization (which we use in the text) are based on a combination of sources, including reports of abortion complications treated in hospitals and clinics which are then extrapolated to the community (see discussion in World Health Organization, 1994:5-9). The estimates, especially of clandestine abortions, should be considered approximate at best.

5

Healthy Pregnancy and Childbearing

An estimated 585,000 women die each year from pregnancy-related causes (World Health Organization and UNICEF, 1996). Such estimates have raised awareness of the fact that women still die in what is perceived by most to be a healthy process (Rosenfield and Maine, 1985). Since there are approximately 180 million pregnancies each year, the overall view of a healthy process is reasonable, but that view hides the huge disparity between women in developed and developing countries: about 1 in 48 women in developing countries dies of complications of pregnancy, delivery, puerperium, or abortion, compared with only 1 in 1,800 in developed countries; see Table 5-1. The risk of dying is highest for women in Africa, for two reasons: on average, they are pregnant and deliver more frequently than women on other continents and each pregnancy is riskier. Because of its much higher population, though, the majority of maternal deaths each year take place in Asia.

The consequences of a maternal death for a woman's family are also profound: if she dies, the chance of death for her children under the age of 5 is as high as 50 percent in developing countries (World Bank, 1993).

MATERNAL AND INFANT DEATH AND DISABILITY

Maternal Mortality

The causes of maternal mortality are divided into direct causes, those which occur only during pregnancy and the peripartum period, and indi-

TABLE 5-1 Maternal Mortality by Major Regions, Circa 1990

Region	Total Fertility Rate (births per woman)	Maternal Mortality Ratio (deaths per 100,000 live births)	Maternal Deaths	
			Lifetime Risk	per year
World Total	3.4	430	1 in 60	586,000
Developed Countries	1.8	27	1 in 1,800	4,000
Developing Countries	3.8	480	1 in 48	582,000
Africa	6.0	870	1 in 16	235,000
Asia	3.4	390	1 in 65	323,000
Latin America and the Caribbean	3.3	190	1 in 130	23,000

SOURCES: Data from World Health Organization and UNICEF (1996) and United Nations (1996).

rect causes, those that are aggravated by pregnancy but may be present even before pregnancy, such as diabetes, malaria, or hepatitis. Approximately 80 percent of all maternal deaths are estimated to be due to direct causes (World Health Organization, 1996). The World Health Organization (WHO) (1993c) estimates that hemorrhage is the most common direct cause, followed by sepsis and complications of unsafe abortion, hypertensive disorders of pregnancy (including eclampsia), and obstructed labor. The relative importance of different direct causes of mortality varies among studies, due in part to differences in reporting and definitions, and in part to real differences in the quality and accessibility of delivery care.

Although the definition of a maternal death includes a woman's death while pregnant or up to 42 days postdelivery from any cause (except accidental), most maternal deaths, excluding abortion-related deaths, occur during labor and delivery or soon thereafter. In a rural area of Bangladesh, for example, more than 70 percent of the nonabortion deaths occur in this short time span: 40 percent during labor or within 48 hours of delivery (primarily due to eclampsia and postpartum hemorrhage) and 30 percent between 3 and 42 days postdelivery, with sepsis and associated diseases leading the list of causes (Fauveau et al., 1988). Extending the definition of maternal death to 90 days postpartum, as has been proposed, would only have increased the number of maternal deaths by 6 percent. The critical period as that of labor and delivery is also supported by a nationally representative study in Egypt (Ministry of Health, 1994): 39 percent of deaths took place during delivery or within the first 24 hours, and 36 percent occurred within 42 days postpartum; only 25 percent took place during pregnancy itself.

Maternal Disability

Between 30 and 40 percent of pregnant women, or over 54 million women in developing countries, are estimated to experience a pregnancy-related complication annually (World Health Organization, 1993b; Koblinsky, Campbell, and Harlow, 1993). WHO estimates that 15 million women per year develop long-term disabilities from such complications as obstetric fistula, prolapse, severe anemia, pelvic inflammatory disease, and reproductive tract infections, as well as infertility.

At the country level, these estimates vary widely. For example, in community-based studies, Guatemalan women reported one in five pregnancies as complicated (Bailey, Szaszdi, and Schieber, 1994); in West Java, one in three women reported complications, not including those experienced in the postpartum period (Alisjahbana et al., 1995); and in Ghana, two of every three pregnant women had some complication, although the serious complications were infrequent (postpartum bleeding, 7 percent, convulsions, 2 percent, and postpartum sepsis, 5 percent (De Graft-Johnson, 1994). A population-based survey in El Salvador found one serious complication alone—intense intrapartum bleeding to the point of losing consciousness—was reported by nearly one-quarter of rural women (Danell et al., 1994). When the definition of complications is broadened to include perineal laceration, prolonged labor not leading to cesarean section, breech, multiple births, retained placenta, and other less severe complications, one-half of women in the Philippines reported a complication, with the most common being perineal lacerations (43% of respondents) (National Statistics Office and Macro International, Inc., 1994).

Reliability and validity of self-reported data on complications and their comparability across studies are likely to be poor (Task Force on Validation of Women's Reporting of Obstetric Complications, 1997). In a validation study undertaken at the Philippine General Hospital, Stewart and Festin (1995) developed algorithms based on reported symptoms to identify women most likely to have experienced hemorrhage, eclampsia, severe infection, and cesarean section due to obstructed labor. The algorithms were then used to identify women in the Demographic and Health Survey (DHS) sample likely to have suffered life-threatening maternal complications: 12 percent of all women in the sample were identified (National Statistics Office and Macro International, Inc., 1994). Hemorrhage was the most common complication (8%), followed by cesarean section due to obstructed labor (3%), severe infection (2%), and eclampsia (1%). The overall estimate is close to the 15 percent of women estimated to suffer "serious" complications based on data from the United States and Canada (Koblinsky, Campbell, and Harlow, 1993; World Health Organization, 1994b). If 12-15 percent of women suffer life-threatening obstetric complications, then approximately 20 million women in developing countries warrant referral care each year.

Millions more women suffer associated illnesses that are aggravated by pregnancy—anemia, malaria, cardiac disease, hepatitis, tuberculosis or diabetes—that can indirectly cause death or further disability for the woman or newborn. WHO estimates conservatively that 12.5 million women each year are affected by these illnesses aggravated by their pregnancies (World Health Organization, 1993b; Koblinsky, 1995). Approximately 20 percent of all maternal deaths in all regions are attributed to these indirect causes (World Health Organization, 1993b). Furthermore, the nonfatal consequences of obstetric complications and associated diseases can severely affect women's quality of life, fertility, productivity, and can result in chronic reproductive morbidities that may become evident only long after delivery.

Anemia

Given its high prevalence and impact on the lives and survival chances of women and newborns, anemia (hemoglobin counts below 11 g/dl) deserves special mention. Dietary iron deficiency is the most common cause of anemia, although malaria, other parasites (schistosomiasis and hookworm), AIDS and sickle-cell diseases may also contribute. Approximately 50 percent of pregnant women throughout the world are estimated to be anemic. A United Nations expert panel considers severe anemia (below 7 g/dl) an associated cause in up to half of maternal deaths worldwide (United Nations, 1991). Severe anemia may be directly associated with maternal morbidity and mortality, although available data do not often allow one to distinguish mild and severe anemia.

The impact of maternal anemia on the outcome of pregnancy—prematurity, stillbirths, spontaneous abortions, perinatal and neonatal mortality—is well documented (Levin et al., 1993). In a sample of 4,434 births in a northern Nigerian hospital, when maternal hematocrit levels measured 2 weeks before delivery were below 18 percent (the cutoff for severe anemia is 23%), nearly 50 percent of the births were stillbirths, and another 15 percent of newborns died in the neonatal period. When hematocrits were between 19-25 percent, stillbirths accounted for 22 percent of all births (Harrison, 1985). Two large studies, one in the United States and the other in Wales, found a U-shaped relationship between hemoglobin levels and the risk of low birth weight, prematurity, and perinatal mortality (Garn et al., 1981; Murphy et al., 1986). In both studies, hemoglobin levels below 10 g/dl and above 13 g/dl were associated with these poor birth outcomes.

One study from Nigeria implicates even mild anemia in 45 percent of maternal deaths of women who also suffered a major obstetric complication (Harrison, 1985). Iron-deficient women have an increased risk of complications during pregnancy, including urinary tract infections, pyelonephritis, and pre-eclampsia (Kitay and Harbort, 1975). Laboratory studies and studies with children have linked iron deficiency with increased morbidity from infectious diseases due to impaired immune function, although this would not explain the association with pre-eclampsia (Srikantia et al., 1976; Stinnett, 1983; Bhaskaram and Reddy, 1975; Enwonu, 1990). Anemia is also associated with reduced capacity to work, affecting both women's productivity and their quality of life (Bothwell and Charlton, 1981).

Besides anemia caused by iron deficiency, folate deficiency, which causes megaloblastic anemia, is also common in developing countries. This deficiency may have independent effects on birth weight, preterm birth, and, possibly, neural tube defects in newborns (Hughes, 1991).

Other common micronutrient deficiencies—particularly iodine and vitamin A—are also known to have similar negative pregnancy outcomes.

Obstetric Fistula and Genital Prolapse

Two chronic conditions warrant attention because of their high prevalence and devastating consequences—obstetric fistula and genital prolapse. An obstetric fistula is a passage in the vaginal wall leading into the bladder (vesico-vaginal fistula), the rectum (recto-vaginal fistula), or both. In developing countries where it has been reported, fistula is associated with prolonged and obstructed labor. Those at high risk of fistulas include very young women of low parity; women whose growth has been stunted by nutritional deficiency and recurrent infection in childhood that led to growth stunting; women in rural areas where health care is not accessible because of distance, lack of transport, and poverty; and women who prefer and have used traditional care and home delivery many times (Lawson, 1992; Murphy, 1981; Mustapha and Rushwan, 1971; Tahzib, 1983). A traditional practice in northern Nigeria, the gishri cut (the cutting of the anterior of the vagina as a way of treating a number of conditions, including obstructed labor, infertility, dyspareunia, and amenorrhea) further contributes to the risk of fistulas (Tahzib, 1983, 1985).

Good estimates of the prevalence of obstetric fistulas are impossible because the affected women do not seek or get care at hospitals, and health interview surveys have not elicited data on the condition. The available reports of fistula in developing countries come from most countries of sub-Saharan Africa and South and Southeast Asia (World Health Organization, 1991; Lawson, 1992).

The consequences of fistulas are devastating, especially for primiparas (women in their first pregnancies). In most cases, the baby is stillborn. The woman becomes incontinent of urine and sometimes of feces, uncomfortable conditions producing a foul odor and leading to feelings of shame and disgrace. The woman may not know about treatment, or she may be unable to seek professional help. Once the condition is seen as chronic, she is often deserted by her husband and has to seek support within her own family. Even there, she is usually segregated and not allowed to participate in certain activities, such as food preparation. In Islamic cultures, the woman may be forbidden to pray because of the requirement of cleansing oneself for prayer, which her condition of incontinence does not allow (Women's Global Network for Reproductive Rights, 1991; Murphy, 1981).

Also borne silently in most countries is genital prolapse, often considered a normal consequence of childbearing. Occurring when the vagina and uterus descend below their normal positions, this condition is associated with high parity and is often the result of damage during childbirth to the muscles and ligaments that support those organs. Genital prolapse is extremely uncomfortable, particularly for women who undertake chores in a squatting position, as is common in low-income and rural settings in developing countries . Prolapse may also be accompanied by backache (Younis et al., 1994) or urinary problems (Otubu and Ezem, 1982). Sexual intercourse may be painful, and pregnancy can lead to fetal loss and further maternal morbidity (Younis et al., 1994; Das, 1971).

As with fistula, there are no reliable large-scale population-based estimates of the prevalence of genital prolapse. A Brazilian hospital study revealed that 40 of every 1,000 women coming to a university hospital for other reasons suffered severe genital prolapse (Pinotti, Brenelli, and Moragues, 1993). Community-based studies have found between one-third and two-thirds of women with prolapse in Lahore, Pakistan, Istanbul, Turkey, and in two rural villages in Giza, Egypt (Omran and Standley, 1981; Younis et al., 1993). Clinically confirmed severe prolapse was found in almost one-third of the women in a study in Giza, Egypt; many were found to be using an intrauterine device (IUD) for contraception despite the fact that IUDs increase the discomfort of the prolapse (Zurayk, Younis, and Khattab, 1995). The Giza study also revealed an association between prolapse and reproductive tract infections (Younis et al., 1993).

Consequences for Infants

The impact of women's reproductive health on the fetus or newborn is immediate and dramatic. An estimated 7.6 million perinatal deaths (stillbirths and first-week deaths) occur each year in developing countries (World Health Organization, 1996). These perinatal deaths are associated to a large extent with their mothers' health and nutritional status prior to and during pregnancy, the management of labor and delivery, and the same maternal complications that can cause women's deaths. About one-half of all deaths of children under age 5 occur in their first month of life. Population-based studies in South Asia and the Philippines suggest that approximately 20-25 percent of perinatal deaths are associated with causes known to threaten the survival of women during pregnancy or delivery, another 20 percent are due to management practices at delivery, and more than one-third are due to women's health and nutritional status (Shah, Pratinidhi, and Bhatlawande, 1984a, 1984b; Fauveau et al., 1990; National Statistics Office and Macro International, Inc., 1994). Programs aimed at improving women's health and nutritional status and at managing obstetric complications and providing appropriate care of the newborn could reduce this enormous death toll (World Health Organization, 1994a).

The consequence of a mother's health and nutritional status, management of delivery, and early newborn care may not be death for the infant, but long-term disability. Obstructed or prolonged labor leads to asphyxia for an estimated 3 percent of newborns, resulting not only in death for nearly a one-quarter of these infants, but also in brain damage leading to cerebral palsy, seizures, and severe learning disorders for another quarter (World Health Organization, 1993b). Women with poor nutritional status (short stature, poor prepregnancy weight, inadequate weight gain during pregnancy, and anemia) or reproductive tract infections or other infections during pregnancy are more likely to have low birth-weight infants. The perinatal mortality rate of a low birth-weight baby is 20 to 30 times higher than that of a fetus or infant of normal weight. Many low birth-weight infants who do not die may suffer serious neurological problems, hearing and visual defects, and may be subject to slow development throughout their lives.

INTERVENTIONS TO REDUCE MATERNAL DEATHS

The most immediate pathway to maternal death begins with conception. The major complications that cause maternal death may be present initially in a mild form, progressing to severe complications in some 12-15 percent of all pregnancies. Interventions can stop this progression at several points:

- prevent unintended pregnancies (see Chapter 4),
- prevent diseases that will complicate pregnancy or detect and treat early signs of complications, and
- treat complications at the mild or severe level with "essential care of obstetric complications."

Prevention and Early Treatment of Diseases and Complications

Prenatal care is primarily preventive, enabling health care staff to identify problems and illnesses that threaten a pregnancy and its outcome, to monitor and treat some conditions, and to give the pregnant woman and her family information about appropriate diet, behaviors, and delivery care.

Most studies of the effectiveness of prenatal care have focused on infant outcomes—perinatal mortality, preterm delivery, and low birth weight. But an association between use of prenatal care and maternal mortality has also been found in hospital case series, case-control studies, and informal surveys, although it is argued that this association is due to selection bias—that is, the women who use prenatal services are also more likely to take better care of themselves and use delivery services (Rooney, 1992). The major direct causes of maternal deaths in developing countries can neither be predicted nor prevented (Maine, 1991; Thaddeus and Maine, 1994).

Prenatal care may be effective in detecting and treating two conditions that underlie the direct medical causes of maternal and perinatal death: anemia and hypertension. For the mother, one of the most important benefits of prenatal care can be the provision of information about obstetric emergencies and linkage to sources of care. For this reason, it is best to consider prenatal care and delivery and early postpartum care as parts of a whole, rather than as separate interventions.

The benefits of adequate prenatal care for the health of the infants are somewhat clearer, but difficult to evaluate, because women who get inadequate prenatal care are more likely to have other risk factors for poor pregnancy outcomes (Kramer, 1987). Some observational studies with reasonable controls for confounding variables have found that better prenatal care is associated with such improved outcomes as lower rates of intrauterine growth retardation and premature delivery (e.g., Coria-Soto, Bobadilla, and Notzon, 1996). Tetanus toxoid immunization during pregnancy has been crucial in reducing neonatal and maternal tetanus (Fauveau et al., 1990). Screening for, and treating, syphilis during pregnancy is beneficial to both mothers and infants.

Risk Assessment

Predicting those pregnancies that will go on to suffer mild or severe complications on the basis of risk factors (as opposed to medical signs or symptoms of complications) has not proved useful. Demographic factors, such as age, parity, or a combination thereof, have not proved to be sensitive and specific enough. In a Philippines' population-based survey, for example, background characteristics of respondents reporting symptoms of major obstetric complications for births in the past 3 years revealed minimal variation among the age or parity groups, suggesting that these demographic indicators are inadequate predictors of risk of an obstetric complication (National Statistics Office and Macro International, Inc., 1994). In a program context, the use of such risk factors as the basis for referral could either overwhelm the maternity care system, or, if only specific ones are used, focus attention on those women who contribute minimally to maternal deaths. In Guatemala, for example, 70 percent of the women would be considered at risk if age and parity were used as risk factors, while the system can only manage 20 percent (Schieber, 1993). In

Egypt, only 16.4 percent of deaths occurred among women aged less than 20 or more than 40 years, two common demographic factors. Although these women have a higher risk of death, the numbers of such women are low in comparison with women who die between 20-40 years of age simply because most pregnancies occur to women aged 20-40 (Ministry of Health, 1994).

Educational background did produce some variation in the proportion of women with any symptom of obstetric complication in the Philippine survey. However, most of the variation could be explained by differences in cesarean section due to obstruction, the one complication that requires hospital treatment. This result has been interpreted to indicate that educated respondents had better access to medical services (National Statistics Office and Macro International, Inc., 1994).

Any woman, regardless of age, parity, socioeconomic status, or education, can develop a complication at any stage of pregnancy, delivery, or the postpartum period. If a complication develops, it may be an emergency (e.g., hemorrhage) or may be taken seriously only when it reaches the stage of being an emergency (e.g., sepsis, eclampsia, obstructed labor).

Anemia

Anemia is targeted for detection (if screening is carried out) or prevention (if iron tablets are given to all pregnant women) during prenatal care. However, three decades of prenatal distribution of iron and folate tablets to pregnant women has had little impact on the levels of anemia. This outcome does not reflect lack of efficacy of iron supplementation: in supervised trials in both developed and developing countries, iron tablets are associated with improved maternal hematologic status (depending on the initial anemia status and dose and duration of supplementation) (Mahomed and Hytten, 1989; Sloan, Jordan, and Winikoff, 1992). The side effects that sometimes accompany iron consumption or women's dislike of the pills themselves (due to smell or taste) often have been blamed for the failure of programs to reduce anemia, although a recent literature review found that side effects accounted for only 10 percent of the noncompliance. Rather, in most cases, women did not take their pills because they never received them or received them in inadequate numbers (Galloway and McGuire, 1994). Not enough pills are purchased by health facilities or governments because of lack of funds or a perception that anemia is not a serious health problem.

Yet even in areas where supplementation trials have taken place, overall prevalence of anemia often remains high. In India, for example, the prevalence of anemia decreased only from 88 percent to 56 percent in the highest iron dose group (240 mg) after a well-conducted trial by Sood et al. (1975). The authors concluded that it is difficult to treat a severely iron deficient woman and provide for increased fetal needs through oral iron supplementation alone during the relatively short period of pregnancy. Thus, in developing countries, prolonged supplementation beginning before women become pregnant may be a more effective strategy to benefit the majority of the population (Sloan, Jordan, and Winikoff, 1992; Galloway and McGuire, 1994). Community-based distribution schemes along with counseling on why, how, and when to take pills and where to obtain refills could increase access and compliance.

Long-term strategies to improve the overall iron status of the general population include increased production and consumption of iron-rich foods, increased family income, fortification of commonly consumed food with iron, and reduction of work for women. Food-based solutions for increasing iron consumption are not promising because most diets are plant-based and contain only small amounts of absorbable iron, except when fermented and germinated foods are added (which reduce the inhibitors of iron in the diet). Even when such additives are provided, food-based solutions seem to require increasing family income or the control of it by women.

Fortification schemes have proved successful in developed countries and have virtually eliminated iron deficiency anemia in small children (Dallman, 1989, 1993). The key to successful fortification is finding a food that all vulnerable groups consume and regulating the private sector to ensure compliance with norms for fortification. These are not easy tasks. Even if an appropriate food is identified, women would still need to take supplements to meet their iron requirements during pregnancy. Reducing maternal workloads may decrease women's overall requirement for iron, and all programs addressing anemia should include counseling of family members so they can help reduce a pregnant woman's activities, particularly during her third trimester.

Hypertension

Eclampsia and pre-eclampsia, the life-threatening complications of hypertensive disorders in pregnancy, have proved difficult to predict or prevent. Although eclampsia is considered the terminal stage of hypertensive disorders of pregnancy, a high proportion of cases occur in women in developed countries who did not have previous hypertension and proteinuria. This may be due to detection and management of patients with classic signs of pre-eclampsia, leaving a higher percentage of atypical eclampsia cases, or it may be that eclampsia can occur so rapidly that prior signs are not noted. At any rate, detection of the classic form of the disease is made difficult because its natural progression is not well understood, and the relative importance of the degree and timing during pregnancy of the symptoms (hypertension, proteinuria, edema, or other biochemical abnormalities) is unclear (Rooney, 1992). Predicting pre-eclampsia is also elusive: only severe obesity and a history of pre-eclampsia have been found to be independently associated with severe pre-eclampsia (Stone et al., 1994). Primary prevention with low-dose aspirin or with calcium supplementation is being studied, although evidence is accumulating against the use of aspirin among low-risk women for prevention of pre-eclampsia (Villar and Bergsjo, 1996).

Blood pressure measurements during pregnancy continue to be recommended, although the minimum number and timing of the measurements to detect cases of severe pre-eclampsia or eclampsia is unknown (Rooney, 1992). Neither edema nor proteinuria detect pre-eclampsia as well as prenatal measurements of blood pressure (Golding, Shenton, and MacGillivray, 1988; Hall, Chng, and MacGillivray, 1980). However, urinalysis for proteinuria is recommended for all women on the first prenatal visit (along with blood pressure measurement) because of the severity of the disease if found in the early part of pregnancy. After the first visit, proteinuria should be detected during all visits only for nulliparous women or those with previous pre-eclampsia or hypertension (Villar and Bergsjo, 1996). Women with moderate or high hypertension with proteinuria require referral and treatment.

The wide variation in case fatality rates for women from eclampsia or pre-eclampsia among countries suggests that differences in care can improve outcomes. Women with pre-eclampsia and eclampsia experience better outcomes when they have access to and use professional care (Rooney, 1992). Rest, antihypertensives, and anticonvulsants are presently considered possible treatments. Evidence is insufficient to determine the effect of bedrest, which in any case is often an unrealistic prescription. Antihypertensive drugs have been shown to prevent further increase in hypertension, but their effect on preventing pre-eclampsia is still uncertain (Rooney, 1992). For women who have already progressed to convulsions (eclampsia), a recent multicenter trial showed that the anticonvulsant drug of choice should be magnesium sulfate rather than diazepam or phenytoin, as it decreases the risk of recurrent convulsions (The Eclampsia Trial Collaborative Group, 1995).

Other Diseases

Approximately 30,000 maternal deaths yearly may be caused by tetanus (Fauveau et al., 1993). Where tetanus is a cause of maternal mortality, adequate protection for mothers may be provided during prenatal care by the tetanus toxoid immunization typically aimed at protecting newborns.

In the Philippines, tetanus toxoid injections have been given to all adolescent girls to increase the probability that they will be adequately protected the first time they give birth. Reproductive tract infections, including sexually transmitted diseases, should also be screened for and treated during prenatal care. As we note in Chapter 3, at a minimum, syphilis should be screened and treated during pregnancy, and newborns should be given prophylaxis for gonococcal and chlamydial eye infections (ophthalmia neonatorum). These eyedrops can be given by traditional birth attendants: they are simple, inexpensive interventions that are highly cost-effective in most parts of the developing world.

Obstructed and Prolonged Labor

Obstructed and prolonged labors are estimated to cause 40,000 maternal deaths each year, with many more survivors suffering obstetric fistulae while their newborns suffer death or brain damage from asphyxia. Prompt detection and management of obstructed and prolonged labor can have a beneficial effect on the outcome of pregnancy for both mothers and infants. Risk factors for this complication during pregnancy (e.g., height, foot size, or history of poor previous outcome) have not proven to be specific or sensitive enough (Fortney, 1995; Maine, 1991). But monitoring during labor allows for early intervention or referral with the consequent reduction in a number of sequelae of severe obstructed labor.

A recent WHO multicenter trial of more than 35,000 women who delivered in eight hospitals in Indonesia, Thailand, and Malaysia found the partograph a beneficial tool for detecting labors that progress too slowly and led to guidelines for labor management (World Health Organization, 1994a). The partograph is a chart to record the progress of labor and other essential fetal and maternal observations. When the partograph shows an abnormal progress of labor, drugs may be used to improve the pattern of contractions for a normal delivery, or a cesarean section may be performed. Through comparison of patients before and after introduction of the partograph, this multicenter hospital study showed that the number of prolonged labors (>18 hours) was halved, the rate of postpartum infection (sepsis) was cut by over one-half, and the number of stillbirths fell from 5 to 3 per 1,000 babies. Fewer drugs were also needed, and caesarean sections for women without complications were avoided, with no adverse impact on the condition of the fetuses.

If labor is followed with the partograph by a medical professional in a home or health center, it is assumed that time would allow for referral to a medical center where prolonged or obstructed labor could be managed. However, there has been no trial on use of the partograph in the home or health center by medical staff.

Essential Care for Obstetric Complications

Since the major causes of maternal mortality cannot be predicted or prevented well enough during pregnancy to allow reliance on primary prevention and screening, improvements in maternal death rates will require that women have access to facilities with trained providers and equipment that can carry out essential care of obstetric complications. Defined by WHO first in 1985 with refinements made in 1995 (World Health Organization, 1995), essential care of obstetric complications consists of:

- the ability to carry out surgery (i.e., caesarean section, treatment of sepsis, removal of an ectopic pregnancy),
- the ability to provide intravenous oxytocin,
- the provision of anesthesia,
- medical treatment (for shock, sepsis, anemia, and hypertensive disorders of pregnancy),
- replacement of blood,
- manual procedures (e.g., removal of placenta, repair of episiotomies and perineal tears and vacuum extractions),
- monitoring of labor (including use of the partograph),
- management of problem pregnancies (severe anemia, diabetes, twins, malpresentation),
- manual vacuum aspiration for treatment of incomplete abortions, and
- provision of special care for neonates (e.g., resuscitation).

Historical experience provides evidence for the effectiveness of this approach. It was not until the mid-1930s, with the introduction of medical technologies to treat obstetric complications, that maternal mortality began to decline in several European countries and in the United States. After antibiotics, blood transfusions, and improved surgical techniques in caesarean sections and safe abortions became routinely available in the industrialized world, maternal mortality all but disappeared (Loudon, 1991). Prior to that time, infant mortality had declined dramatically in the United States and Europe, but maternal mortality had remained constant. While the causes of infant death are extremely sensitive to environmental factors and respond quickly to improved sanitation and nutrition, the majority of obstetric complications that cause maternal deaths cannot be averted simply by improving women's overall health or nutritional status (Loudon, 1991).

In Sweden, where mortality statistics have been kept since 1750, the maternal mortality ratio declined from 900 to 6 per 100,000 live births between 1750 and 1980, with two-thirds of the decrease occurring in the eighteenth and nineteenth centuries. This decline, not reported in other European countries, has been attributed to home-assisted births by trained midwives and the use of aseptic techniques. The decline in the maternal mortality ratio in Sweden in the twentieth century was attributable to the same factors as in the rest of Europe and United States (Hogberg and Wall, 1986; Hogberg, Wall, and Brostroin, 1986).

Implementation of some elements of essential care of obstetric complications in a few developing countries has also resulted in substantial declines in maternal mortality (World Health Organization, 1995). Sri Lanka's maternal mortality ratio dropped dramatically: from 555 per 100,000 live births in 1950-1955 to 239 in the 1960s and to 95 in 1980. A nationwide extension of the health center system and expansion of midwifery skills are credited with this rapid decline. A major shift toward birth with trained personnel occurred over this 30-year period, with a major impact on the proportion of deaths attributed to sepsis.

MATERNITY CARE AND SURVIVAL

Use of Maternity Care

The use of medical services for delivery lags far behind use of prenatal care in most developing countries. Home birth, either alone or with someone from the community, remains a strong preference. WHO estimates that only 37 percent of births in developing countries take place in a health facility; more than 60 percent of births—or 55-60 million infants annually—take place with only the help of traditional birth attendants, family members, or no assistance (World Health Organization, 1993a).

The reasons for the widespread acceptance of prenatal care throughout developing countries were captured nicely by Bolivian women who stated, "because you're in a delicate condition," "to see if the baby's okay" (The Center for Health Research, Consultation and Education and MotherCare/John Snow, Inc., 1991). In 39 of 43 countries covered by DHS surveys between 1985 and 1994, coverage for prenatal care was found to be higher than for delivery care from a trained health provider (doctor, nurse, or nurse-midwife) (Macro International, Inc., 1994). In sub-Saharan Africa, for example, 15 of 22 countries surveyed had achieved over 75 percent prenatal care coverage (women's own definition of prenatal care was used), and only 2 had below 50 percent coverage (Macro International Inc., 1994). But only one country, Botswana, achieved over 75 percent of deliveries with professional health care providers. Between 50-75 percent of pregnant women in one-half of the other countries used medical services for delivery, while in the other one-half of the countries less than 50 percent did so.

Latin American and Caribbean countries have somewhat higher coverage rates than sub-Saharan African countries. In 3 of 11 Latin American countries (Trinidad and Tobago, the Dominican Republic, and Colombia), more than 75 percent of women both used prenatal care and gave birth with the assistance of a professional health care provider. In five countries, prenatal coverage rates ranged between 50-75 percent, and four of these had delivery assistance in the same range. Bolivia had prenatal care coverage in that range, but delivery assistance was slightly lower at 47 percent. In only one country, Guatemala, was coverage for both types of services less than 50 percent (Macro International, Inc., 1994).

In the Asian countries surveyed, three-quarters of pregnant women used prenatal care, covering women in Indonesia, Philippines, Sri Lanka, and Thailand; in Bangladesh and Pakistan, only one-quarter of women used prenatal care. Three of every four Sri Lankan women, one-half of Thai women, and two-thirds of Philippino women had a professional attending their deliveries. In the remaining three countries, Bangladesh, Pakistan, and Indonesia, between one and three out of every ten women had a professional in attendance.

Data on the use of postpartum services are relatively scarce, but the rates are typically lower than rates of institutional delivery. In the African countries for which data are available, coverage for postpartum care has for the most part not exceeded 40 percent, even in urban areas. Latin American rates are slightly higher than those for Africa, and Asian women seem the most likely to attend a postpartum clinic. However, data are sparse, and information is not available on the types of providers who are serving women in this period nor women's reasons for seeking such care (World Health Organization, 1993a). Even rates of coverage provide little information about the quality of care or the reasons for its use.[1] What these coverage rates do show is that a substantial portion of women remain outside delivery and postpartum services for reasons that could range from taboos on mobility to preference to remain at home to the unavailability or inaccessibility of appropriate care. Women living in rural areas or having no education use all these services less than other women, while differences in age, parity, and birth interval are less consistent in determining coverage rates (Govindasamy et al., 1993).

---

[1]When facilities exist, service providers may lack the basic equipment and supplies, the person with the appropriate skills may be absent, or routine monitoring during pregnancy, labor, and delivery or in the puerperium may result in no follow-up of abnormal findings.

Pathway to Maternal Survival

Since most women in developing countries experience labor and delivery outside the formal health care system, we discuss obstetric care under a four-step pathway to maternal survival, assuming that labor begins for a woman in her home (see also Thaddeus and Maine, 1994). From the point that an obstetric or newborn complication occurs, four steps are required to promote survival of the woman or the baby:

Step 1: recognizing a life-threatening complication by the woman, her family, traditional birth attendant, or others in attendance;

Step 2: deciding to seek care, typically by family members if the woman is in poor condition;

Step 3: reaching quality services, which often involves overcoming impediments such as distance, cost of or lack of transport, cost of the services, geographical or weather constraints, and perceived poor quality or attitude of the providers; and

Step 4: obtaining appropriate care for obstetric complications.

Death of a woman, fetus, or newborn is likely to ensue if one of these steps is not taken.[2] This same sequence is relevant when a woman suffering complications has made contact with a health care provider. If the provider diagnoses the problem, decides on the appropriate care, and refers to quality care on a timely basis or provides adequate care, death is more likely to be averted for the woman and her baby.

The family side of this chain of events was followed in a retrospective study in the altiplano in a remote area of Bolivia (Bartlett, 1991). In only one-quarter of the cases resulting in maternal and neonatal deaths were the symptoms of a life-threatening condition recognized by the family in time, and in another one-quarter of cases the symptoms were not recognized at all. The most common response among the families who tried to do something about the problem was to administer home-made remedies to the sick mother or infant; fewer than one-third of families who took any action sought care from a source with at least some appropriate knowledge and resources (9% of the fatal cases).

Step 1: Recognition of Complications

Pregnancy is generally considered a time of well-being. Evidence for

---

[2]The problems we classify under steps 3 and 4 (getting to care, poor quality of care) would also influence the family's decision whether or not to seek care. We discuss them sequentially, though, as a convenient way to classify needed interventions.

this view comes from focus groups with pregnant and recently delivered women in projects in rural areas of West Java, Indonesia, Bangladesh, and Nigeria; in rural and urban settings in Jamaica; and a periurban/urban area of Bolivia (see Appendix B). Labor and delivery, however, are anticipated with some trepidation: it is rightly considered, in the words of an Indonesian woman, the time when she is "caught between life and death." Jamaican women were even more expressive: "Having the baby is life and death . . . is not cutting a slice of cake" (Wedderburn and Moore, 1990:26). When the delivery is over, however, fears for the woman's life generally pass, and attention shifts to the newborn, for whom the first month of life is seen as challenging.

If a complication for either the woman or newborn arises, it is often considered fated, with little that can be done. In Indonesia, most pregnant women are even reluctant to talk about possible complications because they believe talking may be prophetic. Hessler-Radelet (1993), in exploring these issues in West Java, determined that a complication may not be considered serious if it disappears after birth (e.g., as does swelling), does not cause pain (malposition), is treatable with medicine (e.g., fevers and headaches), is common in pregnancy (swelling), is common outside of pregnancy (e.g., fevers), does not restrict daily activities, or is inevitable (fate or the will of God). Bolivian women, for example, consider swelling beneficial, believing it to result from the accumulation of blood that is necessary for the birth to take place. Even fever following delivery is considered a normal part of the birthing process for most women. Bolivian women are the exception, however, greatly fearing complications in the postpartum period; several of the conditions they describe as dangerous include chills and fever. Although Bolivian women with fever are treated first at home, they may also go to the hospital (if referred) because of the perceived seriousness of this complication (The Center for Health Research, Consultation and Education and Mother-Care/John Snow, Inc., 1991).

In Indonesia as well as in Bolivia, malposition is viewed by women and traditional birth attendants as the domain of the attendants. Following the seventh month, Indonesian women visit the attendants regularly for checks on the baby's position. Soothing massage is given to help pregnant women maintain the inner calm deemed necessary during pregnancy, labor, and delivery and to "correct" the baby's position (Ambaretnani, Hessler-Radelet, and Carlin , 1993). Referral may not take place until prolonged or obstructed labor is already under way. Bolivian women also seek attendants to correct the position of the baby through massage as well as *manteo*, a gentle rocking of the woman in a blanket (The Center for Health Research, Consultation and Education, and MotherCare/John Snow, Inc., 1991).

Bleeding stands out as the one maternal complication that commands attention almost everywhere. During pregnancy, or in the intrapartum or postpartum periods, the extent of bleeding is watched apprehensively—"bad" blood must leave the body, but "good" blood must remain. But there are exceptions even to this rule: Yoruba women of Nigeria stated that bleeding causes a pregnancy only to be interrupted, and the woman will take more than nine months to deliver (Public Opinion Polls, 1993).

The Quechua and Aymara women of Bolivia believe they must watch what enters their bodies to control the necessary shedding of blood. A balance of hot and cold must be achieved after delivery, as "dirty blood" of childbirth must be lost, but not to the point of excessive bleeding. Cold air and being unclothed, or underclothed, as is often the case in a hospital delivery, are feared, as coldness suspends the expulsion of the "dirty blood" and can cause swelling of the body and a series of very dangerous puerperal illnesses according to women (The Center for Health Research, Consultation and Education and MotherCare/John Snow, Inc., 1991).

Since traditional birth attendants oversee many deliveries, their recognition of symptoms of complications and knowledge of what to do about them can be critical for maternal and infant survival. In focus groups with attendants in Bolivia, Indonesia, and Nigeria, discussion of complications during any period of the reproductive process did not elicit much reaction. Their major role, as perceived by themselves, is the appropriate positioning of the baby. In West Java, for example, malpresentation was the major discussion topic. Malpresentations are managed by the attendants unless labor is prolonged, which one considered to be more than 8 hours. No attendant admitted a "difficult labor." Traditional birth attendants occasionally referred a patient to a health center or hospital, but most often the referral is declined, they stated, for reasons of expense, distance, and fear of being away from family and friends. In Indonesia and among the Fulani and Hausa of Nigeria, attendants said they will not even advise referral if they believe that the family will not comply.

Bolivian attendants mentioned pain in the back, vagina, and belly and vaginal bleeding as pregnancy-related complications, and almost all of them attributed these symptoms to the poor position of the baby. Management includes massage of the abdomen or advice on rest; a few attendants do refer women to formal health services. Delivery complications they mentioned include a bad position of the baby, emergence of the umbilical cord, arm, or leg prior to the head, and the umbilical cord wrapped around the baby. These complications mean that women have not taken care of themselves or pushed too early, stated the attendants, and referral to a doctor is in order, although some mentioned they try to accelerate delivery by cutting the amniotic sack with a razor blade or massaging the abdomen. Most said a normal delivery is 4 to 14 hours, but others said 1 to 3 days. If labor lasts longer than normal, the woman is given hot teas and massage.

From these qualitative studies it can be concluded that neither women nor traditional birth attendants perceive obstetric complications as necessarily requiring medical assistance. Apart from bleeding, problems are generally explained by and thought to require other types of more spiritual interventions, described below. The attendants' role is primarily involved with the baby's position, and to her most other problems are explained by this central factor.

Step 2: Deciding to Seek Care

Use of formal health care for delivery is rare not just because of perceptions about the services, lack of transport, distance, or funds. Home is strongly preferred as the place of birth for a variety of reasons. The decision to seek professional assistance for women suffering with complications is made even more complex by what is considered "appropriate care." Appropriateness depends on the perception of the interpreter as to the nature of the complication (physical versus spiritual) and of the seriousness of the condition. For bleeding, women most often seek medical care. But for other complications, such as obstructed labor—which is believed in one country to be caused by adultery during pregnancy—it is perceived to be more "appropriate" to consult a diviner and confess one's sins than to seek care from the formal health care system. According to the available qualitative studies, the demand for delivery services can be weak, even when other obstacles to access are absent.

In Indonesia, the period of labor is seen to place women in a vulnerable position between life and death—death may come to her as life is entering this world. However, the forces that keep a woman in labor on the side of life are linked to the home and the inner calm that is found there, not to a health facility. Because Indonesian women do not want to think about negative events or plan ahead for such (which will disrupt their sense of inner calm), they instead plan for the best-chance scenario, hoping that a complication will not arise. Should a complication arise during delivery with a traditional birth attendant (who assists with 85% of deliveries in Indonesia), she may or may not be referred, depending on whether the attendant believes the woman will accept referral. For bleeding, however, most Indonesian women state they would seek help at the health center from a midwife or doctor (Ambaretnani, Hessler-Radelet, and Carlin, 1993).

In Bolivia, the home provides privacy; no strangers to look, laugh, and touch the woman. As Bolivian women said (The Center for Health Research, Consultation and Education, 1991:23):

> At home it's private, you don't pay anything. . . . They don't under-
> stand us well in the hospital; besides, my friends tell me that they touch
> everything—our genitals—and also there's a lot of health staff.

Although the complications of delivery that can kill may be recognized by
Bolivian women, they are not considered amenable to medical intervention (The Center for Health Research, Consultation and Education, 1991).
Locally recognized causes of maternal death include *arrebato*, a disease
caused by failing to bind the woman's head, and the rising up of the
magre, an organ formed behind the navel during pregnancy that should
be "lowered" during childbirth with the womb, baby, placenta, and blood.
There is no organ equivalent in biomedical anatomy, but the fear of the
magre rising is so great that women bind their abdomens to keep it down.
To prevent these complications, Bolivian women not only bind their bellies, but also wrap their heads, drink teas and other home preparations,
and massage bellies (both to apply heat and to assure the proper position
of the baby). Few women believe that these problems could be prevented
by going to prenatal care and to the hospital for delivery.

The "secret of pregnancy," the feeling of shame, and the uncertainty
about the outcome are so strong among the Fulani and Hausa in Nigeria
that no preparation is made concerning labor and delivery by women and
their husbands. The home is the natural place for delivery, more familiar
and less threatening than a medical facility, and does not expose one to
shame. Little or no assistance is sought by these women during delivery,
even in their home (Public Opinion Polls, 1993).

The postpartum period, described most often by women as non-life-
threatening, is generally filled with traditions and taboos. Many are harm-
less or beneficial, but some can interfere with the use of valuable postpartum services. Women in Indonesia are prohibited from leaving their
home for 40 days, so they do not seek postpartum care from a formal
health provider unless and until the situation becomes very grave
(Ambaretnani, Hessler, and Carlin, 1993). Nigerian women go through a
period of hot baths or massage with a hot napkin after delivery. Most
Yoruba women claimed that this will rid the body of blood that has co-
agulated inside the woman during delivery. Failure to observe the hot
bath period (7 to 40 days) is believed to meet with dire consequences—
swelling and smelly vaginal discharge (Public Opinion Polls, 1993). Medical providers are not seen as beneficial at this time.

Step 3: Reaching a Facility that Can Provide Care

There are many logistical and provider barriers to access for women
trying to reach appropriate services once they and their families have
determined to do so (Leslie and Gupta, 1989; Sundari, 1992; Kutzin, 1993;

Thaddeus and Maine, 1994). Lack of facilities with skilled personnel and equipment and supplies to support essential obstetric care, poor attitudes of providers, unavailability and cost of transportation, and the high costs of services are referred to repeatedly as the major obstacles to using services. Specific country-level efforts aimed at detailing these barriers to access essential obstetric services have only recently begun. The lack of services (including facilities, skilled personnel, drugs, and equipment) has been underscored in India, Bangladesh, Indonesia, Guatemala, and Bolivia, as well as in the African countries of Nigeria, Ghana, and Sierra Leone.

A UNICEF survey in three districts of India in 1993 found that two districts had a deficit of emergency obstetric care beds (those assigned for patients with emergency obstetric complications), assuming one bed is needed per 1,000 births. (Emergency obstetric care in their definition is a subset of what we have termed essential care for obstetric complications, consisting of caesarean sections, blood transfusions, as well as the availability of oxytocin, sedatives, and antibiotics.) In all three districts, the emergency obstetric beds were concentrated in district hospitals, resulting in a very high bed occupancy rate (110 percent in one of the districts). Between 4 and 10 percent of births were taking place in these first referral units, although 15 percent of births are expected to have serious complications (as described above). Actually, only 3.0 to 6.5 percent of complicated births were managed in these facilities.

Using a list of 38 drugs as essential for effective management of common obstetric complications that can lead to maternal death (World Health Organization, 1995), the UNICEF survey found that not one of the 18 facilities observed had all the drugs. In fact, less than one-half of the essential drugs were available in most sites. Trained personnel to provide caesarean surgery was missing in 14 of the 18 facilities, and none of the first referral units had staff with neonatal resuscitation skills. Most sites did have anesthesia capability or a surgical specialist who might need only a short orientation; all but three of the sites needed staff training in blood transfusion services.

Similar results were found in Indonesia and Bolivia. Each of three districts in South Kalimantan, Indonesia, had one or more government hospitals, but obstetricians were absent in two of the three districts. Although one midwife was available per 100-200 pregnant women, the midwives did not have the supplies or equipment (or the regulations to support them) to manage serious complications. Resuscitation equipment and skills were notably lacking, as was the skill to remove retained placenta, a common complication. Less than 5 percent of pregnant women delivered in the hospitals of the two districts for which there were data (Achadi et al., 1994).

In five districts in Bolivia, no obstetricians or anesthesiologists were found in two of the district hospitals. In a large urban district, no blood bank was available to support the district hospitals. There was a general shortage of client education materials. Privacy for provider-client counseling was lacking in the district hospitals (Seoane and Castrillo, 1995).

In Nigeria, Ghana, and Sierra Leone, there were declines in deliveries in seven referral facilities from 1983 to 1989, paralleling increased costs to patients for drugs and services (especially in Ghana and Nigeria). These declines are believed to coincide with the introduction of fees in five of the seven sites. The effect of user fees on the number of complicated obstetric cases seen at a referral site is mixed, although the scant data suggest that the patients with complications are continuing to come in for management (Prevention of Maternal Mortality Network, 1995).

In Indonesia, however, the obstacle of cost cannot be overestimated. According to one Indonesian woman: "I have to live through today, before I can think about tomorrow. I can't put away money for a hospital birth, because if I do, we may not be able to eat tonight" (quoted in Ambaretnani, Hessler-Radelet, and Carlin, 1993) Traditional care in Indonesia for prenatal and postpartum massages and child care plus delivery costs a total of U.S. $7.50 (1994), but a complicated delivery at a health center would cost nearly three times as much. If a hospital delivery with caesarean section is required, it could cost even 100 times the rate for traditional care (Achadi et al., 1994). Yet if a recognizable complication arises during delivery, most Indonesian families say that they will spare no expense to ensure that the woman and her baby are safe. But one husband expressed anger that his wife was referred to a hospital and then had a normal delivery there. He felt that they had spent a tremendous amount of money on something that they did not really need (Ambaretnani, Hessler-Radelet, and Carlin, 1993).

It is not only the lack of supplies, logistics, or costs that create barriers. Provider attitudes remain a major hurdle. An example is seen from a focus group report from Nigeria. Doctors in the Yoruba community believe that good prenatal care could prevent many of the complications they see, but that "pregnancy is considered to be a natural thing . . ." and "ignorance" is pervasive. Hence, women obtain prenatal care only late in pregnancy. Nurses and midwives claim this late registration is due to the fact that attendance for prenatal care is very expensive, and women want to delay registering as long as possible (Public Opinion Polls, 1993).

Step 4: Provision of Appropriate Care

The few studies of the quality of maternity care point to major deficiencies in the systems of care available and to a large gap between what facilities and life-saving skills are available and what is needed.

Indicators of the quality of emergency care for obstetric complications at a facility include the time interval between admission to treatment, facility trends in case-fatality rates for all complications, the caesarean section rate, and trends in numbers of deaths (maternal and perinatal); the proportion of perinatal deaths contributed by stillbirths or early neonatal deaths and proportion contributed by full-term babies may also be useful. Such data have only recently begun to be collected in most places. Medical records are typically the source of such information, and they are notoriously lacking or incomplete. Medical or verbal autopsies of maternal deaths, in which causes of death and avoidable factors are determined by a medical team that reviews each death, have proven to be a very useful way to monitor deficiencies.

Trends in the time from admission to treatment for emergency obstetric cases were observed in three referral sites in two African countries, Ghana and Nigeria. From a review of medical records, it was found that waiting time had increased from an average of 5 hours in 1983 to 15.5 hours in 1988 in Calabar (Ghana) for women who died of hemorrhage. In Zaria (Nigeria) the waiting increased from 3.5 to 6.9 hours between 1983 and 1988 (Prevention of Maternal Mortality Network, 1995).

Although data on admission to treatment for most complications is often lacking, caesarean sections require an operating theater; typically, the dates and times of procedures are recorded. The average admission-to-treatment interval for emergency caesarean sections for six referral facilities in three districts of India was 1.5 to 5 hours. These long intervals were caused by the need to locate doctors who were on call and time for them to come to the facility. In another setting, a delay was caused by a patient's relatives having to purchase anesthetics outside the facility. Case fatalities in these sites ranged from 2.8 percent to 6.9 percent. Low case fatality rates were found in some cases because the most serious cases were referred to another facility or left the facility against medical advice.

In Quetzaltenango, Guatemala, only 8 percent of patients had no wait upon arrival at the referral hospital; 45 percent waited up to 1 hour, and 47 percent waited more than 1 hour. Women in a study indicated that they would not accept referrals from traditional birth attendants to hospitals because of long waiting periods (O'Rourke, 1995).

Most incriminating of the quality of care is a nationally representative study of 718 maternal deaths in Egypt in 1992 (Ministry of Health, 1994). Avoidable factors were assigned by a local advisory group of a panel of doctors for each governorate that met weekly to review each maternal death in that area; their decisions were reviewed by a central advisory group at the national level. The leading avoidable factor was poor management and diagnosis by obstetric teams—47 percent. Patient factors, particularly delay in seeking (or compliance with) medical care, were blamed in 42 percent of deaths studied.

Review of the maternal deaths revealed that there was no referral system in place in the Egyptian health care system, and that this gap affected when and where cases were referred. A disproportionately large number of the women had seen a private practitioner who delayed referral to a hospital. No protocols for managing complications were available, and most cases were managed by junior staff. Both traditional birth attendants (*dayas*, who deliver nearly 60% of all births in Egypt) and general practitioners (who are sought only infrequently) played minor roles in the avoidable factors (12% each) (Ministry of Health, 1994).

A similar investigation of 1,173 maternal deaths in China in 1990 also pointed to maternal services as the highest contributor to avoidable factors (48%), followed by individual and family delays in using health care and transport problems. All factors occurred more frequently at village and township level (68 percent) than at county or provincial level (32 percent) (World Health Organization, 1994b).

In Guatemala, four departmental hospitals appear to have adequate numbers of beds and skilled staff available to manage serious complications, but they are highly underutilized for several reasons: traditional birthing positions (squatting, kneeling) are not permitted; no provision is made for respecting women's privacy; and language barriers make communication between providers and women and their families virtually impossible. Technical skills could also be questioned, as two cases of postsurgery tetanus had been reported in a previous year (Colgate-Goldman et al., 1994).

LESSONS FOR SAVING LIVES

Each of the steps in the pathway to survival may require one or more intervention(s), especially in rural settings where home birthing is not only preferred, but may be a necessity given the distance and adequacy of available health services infrastructure to respond to life-threatening complications. In urban and periurban sites, where women intend to deliver in a health facility, and do so to a large extent, interventions may aim at promoting more selective use of facilities. In both rural and urban areas, efforts to improve the quality of care are needed to complement community efforts to overcome the barriers to access. Appendix B presents more details of the setting, implementation, and results of selected interventions at each of the four steps discussed below.

Step 1: Recognition of a Problem

What seems like a simple and obvious lesson comes from projects in West Java, Indonesia (Alisjahbana et al., 1995), Bolivia (Howard-Grabman, Seoane, and Davenport, 1993; Bower and Perez, 1993), and Forteleza in Northeast Brazil (Janowitz et al., 1988; Bailey et al., 1991): focus on families because they are most involved in observing the progress of pregnancies and the ones who will benefit most by a good outcome of pregnancy for both the mother and newborn. Families and those who influence families, not just pregnant women, should be the focus of efforts aimed at recognition of obstetric and newborn complications. They should also be informed about where to take a woman when such complications are recognized. The woman herself often can tell if she has a problem, but she may not be in any condition to advise or influence others. Specific groups—husbands, mothers-in-law, sisters—as well as pregnant women and traditional birth attendants, may be targeted. Providing messages through different media and consistently over time may emphasize the seriousness of the message. Caution must be exercised in crafting locally appropriate messages, however. For example, pregnant women in Indonesia did not want pictures of possible complications near them as they believed they were sure then to have the complications (Hessler-Radelet, 1993).

Traditional birth attendants provide labor, delivery, postpartum, and newborn care for the majority of women in many developing countries. Hence, it is tempting to train them in recognition of the danger signs of complications, but the results of such efforts have been mixed. Where women use formal medical services for birth if they have a complication, as appeared to be the norm for one-half the Guatemalan women in a study near the town of Quetzaltenango, training traditional attendants did not seem to improve the use of services for care of complicated cases (Schieber, 1993; Bailey, Szaszdi, and Schieber, 1994). Similarly, a randomized controlled trial in four cities of Latin America showed that an intensive intervention of home visits for health education had no impact on pregnancy outcomes—or even on use of postpartum services for women with complications—where women are already using services for labor and delivery and making a high number of prenatal visits (Villar et al., 1992). A home visit program with health education is probably not the answer to changing the behaviors of women who are already using services.

However, where women do not use formal services even when they suffer a complication, training traditional attendants may increase the use of services when needed, as shown in a rural area of West Java (Alisjahbana et al., 1995). However, there can be a backlash, whereby women no longer seek assistance because it is known that many women will be referred to an expensive setting. This problem must be addressed through a communications effort directed to women and their families. It is important that traditional birth attendants—and those who use their services—believe that making a referral adds to their credibility rather than detracts from it. Connecting attendants to medical facilities, and making them welcome at the facilities with the women, has also proved beneficial.

Step 2: Deciding to Seek Care

Little is known about the decision making in families with regard to seeking care for complicated obstetric or neonatal problems. However, it appears that it is families that make the decisions. They may be influenced by traditional birth attendants, but as seen in the periurban Quetzaltenango project (Bailey, Szaszdin, and Schieber, 1994) and in the rural areas of Forteleza, Brazil (where a project to connect attendants and their clients with hospital back-up had been operating for 10 years) (Bailey et al., 1991; Janowitz et al., 1988), attendants were usually by-passed (as was the health center level staff) when a complication occurred.

Hence, interventions should focus on families not only for recognition of problems, but also because they are the primary decision makers for determining whether and where they will seek care. While we know of only one effort to date to involve men directly in such efforts, in Inquisivi, Bolivia (Howard-Grabman, Seoane, and Davenport, 1994), men are the obvious target audience in many places because they control the cash reserves of the household or their permission must be sought for movement of women.

A positive image of the referral site has proven effective in increasing use in Quetzaltenango, Guatemala (Bailey, Szaszdi, and Schieber, 1994). With training on protocols to manage complications and a sensitization of staff to cultural issues so that the hospital doors were opened to families and traditional birth attendants, more women began to use these services. There was no advertisement of these changes, but the news passed rapidly by word of mouth: a "woman-friendly" hospital appears to generate its own demand. The reverse of this was confirmed in the Danfa project in Ghana: women preferred traditional birth attendants because of their fear of anticipated treatment, described as painful and disrespectful, in the hands of medically trained staff (Eades et al., 1993).

Step 3: Reaching a Source of Care

The barriers to reaching services are manifold even if the family is positively disposed to using them. Distance to a referral site may be an obstacle, but three experiments aimed at ensuring transport, with taxi subsidies (Poedje et al., 1993), an ambulance (Alisjahbana et al., 1995), and a revolving fund for transport (Prevention of Maternal Mortality Network, 1995), did not alone increase the use of services. Transportation was not seen as the major obstacle in any of these three settings; rather, it was the costs or the perception of poor care at the end of the journey that proved more formidable. But improvements in transportation have been found useful in some settings. A low cost system of ambulances, relying on country boatmen to get women with complications to a hospital in rural Bangladesh, was an important part of a successful maternity care intervention there (Fauveau et al., 1991; Maine et al., 1996).

Posting certified midwives in rural health centers to provide obstetric care in times of emergencies has appeared to be effective in reducing maternal mortality in rural Bangladesh, where use of formal health care for labor and delivery is exceedingly low (Fauveau et al., 1991). However, posting certified midwives in rural health centers on provincial or national level is costly and difficult, as is shown by efforts in Indonesia. Certain obstetric problems may be managed or stabilized at a peripheral level prior to referral (e.g., antibiotics for infections, sedatives for eclamptic patients), but severe cases may by-pass the midwife anyway and be taken directly to a hospital, and midwives may not see enough cases of severe complications each year to make the investment worthwhile. In Indonesia, for example, one midwife serves approximately 2,000 people. With a birth rate of 28 per 1,000 population and assuming a level of severe complications at 15 percent of all pregnancies, a village-based midwife would see 10-20 complicated cases per year—if *all* complicated cases in her catchment area came to her. If a village-based midwife's tasks also included such efforts as improvements in women's health (e.g., family planning, iron/folate tablet distribution) and newborn and infant survival and health (breastfeeding promotion, cord care, eye care, warming of the newborn, as well as assistance for diarrhea and respiratory infections), however, it might make the investment worthwhile. Determining the most useful role for health centers and their staff in safe motherhood interventions is an important topic for further research.

Maternity waiting homes are another intervention that has been tried to address the problem of distance. Such homes provide a site where women who live far away or who have had a prior poor birth outcome can stay within reach of the hospital before labor begins. Studies in Ethiopia and Zimbabwe have reported improvements in maternal mortality for women who use them (Poovan, Kifle, and Kwast, 1990) and in perinatal mortality (Chandramohan, Cutts, and Millard, 1995). But as Chandramohan, Cutts, and Millard (1995:266) state: "For a maternity waiting home to be effective, a high proportion of women must attend an prenatal clinic, there must be an effective screening and referral system in place, and hospital delivery must be acceptable to mothers."

Yet another alternative, birthing homes, where medically trained personnel can be called to assist in a difficult delivery at some distance from a hospital, have been tried in Forteleza, Brazil, as well as in Tanjungsari in West Java. The birthing homes with traditional birth attendants did not appear as attractive to women as either home or hospital delivery. Even 10 years after the initiation of a birthing home in Forteleza, only one in ten women sought to deliver there. Traditional birth attendants at the birthing homes in Fortaleza did prove to be effective in screening appropriate cases for referral to the main hospital, so an intermediate care facility like birthing homes may help promote a cost-effective system of referral (Bailey et al., 1991).

Step 4: Obtaining High-Quality Care

From efforts in Guatemala, Nigeria, and Uganda, the lesson is simple and repeats lessons from other areas of public health: high-quality care generates demand. Use of delivery services increased where training of medical providers in advanced obstetric care was available (O'Rourke, 1995; Payne, Hooks, and Marshall, 1993; Mantz and Okong, 1994). This occurred although there had been no formal advertising of the improvements; word of mouth seemed to spread quickly, resulting in increased numbers of clients at a hospital within a matter of months.

Training has been the major intervention to improve quality of care—training in life-saving skills (Marshall and Buffington, 1991) and interpersonal skills communication for midwives (Family Health Services et al., 1993). While highly appreciated among midwives, training of one cadre of workers is not enough to sustain the practices taught. Programs must also support the use of these skills with policies that allow the trainees to carry out their new skills, improved management and supervision, an information system that allows them to monitor their own progress, logistics and supplies, and training of those to whom the midwives will refer women (typically, specialist doctors).

Protocols for the management of obstetric and neonatal complications have proved necessary (but not sufficient) for medical care providers to guide and coordinate their actions and know their limits and next steps. They have provided the standard against which to measure appropriateness of actions, especially if a maternal or perinatal audit is in place. Following institutionalization of neonatal care protocols in a referral hospital in Quetzaltenango, Guatemala, the hospital early neonatal mortality rate decreased from 33 to 26 per 1,000 women between 1989 and 1992, with a remarkable drop in avoidable factors assigned to the staff, emphasizing the pediatric staff's improved response to newborn problems (Schieber et al., 1995).

Audits themselves can provide an internal mechanism to monitor and change provider practices. Where they have been implemented, as in India (Bhatt, 1989) and Egypt (Ministry of Health, 1994), they have proved a powerful tool, going beyond raising awareness of the problems. Factors determined to be avoidable can be used in monitoring on-going services. Using both audits and obstetric rounds for on-going services, and bringing together all levels of providers responsible for emergency obstetric clients might suffice to prevent future maternal deaths due to avoidable factors.

Governments, in consultation with private-sector providers, need to establish a regional or national framework for maternity care, including the allocation of resources for each level of care. Many previous efforts to reduce maternal mortality in developing countries have foundered because they relied on attempts to train traditional birth attendants and screen high-risk pregnancies and refer women to expensive, distant, and ineffective sources of treatment. To save lives and reduce morbidity will require expenditures to upgrade facilities and train and supervise providers, as well as efforts to raise awareness at a community level of the signs of obstetric complications and how and where to seek appropriate care.

6

Program Design and Implementation

This chapter addresses issues of design and delivery of health and related services to improve reproductive health. We start by reviewing data showing the great variation in existing capacity and utilization of reproductive health services. Next we discuss organizational issues for reproductive health programs. Finally, we discuss an illustrative, generalized strategic plan for measures to improve reproductive health and describe steps that are being taken in two countries.

No one program design or service configuration can be formulated to promote reproductive health in all settings. Instead, given the limited empirical research available, we review and discuss the features of effective interventions. The chapter emphasizes the organizational setting for effective reproductive health initiatives, including the selection of prevention and treatment approaches, the advantages and disadvantages of service integration, and management by governmental and nongovernmental institutions. The experiences of past and ongoing large-scale health initiatives, in such areas as family planning, primary health care, child immunization, infectious disease control, and environmental sanitation, offer lessons in how to define and develop reproductive health programs. There is no technological or programmatical "magic bullet" for reproductive health care.

EXISTING SERVICE CAPACITY AND UTILIZATION

Almost all countries have some infrastructure in place to deliver related maternal and child health (MCH) and family planning services at different levels of facility. Some have services for the prevention, diagnosis, and treatment of sexually transmitted diseases (STDs), though these are typically weak and poorly coordinated with other health services. Most countries also have health education or communication programs, though again the quality and funding is often low, and these efforts are poorly coordinated with other prevention and treatment services. Hence, organizing delivery for reproductive health services does not typically start from a zero base; rather, it requires strengthening coordination, linkage, or integration and diversifying existing services, as well as adding new ones.

Table 6-1 presents information on existing MCH and family planning service capacity obtained through the Demographic and Health Surveys (DHS) service availability module (SAM) administered either through direct facility visits or to key informants in sample clusters (communities).[1] In the eight countries, services are reasonably accessible to most clusters, at a facility within 30 kilometers. Coverage of basic services ranges varies widely across countries: for example, residents in 93 percent of the sampled clusters in Thailand have access to immunization services at a hospital, compared with only 35.2 percent of the Nigerian DHS clusters. In approximately one-half of the 624 clusters in Bolivia, residents have access to a constellation of six types of MCH services, as well as contraception, from a nearby hospital.[2] These aggregate data only show availability of services at the community level, of course; they do not show the great variation in quality of services (Fisher et al., 1994) or in barriers to access that may exist.

The availability of contraceptive services is highly associated with the availability of MCH services. This pattern reflects the common practice of integration of contraceptive with MCH services in health facilities. These

---

[1]The DHS SAM (Wilkinson, Njogu, and Abderrahim, 1993), as well as the situation analysis tool used in several regional operations research programs (Fisher et al., 1994), obtains information about services at the nearest facility of four to five main types, located within a specified radius of the sampled cluster. Although not a probability sample of facilities, the information from the DHS SAM is presently the most standardized and systematic available for a cross-national comparison of MCH and family planning services. Often the SAM is restricted to rural areas. The DHS SAM has not yet included data on STD diagnosis and treatment services. Some include information on information, education, and communication activities and other community-based services carried out in sample clusters. To monitor and evaluate the effectiveness of reproductive health programs, the content of existing facility-level surveys would need to be modified.

[2]These data are not weighted or linked to the individuals interviewed; thus, one cannot generalize about the areas or population covered by the clusters.

TABLE 6-1 Maternal and Child Health and Family Planning Service
Availability to Sample Clusters of Eight Selected Countries with DHS
Data: in percent

Country and Year	Number[a] (and type)	Facility[b] type	Maternal and Child	
			Prenatal	Delivery
Bolivia	624	Hospital	54.3	54.6
1989		Health center	72.4	50.3
		Clinic	30.1	38.0
Colombia	181	Hospital		
1986		Health center		
		Clinic		
Philippines	744	Hospital[d]	93.3	92.6
1993		Other facility	96.9	65.6
Thailand	192	Hospital		
1988	(rural)	Health center		
		Clinic		
		Pharmacy		
Egypt	120	Hospital	29.2[e]	33.3[e]
1989	(rural)	Government center	88.3	85.8
		Government family planning clinic	43.3	40.0
		Private family planning clinic	10.0	1.7
Kenya	508	Hospital	71.6	71.5
1993		Health center	78.5	60.0
		Dispensary	40.2	5.5
Tanzania	319	Hospital	50.2	50.8
1991	(mainland)	Health center	54.9	46.7
		Dispensary	81.2	73.0
Nigeria	165	Hospital	39.4	39.4
1990	(rural)	Health center	33.3	27.9
		Clinic[g]	37.6	36.9

[a]See text and footnote 1 for explanation of community (cluster) samples.

[b]Nearest facility of each type within 30 kms. of cluster; in Bolivia, family planning services at nearest facility where available.

[c]Any service.

[d]Nearest hospital or nearest other health facility if nearest was not a hospital.

Health Services Offered

Postnatal	Immun-ization	Rehy-dration	Growth	Other	Family Planning
54.6	46.2	52.1	49.4		54.8
67.8	68.3	58.0	70.2		58.8
37.5	10.1	24.2	23.6		28.5
		74.6		76.8^c	76.8
		59.1		59.1	86.2
		37.0		44.8	30.4
93.0	90.6				90.0
93.5	97.3				94.2
	93.2			95.3^c	95.3
	69.3			69.3	69.3
	58.3				72.4
	79.2				90.6
	13.3^e	34.2^e		39.2	77.5
	82.5	88.3		92.5	66.7
	37.5	41.7		45.8	90.8
	2.5	7.5		17.5	49.2
	72.0				67.3
	79.3				76.6
	43.1				40.7
48.3	53.0	45.8	52.0		50.8
45.8	53.6	0.0	54.2		55.2
54.9	82.1	0.3	80.9		79.3
39.4	35.2	32.1	20.6	26.1^f	37.6
30.3	41.2	36.9	23.6	30.3	21.8
31.5	29.1	27.3	16.9	18.8	20.0

^{e}For all Egyptian facilities, availability of services based on reported number of clients for service type in past month.
^{f}Nutrition demonstration.
^{g}Health clinic, maternity center, or maternity home.

data do not necessarily reflect the full availability of contraceptive supplies, which are often distributed through private stores and pharmacies and providers. Still, the concurrent availability of family planning and MCH care suggests that efforts to ensure availability of treatment for reproductive tract infections (RTIs), along with targeted information, education, and communication services, can be built on an existing service capacity.

Table 6-2 shows recent estimates of total fertility rates, infant mortality rates and perinatal mortality ratios, maternal mortality ratios, and service utilization for countries and subnational regions where there have been DHS surveys. Along with wide variation of mortality rates, there is wide variation in estimates of service utilization. Prenatal care coverage

TABLE 6-2 Selected Reproductive Health Outcomes and Service Utilization for 51 Demographic and Health Surveys

Country	TFR	MMR	IMR	ANC	DEL	CPRM	PMR
Botswana	4.9	250	37	92	77	32	25
Burkina	6.9	930	94	59	42	4	80
Burundi	6.9	1300	75	79	19	1	60
Cameroon	5.8	550	65	79	64	4	75
Central African Republic	5.1	700	97	67	46	3	80
Eritrea	6.1	—	—	49	21	4	—
Ghana	5.5	740	66	86	44	10	90
Ivory Coast	5.7	810	89	83	45	4	55
Kenya	5.4	650	62	95	45	27	45
Liberia	6.7	560	144	83	58	6	130
Madagascar	6.1	490	93	78	57	5	65
Malawi	6.7	560	134	90	55	7	70
Mali	7.1	1200	108	31	18	1	100
Ondo Nigeria	5.9	—	56	80	59	4	—
Namibia	5.4	—	57	87	68	26	60
Niger	7.4	1200	123	30	15	2	100
Nigeria	6.0	1000	87	57	31	4	90
Rwanda	6.2	1300	85	94	26	13	65
Senegal	6.0	1200	68	74	47	5	80
Sudan	4.7	660	70	70	69	6	55
Tanzania	6.3	600	92	92	53	13	65
Togo	6.4	420	81	82	46	3	90
Uganda	6.8	1200	—	91	38	8	70
Zambia	6.5	940	107	92	51	9	70
Zimbabwe	4.3	570	53	93	69	42	40
Bangladesh	3.4	850	87	26	10	36	85
Egypt	3.6	170	—	39	46	46	45
Indonesia	2.9	650	57	82	37	52	45
Jordan	5.6	150	34	80	87	27	30
Kazakstan	2.5	60	—	92	99	46	30

TABLE 6-2 Continued

Country	TFR	MMR	IMR	ANC	DEL	CPRM	PMR
Morocco	3.3	320	62	45	40	42	45
Pakistan	5.4	340	91	26	19	9	70
Philippines	4.1	280	34	83	53	25	25
Sri Lanka	2.7	140	25	97	87	41	25
Thailand	2.2	200	35	77	66	64	20
Tunisia	4.2	170	50	58	69	40	40
Turkey	2.7	180	53	62	76	35	50
Yemen	7.7	1400	83	26	16	6	70
Bolivia	4.8	650	75	53	47	18	55
Brazil	3.4	220	76	74	—	57	45
Northeast Brazil	3.7	—	75	64	70	54	—
Colombia	3.0	100	28	83	85	59	25
Dominican Republic	3.3	110	43	97	92	52	35
Ecuador	4.2	150	58	70	61	36	45
El Salvador	4.2	300	71	—	86	45	35
Guatemala	5.1	200	51	53	35	27	45
Mexico	4.0	110	47	71	70	45	40
Haiti	4.8	1000	74	68	46	13	95
Paraguay	4.7	160	34	84	66	35	40
Peru	3.5	280	55	64	53	33	35
Trinidad and Tobago	3.1	90	26	98	98	44	—

NOTES: TFR = total fertility rate; MMR = maternal mortality ratio; IMR = infant mortality rate; ANC = antenatal care; DEL = proportion of births delivered by medically trained attendant; CPRM = modern contraceptive prevalence; PMR = perinatal mortality rate.

SOURCE: Data from Demographic and Health Surveys and World Health Organization and UNICEF (1996).

is notably high, but these estimates do not gauge the quality or adequacy of that care (see Chapter 5). Some countries, such as Trinidad and To-bago, the Dominican Republic, and Kazakstan, have already achieved very high rates of attended deliveries, while rates are far lower in countries such as Mali, Niger and Pakistan.[3] Utilization of reproductive health

---

[3]Unfortunately, reliable direct estimates of maternal mortality ratios are available for only a small, unrepresentative sample of the countries shown in Table 6-2. The estimates reported here were imputed, or were adjusted, using models with fertility rates and proportions of births attended by trained personnel as independent variables (World Health Organization and UNICEF, 1996). Likewise, perinatal mortality ratios are imputed for many of these countries as proportions of total infant mortality, using variables highly correlated with those shown in Table 6-2. Because of this lack of independence of measurement or estimation, we cannot use these aggregate data to show how the service utilization models affect the demographic outcomes; nevertheless, the data suffice to illustrate the range among countries.

services, particularly for RTI/STD treatment and prevention, is only superficially known, largely due to difficulties of measurement and incomplete reporting of service statistics.

As the limitations of these DHS SAM and household data indicate, national assessments are needed of the distribution, accessibility, quality, and acceptability of existing services for reproductive health concerns. Countries vary by mortality and morbidity conditions as well as levels of economic well-being.

LESSONS LEARNED FROM
LARGE-SCALE HEALTH PROGRAMS

Reviews of effective organizational models for health programs often cast their conclusions in terms of lessons learned from what are considered "best practices." Reviews of health program development in developing countries over several decades (e.g., Simmons and Lapham, 1987; Mosley, 1988; Bulatao, 1993; Liese, 1995) suggest that at least two factors can influence successful performance: a focused commitment to achieving program objectives and access to adequate resources. (Public-private partnership in service provision, a third important condition, is discussed in the next chapter.)

Focused Objectives

Commitment to promote and support a new health initiative can be demonstrated in different ways, such as vesting the health initiative under the authority of strong, capable and senior leadership; formulating or reformulating national policy; undertaking highly visible strategic planning, including the adoption of clear, explicit goals and objectives; or implementing an active and comprehensive agenda to achieve those program goals and objectives. The governments of Malaysia, Indonesia, Kenya, and Egypt, for example, elevated the visibility of their support for family planning services by placing them under the supervision of national coordinating boards or councils. In Egypt, India, and Indonesia, these programs eventually acquired ministry status. In Thailand, China, Brazil, and Uganda, HIV/AIDS, schistosomiasis, tuberculosis, malaria, and other communicable diseases have received specialized status in central ministries of health. Such commitment to program visibility, strategic management and institution building will be required for reproductive health programs to achieve their goals.

As much as political or managerial commitment can influence health program performance, the ability to monitor results appears to be equally important. As Liese (1995:352) comments, "Successful disease control organizations would tend to be production organizations" which adopt a "clear result orientation and a sharp focus on measurable disease control activities." Measurable results provide program management with an unambiguous means of gauging performance. Access to trend information on performance indicators provides decision makers with a standard basis by which to determine the adequacy and efficiency of their efforts. Other large-scale health programs focused on disease control—STDs/HIV, malaria, and tuberculosis, for example—have benefitted from registry data on new and recurring infection cases to calculate incidence and fatality rates. Child immunization programs have diligently monitored levels of immunization through rapid assessment and national health surveys (UNICEF, 1995). Family planning programs similarly monitor the contraceptive prevalence rate and method mix to assess the extent of contraceptive practice, while MCH programs have emphasized infant and child mortality rates, antenatal and delivery care coverage, and children's nutritional status as the key indicators of their performance.

Reproductive health programs will likewise benefit if their achievement can be defined and measured. Given the diversity of programs, a single comprehensive indicator is unlikely to prove useful. Reproductive health programs may target outcomes, such as reduction in STD/HIV prevalence, increased contraceptive practice, universal prenatal care and child immunization, increased levels of obstetrical complications managed by medical staff, and elimination of maternal mortality.

An emphasis on measurable program achievements does have some risks. The pressure on workers to achieve simple targets could lead to coercion of clients and distortion of fundamental objectives. For example, family planning workers given method-specific targets, or targets for numbers of acceptors of all methods, may not have direct incentives to ascertain client needs and inform them about all options. They may even have perverse incentives for fraud or aggressive promotion of contraceptives. Effective reproductive health programming will require a reorientation of existing MCH, family planning, and STD services toward the health needs of women, newborns, and men in terms of service quality standards. An example is India's experience with replacing contraceptive acceptors targets for its family welfare program (see Townsend and Khan, 1996).

The program evaluation literature suggests that managerial focus on achieving measurable results will tend to strengthen the chances of effective program implementation. An initial challenge to reproductive health programs is for them to determine which synergistic, measurable results can be feasibly pursued.

Adequate Resources

Health initiatives have foundered because insufficient resources were allocated. Some, like the primary health care movement and safe motherhood, seem to have stalled for lack of organizational and financial resources. Obstetric care has been an underemphasized component of MCH programs. International assistance has traditionally given priority to contraceptive services, MCH (primarily for antenatal care and traditional birth attendant training), and nutrition, with less than 1 percent going toward obstetric care (Nowak, 1995).

In order to build the institutional and administrative capacity to implement an effective reproductive health program, new or re-invigorated health initiatives must be sufficiently supported in terms of personnel, financing, materials and equipment, medical supplies, and information. Costa Rica, for example, increased its public expenditure on health care coverage from 4.5 percent in 1972 to 7.5 percent in 1981 and 8.0 percent in 1991 (World Bank, 1985, 1993). Between 1970 and 1980 Costa Rica enjoyed a 71 percent decline in infant mortality from 68 to 20 deaths per 1,000 births (Rosero-Bixby, 1986). As Chapter 7 shows, a package of reproductive health services can be provided at a per capita cost that is within the reach of many governments.[4]

ORGANIZATIONAL ISSUES FOR
REPRODUCTIVE HEALTH PROGRAMS

Three organizational issues cut across the types of reproductive health services we have discussed in preceding chapters: the scope or breadth of services, service intergration, and the need to inform potential clients and create demand for unfamiliar services.

Breadth of Services

Several international organizations have recently proposed combinations of services for reproductive health programs, either generic programs or for particular countries (e.g., World Health Organization, 1994; Measham and Heaver, 1996). A prominent example is the Mother-Baby Package, a package of reproductive health services (described in Chapter 7 and Appendix C). The breadth and scope of the services to be delivered presents a formidable challenge in design, execution, administration, and evaluation.

---

[4]Rosero-Bixby (1986) notes that Costa Rica's ability to allocate significant resources to health programs was in part aided by its constitutional renunciation of a military.

Table 6-3 shows a possible allocation among community-based activities and levels of facility in the health system of the major health-sector interventions discussed in the preceding chapters. For this table (and for the cost models described in Appendix C), we assume that there are three levels of health care facility, although in several countries, particularly for urban populations, a two-tier system is used. Each of the major categories of reproductive health intervention involves tasks for each of the levels of the system; the higher level facilities need to be able to perform the functions of lower-level facilities as well, since in practice very few hospitals exclusively treat serious cases referred from health centers.

Several interventions and treatments listed are known to be effective in addressing a number of key sexual and reproductive morbidities. Some of these services are needed continuously over an adult's reproductive lifetime, while others are necessary only during various stages of reproduction, such as after conception, during and after pregnancy, or for the newborn. For example, postconception services may include pregnancy testing and counseling and induced abortion, as well as postabortion services for family planning and STD prevention. Postabortion care is important for the treatment of complications and prevention of additional unwanted pregnancies. Coordination could also require training staff, especially at the field level, in multiple technical areas to provide high-quality, competent and comprehensive reproductive health care to clients. In some cases, this may best be accomplished by using MCH/family planning workers to emphasize specific tasks known to be effective, while deleting other less effective ones.

The interventions shown in Table 6-3 will require coordination and linkage across levels and within the relevant service clusters. Those addressing fertility through postconception services should be coordinated with those addressing pregnancy health. For example, the latter might involve three clusters of services: (1) prenatal care, such as nutrition counseling and supplements, screening for syphilis and other STDs, treatment of these infections, maternal tetanus immunization, fetal monitoring for intrauterine growth, and delivery planning; (2) delivery care, particularly, referral for complications, attended delivery by trained personnel especially for complications, appropriate instrument delivery, and immediate newborn care, including prophylaxis for neonatal ophthalmia; and (3) postpartum care, such as lactation and nutrition counseling, infection control, and family planning.

The simultaneous delivery of different clusters of services at different levels of the health care system imposes major demands on clinical and nonclinical training, acquisition and distribution of essential drugs, contraceptives, nutrition supplements and equipment, worker supervision, and client record-keeping. Program planners must achieve an opera-

TABLE 6-3 Illustrative Division of Reproductive Health Interventions Among Levels of the Health Care System

Health Intervention	Community Level	Health Post	Health Center	District Hospital
Prevention of Violence, Promotion of Healthy Sexuality[a]	IEC[b] about violence, sources of support IEC about health effects of female circumcision (where needed)	Treatment of victims, referral to sources of legal and community support	Treatment of victims, referral to sources of community support	Treatment for severe cases
Prevention and Management of RTIs/STDs	IEC messages on symptoms Promotion of safe sex, partner reduction Condom distribution	Syphilis testing and treatment for pregnant women Partner notification and referral Syndromic management (vaginal discharge, lower abdominal pain, genital ulcers, etc.) Infection control	Syndromic management (vaginal discharge, lower abdominal pain, genital ulcers, etc.) Infection control	Laboratory diagnosis and treatment of RTIs Infection control
Prevention and Management of Unintended Pregnancies	IEC for contraceptive methods Community-based distribution; social marketing of condoms, oral pills	Counseling/screening for contraception Counseling and referral for menstrual regulation or abortion Provision of injectable contraceptives, IUD insertions Counseling and treatment of contraceptive side effects	Menstrual regulation/ MVA abortion Performing surgical contraception on set days Post-abortion counseling and contraception Counseling and treatment of contraceptive side effects	Surgical contraception Abortions through 20 weeks, where indicated Post-abortion counseling and c ontraception

Maternity and Newborn Care	Breastfeeding promotion and support Iron and folate supplementation Tetanus toxoid immunization IEC for warning signals of complications; sepsis; where to seek care IEC for newborn care (drying/warming; resuscitation) Transportation arrangements for pregnancy and labor complications	Prenatal visits/nutrition and health education Malaria prophylaxis Labor management via partograph; referral and transport for complications Prophylaxis for gonococcal eye infection First aid for newborns (resuscitation, hypothermia)	Manual procedures Oxytocin for hemorrhage Antibiotics for sepsis Sedatives for pregnancy-induced hypertension Treatment of incomplete abortion Management of shock	Complete essential care of obstetric complications, package includin caesarean section, blood transfusions

[a]Note that most interventions for prevention of violence and promotion of healthy sexuality are outside the health sector.
[b]IEC, information, education, and communication programs.

tional compatibility among service clusters, availing themselves of possible arrangements for linkage, coordination, or integration. Their decisions can be guided by establishing targeted levels of effectiveness in terms of outreach and coverage and by defining measurable outcomes and developing protocols to guide activities of staff by type of facility.

Hardee and Yount (1995) identify potential linkages among traditional health programs that can strengthen access to reproductive health services. For example, an aim to reduce the level of unsafe abortion could explicitly involve linking family planning and maternity care services with information, education, and communication programs to generate demand for family planning prior to conception. Clients obtaining induced abortions or postabortion care would be provided or referred to family planning services. This linkage would mean coordinating the service provision of the two programs, including defining referral guidelines for abortion clients. Similarly, because STDs increase the probability of a potentially fatal ectopic pregnancy, STD management services could be coordinated with family planning by having former STD clinics automatically provide contraceptive counseling and supplies to male and female clients at risk of unwanted conceptions and having family planning clinics screen for gonococcal and chlamydial cervicitis.

Integration of Services

To what extent services should be integrated is a central issue in reproductive health care (e.g., Hardee and Yount, 1995; Pachauri, 1995). By virtue of its broad definition, reproductive health includes services traditionally offered through a number of categorical programs, particularly those responsible for managing STDs and pregnancy and maternal health problems.

Smith and Bryant (1988) illustrate two types of integration, using malaria and family planning programs as examples (see Figure 6-1). Both kinds of programs have enjoyed a certain degree of autonomy within public health programming, largely due to their access to financial and material resources, some of which has been externally available from international donors. In panel (a), malaria and family planning programs are two of three (with general health services) program blocks; each is administered and implemented somewhat autonomously and has different field staff. In panel (b), the two programs are independently administered at the central level, but their services are delivered in an integrated manner by multipurpose field staff. Reproductive health programs, if organized along highly vertical lines, might resemble one of the columns in panel (a). In the configuration shown in panel (b), in contrast, reproductive health would maintain some separate identity near the central

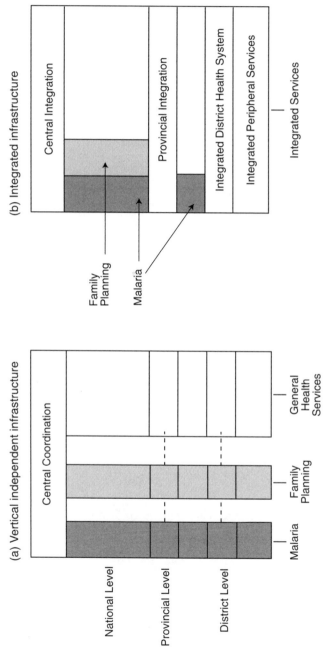

FIGURE 6-1 Two types of integration of health services: (a) vertical independent infrastructure; (b) integrated infrastructure. SOURCE: Smith and Bryant (1988:913). Reprinted with permission.

level of administration but have its services delivered by the same field personnel who are responsible for other general health services. These two forms of service organization have been variously called the "hour glass" shape (b) or "broken zipper" model (a) (Cleland et al., 1994). The question of which structural configuration provides the most synergistic and efficient use of resources is often cast in terms of verticality versus integration.

Integrating formerly categorical programs in an overall reproductive health program may require little more than a reorganization of administrative authority and reallocation of resources for the delivery of relevant services. Such rearrangements could demand a greater degree of political and administrative support than is required to deliver a completely new medical treatment or technology. Bureaucratic inertia or territorial priorities may resist or thwart reorganization efforts (Simmons and Phillips, 1987). To the extent medical protocols are involved, physician versus nonphysician control of relevant technologies and therapies within programs can inhibit efforts to combine them. In Bangladesh, for example, attempts to link child immunization and other health functions to family planning outreach—to make outreach sites better known and used by rural women—have been only moderately successful because at the operational level they require a great deal of coordination of plans between physicians in the health wing of the Ministry of Health and Family Welfare and nonmedical family planning officers in the family planning wing (Haaga and Maru, 1996).

Some services need to be organized as vertical programs because they are meant to reach geographically concentrated or otherwise distinct populations. Programs for persons at high risk of STDs, such as sex workers, for example, would benefit little from integration into general health services. Programs for adolescents and for men may include some that benefit and others that do not benefit from linkage to programs reaching married women. The perceived needs of clients, their convenience, and concerns for privacy, have to be considered, not just operational efficiency and administrative convenience. In contrast, programs designed to provide complementary services for neglected health problems to populations already in contact with the health or family planning services would be particularly good candidates for integration into existing programs, rather than the setting up of new vertical programs. Detection and treatment of syphilis in pregnant women and syndromic management of RTI symptoms are clear examples.

Some of the functions discussed in the preceding chapters might usefully be considered as partially integrated. For example, the provision of essential care of obstetric complications requires facilities, equipment, and trained personnel that will not be available at sites providing the first level of care in family planning or prenatal care. But implementation of that essential care is likely to require efforts to stimulate community awareness of complications and of where to seek treatment; all first-line health care providers, for both women and men, could usefully have this educational role added to their duties.

Inevitably, additional integration issues will be confronted at the field level, where health personnel and facility resources do not usually expand in proportion to the service demands entailed by new or combined categorical programs. Smith and Bryant (1988:917) note:

> It is also here [at the district health system] that the multitude of special programs found at the national level often falls on the shoulders of a small team charged with numerous responsibilities for promotive, preventive, curative, and rehabilitative services for a local community. It is thus here that integration usually occurs by necessity, if not choice. It is also often at the health center or clinic that the conflicting demands of many specialized programs are resolved, for better or worse, by arbitrary decisions.

Mercenier and Prevot (1983) similarly view integration as the assumption of operational responsibility by the health workers who are best suited for particular tasks. They suggest that the process of integration too often has been considered an administrative problem of structures, while complex human resources issues—such as the orientations and practices of health workers—have been overlooked. Thus, integration of services, while appealing as an organizing rationale for reproductive health care, is not a panacea. The quasi-experimental literature on integration of services shows mixed results (Simmons and Phillips, 1987).

A number of service delivery issues can arise with integration (Hardee and Yount, 1995): (1) adequacy of the existing health infrastructure and referral procedures to overcome weaknesses; (2) need for continuous medical support, supplies, and logistics; (3) provision of accurate and up-to-date service delivery guidelines; (4) integration of records systems, primarily at the district level and below; (5) delegation of tasks downward to overcome staff shortages and decrease the physical distances to reaching women; and (6) ensuring the adequacy, competency, and supervision of service personnel. The capacity-building aspects of reproductive health programs will need to address escalating demands for cross-training of field health personnel with the lateral inclusion of more technical and specialized services.

Although the need for reallocation of resources for such program or service combinations seems self-evident, relatively little empirical research is available on how to effect compatible structures. Cates and Stone (1992) note fundamental differences in the characteristics of clients receiving RTI and family planning services, from those receiving other services and variation in service "cultures": the risks of RTIs and of unintended pregnancies both involve sexual contact and both are higher for younger than for older individuals. Important gender differences exist in that women bear the physiologic responsibility of pregnancy, are more susceptible to sexually-transmitted infection by men than the reverse, and are less symptomatic than men. Yet men make up three-quarters of the clients at STD clinics, since they are more likely to recognize symptoms and more likely to seek health care. Sensitizing clinic and outreach staff to the varying profiles of populations at risk of RTIs and STDs and unwanted pregnancies will be necessary.

Health services to prevent RTIs and STDs have different orientations. Family planning counseling tends to be less directive than STD counseling. Because STDs are communicable diseases that can spread rapidly in subpopulations, STD clinics are more likely to operate as urgent care facilities, providing immediate, short-term treatment to infected clients and their sex partners. Family planning clinics, in contrast, adopt a stance more appropriate to preventive care: they exist to support clients' proactive efforts to avoid unintended conception. Different therapies (antibiotic versus hormonal or surgical treatment) for the two types of services also require different technical skills on the part of providers. There can be conflicting goals, as well. Barrier contraceptive methods, which are not considered particularly efficacious for prevention of unwanted pregnancy, offer the greatest protection against STDs. Until female-controlled contraceptive methods are developed that can protect against both STDs and unwanted pregnancy, encouraging clients to use barrier methods exclusively may challenge the operating philosophies, service attitudes, and policies of many family planning providers (Daley, 1994). The likelihood of achieving full-scale, service-level compatibility in family planning and STD clinics, or similar linkages, ultimately may depend on the degree to which interest in and commitment to comprehensive reproductive health care permeate all levels of the program infrastructure.

A key question concerning integration is whether separate services are needed for women and men, young people, (particularly unmarried young people), and married couples. Again, no simple generalization is possible; both integration and separation have their advantages, and they have different weight in different cultures. There are advantages to specialization by clinic staff and counsellors, comparable to the advantages of "audience segmentation" in mass communications. Clients' (and sometimes providers') embarrassment and stigmatization are often barriers to the use of reproductive health services, but only local experience can show whether these are minimized by having separate waiting areas, clinic times, or buildings, or whether separating services in this way actually increases embarrassment for those seen to be using the services. Young people may have fewer opportunities or socially acceptable reasons for trips to specialized health facilities or pharmacies, and so would have to be reached in fixed or mobile clinics located in or near schools or workplaces. Where there is significant opposition to particular services, like abortions, contraception, and STD treatment for unmarried people, their health rationale may be emphasized by integration with other health services.

Concern with minimizing the social burden on clients is not only important for overall questions of strategy and program design; it should also influence management and quality assurance. Family planning clinics have been criticized for a lack of concern about privacy and waiting times and places (Bruce, 1990), and the same criticism could be directed against other health facilities in many countries. Program managers need not take embarrassment and stigmatization as givens in the social environment in which they are working; rather, need to understand it can be reduced by the arrangements of waiting spaces and consultation and examination areas, and by improving patient and record flow. For example, Marie Stopes clinics providing women's health care in several developing countries, including some where other health services pay little heed to client privacy and confidentiality of records, have shown that this is possible (Toubia, 1995).

The reproductive health movement has emerged out of a microlevel orientation, namely, providing care for all reproductive concerns of women. Hence, issues of service integration for reproductive health may revolve more around organizing services to be client-oriented and accessible in one place at one time or through referral links. To what extent these are the service utilization preferences of women and men needing and seeking such care is an important research issue.

Decentralization

Like service integration, decentralization, popularized during the primary health care movement, has both advantages and disadvantages (Smith and Bryant, 1988). Among the former is that it puts authority in the hands of managers, often at the district level, who are better acquainted with local conditions than managers in central organizations. A lower tier administrative unit may be more responsive to the needs of local users and accountable for the consequences of the unit's decisions. Decentralization may offer resource flexibility and facilitate capacity building by adapting training investments to local needs. Decentralization shifts accountability to district managers and planners, providing them with increased authority and responsibility to address local needs.

Among their disadvantages, decentralized services do not exploit economies of scale, and they require greater management capabilities. Evidence of the overall effectiveness of decentralization schemes is mixed (Heaver, 1995). Smith and Bryant (1988) argue that the district health system is a useful compromise between centralization and complete decentralization. They recommend that authorities at the district level set priorities and design and implement centrally defined health interventions. Yet as population needs in STD management and treatment and pregnancy and nutrition care are likely to vary geographically, some degree of decentralization may be useful for reproductive health program design.

Neither integration nor decentralization guarantees an effective program. A strong achievement orientation can produce success in a variety of service configurations:

> What the study could *not* [author's italics] find was that organizational structure in itself influences effectiveness. . . . Based on the empirical research, the main conclusion was that there is no best structure to organize disease control programs (Liese, 1995:357).

> The differences between these approaches [vertical or integrated] frequently seem exaggerated and misconstrued. . . . As such it is a bureaucratic argument and the divisionary effects of a selective approach on the development of sustainable and efficient health services have been overlooked (Gish, 1992:183-184).

Generating Demand for Reproductive Health Services

Partly due to past neglect of many needs in reproductive health, services are often unfamiliar and poor in quality. Reproductive health care providers need to stimulate the demand for services at the same time that they are meeting the demand. This is especially true for essential care for obstetric complications, but it also applies to better quality family planning services and programs for prevention and treatment of RTIs. Processes surrounding sex and reproduction are especially likely to be considered natural and unalterable, not as symptoms of treatable illness. Because women tend to suffer many reproductive morbidities—sexually transmitted disease, pregnancy and delivery complications, and unwanted sex—in a "culture of silence" (Khattab, 1992), effective demand for treatment may be very low in the initial stages of the reproductive health programming. Individual awareness of symptoms, available services, and motivation to treat any infections or undesirable outcomes may be fairly minimal.

An important lesson from the history of family planning programming is the social legitimation of new types of health care that can be conferred by high levels of political commitment and by specific demand-generation activities. As Cleland and Wilson (1987) point out, ideational change was crucial for the fertility transition in developing countries, as couples became aware of their ability to regulate childbearing. Whether through commercial mass media or public information, education, and communication campaigns, exposure to family planning and health messages can influence reproductive attitudes and preferences and promote healthy behaviors. Interpersonal contact with outreach workers from social and health programs may help form and crystallize latent demand for reproductive health improvements. Significant results from this type of program intervention have been observed for family planning in some countries (Simmons and Phillips, 1992).

Reproductive health programs would benefit from population-based evidence of clients' needs for reproductive health care. Informational, educational, communication, and promotional activities are needed to strengthen and motivate health-seeking and help-seeking behavior on the part of client populations. A significant disparity between the projected prevalence of reproductive health morbidities and individual recognition of and motivation to seek treatment can be a costly problem. Early investments in coordinating, linking, or establishing various service infrastructures, such as STD and family planning clinics, may take place but quickly be seen as an inefficient use of resources if adults at risk do not seek care through these facilities. Clients must be able and want to connect their ailments to available care and obtain effective treatment. Awareness-raising and demand creation activities could target health practitioners and service providers as well, since too often the latter's own technical limitations, attitudes, and predispositions toward particular therapies prevent women and men from receiving appropriate care and referral. For example, maternity care providers may blame women for seeking late treatment for health problems, such as obstetrical complications.

An advantage of having a full complement of reproductive health services can be the increase in the number of opportunities for contact. A health care worker's visit with a new mother for postpartum counseling is an opportunity to speak with her about her own nutritional needs, family planning in the context of STD prevention needs, breastfeeding, child immunization, and so on. This outreach, through childhood and the sexual and reproductive lifetime of adults, exposes household members to reproductive health information and counseling. As a result, demand and motivation for such care may increase.

Quality assurance for more complicated services should become easier once both the public and the providers learn to expect decent services and accountability. Creation of demand for services should be seen as a concomitant to the "supply-side" interventions, not as a precondition for them.

IMPLEMENTING REFORM OF HEALTH SERVICES

How then should program designers and managers proceed to select among possible interventions to improve reproductive health? Given the lack of detailed empirical studies in a wide variety of settings, judgment must be informed by professional experience, practical considerations, and broad generalizations. McGinn et al. (1996) suggest a framework for setting priorities in international reproductive health programs that includes six key factors: (1) the severity, magnitude and consequences of the reproductive health problem; (2) the relative efficacy of potential interventions; (3) the program requirements, in terms of appropriate sites or facility levels; (4) the marginal costs of introducing and sustaining the interventions relative to population covered; (5) the capacity of four components of the health system—human resource management, support and supervision, logistics, and financial management; and (6) the context of cultural, policy and legal constraints.

One approach that has proved useful in public health both in calling attention to goals and in translating broad goals into a sequence of actions for which managers can be held accountable is to set out measurable objectives, with a timetable for reaching them. The "Healthy People" objectives for the year 2000 for the United States are an example. Some of the objectives have been achieved or will be achieved before that year; others almost certainly will not be achieved. In a federal system where subnational levels of government have significant roles in public health, the private sector provides most health care, and education and other sectors must be involved, there is an advantage to having such objectives clearly stated so all the participants can refer to them over the course of a long effort. Such objectives have been set at a global level as well, for example, at the world summit for children in 1990, when representatives of governments and international agencies committed to trying to achieve reductions of specified percentages in infant and child mortality rates, maternal mortality rates, and prevalence of protein-energy malnutrition and micronutrient deficiencies.

The International Conference on Population and Development in 1994 did not specify new global objectives for reproductive health. Likewise, we do not believe that such a global effort would be useful at this stage. As we argue in the preceding chapters, there are common goals for reproductive health, but the nature and severity of specific problems, and the resources to overcome them, vary greatly across settings. Without meaning to detract from commitment to global objectives already adopted, we recommend that governments of developing countries adopt a national-level process to specify objectives and timetables, specifying the strategies to achieve them and the agencies and communities that are expected to help achieve them.

Table 6-4 gives an example of what the outcome of the process could be. The first column lists the positive goals of reproductive health that were used as the vision for this report. The second column lists specific objectives, which can be either instrumental, intermediate steps toward these goals, or measurable changes in indicators of reproductive health in the population at large. These objectives should have some target date attached. The third column lists examples of strategies designed to achieve the objectives, and the fourth lists "critical partnerships," agencies and segments of the population needed to put the strategies into action. This last column highlights the importance of intersectoral involvement for the success of an expanded concept of reproductive health. The partnerships need to be specified, since most of the strategies would be unworkable as "top-down" or single-agency missions. Each of the strategies listed here would also have implications for applied research and training needs.

The advantage in linking goals, objectives, and strategies this way is partly that it helps synthesize what could otherwise be a long, incoherent list of isolated actions. It also helps avoid the problem, called suboptimization by economists, whereby agencies focus on objectives too narrowly defined, or stated only in terms of their own outputs, to the detriment of the larger social goals they were meant to serve.

The process of tailoring and completing such a table to make it relevant to local conditions itself could be valuable by stimulating new collaboration and data-based decision making. Leadership and political commitment would be required, but a purely top-down process would be unlikely to achieve much, since most countries already have a sufficient stock of policy pronouncements, plan documents, similar materials. Any such table would need to be revised periodically. There is hope that technical advances—diagnostic tests for STDs, microbicides, new contraceptives—will radically change the "menu" of cost-effective interventions in ways we cannot now foresee. If the reproductive health movement gains strength in a country, the list of relevant actors would also change, to include new nongovernmental organizations, community groups, and professional associations, new agencies or interagency task forces, and the like. A table like this would be put to good use if the first column changed not at all, the second column changed only very slowly as old objectives are achieved or new ones set, and the other columns are updated continually.

Table 6-4 is illustrative; the panel anticipates that the entries in this

TABLE 6-4 Illustrative National-Level Objectives for Reproductive Health

Goal-Specific Objectives	Strategies to Achieve Objectives	Critical Partnerships
(1) Reproductive Health Goal: Every sex act free of coercion, and based on informed and responsible choice		
Eliminate commercial sex involving children, by [year]	Enforcement of existing laws and penalties for sexual exploitation of children	Police and judicial system, Newspaper editors and reporters, parent groups, religious leaders, nongovernmental organizations working for children
Reduce incidence of female genital mutilation by [proportion], by [year]	Information campaign about health consequences of female genital mutilation	Public- and private-sector health care providers, religious leaders, social-science and communication researchers
Reduce percentage of women beaten by husband or partner by [proportion], by [year]	Enforcement of laws; promotion of awareness of violence; better detection and treatment referrals in health and family planning clinics	Police and judicial system, religious and other community leaders, health care providers, teachers
Provide sexuality education appropriate to grade level in all schools, by [year]	Develop and adopt appropriate curricula and other materials; train teachers and principals	Parent associations, private-school associations, curriculum researchers and evaluators, religious leaders
(2) Reproductive Health Goal: Every sex act free of infection		
Subgoal: Reduction of the number of sex partners		
Increase average age of coital debut to 17 years, by [year]	Health promotion via mass media; health education in schools (with component to build sexual negotiation skills); community-based peer intervention programs; legal sanctions against marriage at younger ages; legal sanctions against adults engaging in sex with minors	Religious and lay community leaders; mass media (TV, radio, print media); community-based organizations; ministry of education, teachers; behavioral interventions experts; judicial system; medical and family planning communities

| Decrease percentage sexually active persons who have had >1 sex partner in last 12 months by [proportion], by [year] | Health promotion via mass media; health education in schools (with component to build sexual negotiation skills); targeted community-based intervention programs | Religious and lay community leaders; ministry of education, teachers; mass media (TV, radio, print media); community-based organizations; behavioral interventions experts; medical and family planning communities |

Subgoal: Increased condom use

| Increase percentage consistent and correct condom use among sexually active persons <30 years old who have had >1 sex partner in last 12 months by [proportion], by [year] | Condom social marketing; targeted, community-based intervention programs; health education in schools (with component on condom use); assure adequate condom supplies at all clinical and community distribution points | Religious and lay community leaders; mass media (TV, radio, print media); community-based organizations; ministry of education, teachers; behavioral interventions experts; agency that sets import tariffs; pharmaceutical companies; medical and family planning communities |

Subgoal: Improved health education

| Increase percentage of population >12 years old who can correctly describe 2 ways to prevent STDs/RTIs by [proportion], by [year] | Health promotion via mass media; health education in schools (with skills building component); targeted, community-based intervention programs | Religious and lay community leaders; mass media (TV, radio, print media); community-based organizations; ministry of education, teachers; behavioral interventions experts; medical and family planning communities |

continued on next page

TABLE 6-4 Continued

Goal-Specific Objectives	Strategies to Achieve Objectives	Critical Partnerships
Subgoal: Improved counseling		
Increase the percentage of clients seeking family planning, STD, postpartum or primary health care services who also receive STD risk assessment and contraceptive method counseling for prevention of both infection and pregnancy by [proportion], by [year]	Development and dissemination of guidelines on risk assessment and counseling for both pregnancy and infection tailored to local sociocultural context	Behavior intervention experts and medical and family planning communities
Subgoal: Improved STD/RTI management		
Increase the percentage of family planning, prenatal, and primary health care clients who are appropriately tested and treated for STDs and other RTIs by [proportion], by [year]	Development and dissemination of STD/RTI detection and treatment guidelines at a minimum: abdominal, pelvic, and genital exams; syndromic management of STDs in symptomatic men and women using WHO algorithms; prenatal syphilis screening. Whiff (KOH) test; pH and microscopy of vaginal secretions strongly recommended for women with signs or symptoms of abnormal discharge. Tests for chlamydia and gonorrhea should be included if feasible. Development and dissemination of guidelines for notification of sex partners of patients diagnosed with STDs. Assure adequate laboratory and anti-microbial supplies in all clinics	Medical and family planning communities, agency that sets tariffs, pharmaceutical companies, pharmacists, public and private laboratories, and behavioral interventions experts

Subgoal: Infection Control

Increase percentage of providers of delivery, IUD insertions, and abortion services who can document adherence to infection control guidelines by [proportion], by [year]	Development and dissemination of infection control guidelines; assure adequate supplies and equipment	Medical and family planning communities

(3) Reproductive Health Goal: Every pregnancy and birth intended

All couples have access to more than one method of effective contraception, by [year]	Train providers in clinical methods; strengthen logistical system for resupply methods	Public and private health care providers, family planning nongovernmental, pharmacists
Young adults know about contraceptive options, where to obtain supplies/services and information about effective use, health effects, by [year]	School health curricula; mass media (information, education, and communication efforts; public service announcements); health care/family planning provider training (initial refresher); packages for emergency contraception, train providers	Family planning nongovernmental organizations, health care providers, social marketing agencies/mass media, teachers/principals/school administration, pharmacists
All sexually active women have access to safe legal abortion in first trimester, by [year]	Legalization of abortions; health care provider training and quality assurance	Legislators; health administrators, quality assurance managers; health care providers
Contraceptive supplies and services, and safe abortion and post-abortion care, affordable to the poor, by [year]	Implement and monitor sliding-fee scales, outreach services in poor communities	Legislators/taxpayers, health sector planners, hospital/clinic administrators, family planning program administrators

continued on next page

TABLE 6-4 Continued

Goal-Specific Objectives	Strategies to Achieve Objectives	Critical Partnerships
(4) Reproductive Health Goal: Every pregnancy/birth safe		
Increase percentage of women with complications attended by trained medical staff by [proportion], by [year]	Increase knowledge of warning signals, where to go in emergencies; increase availability of reliable transport to essential care for obstetric complications facilities; increase number of hospitals/clinics trained/equipped to provide essential care for obstetric complications; institute targeted subsidies, reduce unauthorized fees	Community leaders, teachers; first level health care providers; family planning workers
Increase percentage of women with complications correctly managed by [proportion], by [year]	Quality assurance/provider training (competency-based); eliminate financial incentives for inappropriate obstetric interventions	Hospital/clinic administration
Decrease clinic/hospital care fatality rate for women and newborns by [proportion], by [year]	Quality assurance/provider training (competency-based); develop protocols	Hospital/clinic administrators, medical education and licensing authority, health care providers
Reduce prevalence of anemia among women aged 15-49 by [proportion], by [year]	Distribution of iron/folate supplements in adequate amounts to all pregnant women; information, education, and communication campaign about iron-rich foods	Health educators, mass communications, first-level prenatal care providers

sample table will not prove to be the agreed reproductive health strategy for every country. In this spirit, we have avoided giving real target dates; these must be determined during the national-level process. The rationales for our choice of objectives and strategies is given in the chapters above; the table provides an overview to help in translating concepts to implementation steps. This is certainly not meant to be a comprehensive design for the health sector, nor an exhaustive list of current programs that promote one or another goal of reproductive health. However, it may be useful as a checklist or point of departure to ensure that a comprehensive reproductive health strategy is being built.

We have argued that the process of externalizing and reforming existing services and creating new ones to meet reproductive health needs will vary among countries. This process has already begun in many countries, of course. In the rest of this section we discuss examples of government efforts to implement a reproductive health agenda in Mexico and Uganda. The Mexican case highlights how organizational issues have been addressed to raise the visibility of reproductive health; the Ugandan case highlights steps taken to strengthen existing services in a very poor country.

Implementing a Reproductive Health Program in Mexico

Since 1974 the Mexican government has been strongly committed to achieving fertility reduction through a national family planning program (Riquer Fernandez, 1995). Currently, the public sector provides the majority (71%) of contraceptive users with their family planning methods (Pathfinder International, 1995). At the ICPD, Mexico endorsed the Programme of Action without reservations (unlike several other Latin American countries, which expressed reservations about some controversial sections dealing with reproductive rights and health) (United Nations, 1994).

After the ICPD, two formerly separate divisions of the Ministry of Health—maternal and child health and family planning—were merged into a new General Directorate of Reproductive Health. In addition, an intersectoral body that sets family planning priorities and monitors programs changed its title from the Interinstitutional Group on Family Planning to the Interinstitutional Group on Reproductive Health (GISR). The GISR includes all national institutions that provide health services, as well as the National Population Council, the Education Ministry, the family welfare program, and six nongovernmental organizations that are active in the women's health and rights movement—the Information Group on Reproductive Choice and the Safe Motherhood Committee. The GISR is the most recent incarnation of a coordinating body on family planning that dates back to 1976 (Martínez Manatou, 1994).

In 1995 the GISR issued a 5-year plan that incorporated several key aspects of the ICPD agenda—the Reproductive Health and Family Planning Program (Grupo Interinstitucional de Salud Reproductiva, 1995). The program defines reproductive health as "the capacity of individuals and couples to enjoy a satisfactory, healthy and safe sexual and reproductive life, with the absolute freedom to decide in a responsible and informed manner on the number and spacing of their children." This definition comprehends a broad range of services: family planning; perinatal health; adolescent reproductive health; women's health; early detection and treatment of infertility and reproductive cancers; and prevention, detection and treatment of STDs, including HIV/AIDS. The document emphasizes improving quality of services, instituting a gender perspective in service delivery, ensuring reproductive rights, providing a wide range of method choices, and attending to previously ignored populations (adolescents, men, and indigenous peoples).

Several steps have been taken toward implementing an ambitious agenda. At least one of the major public health care providers, the Mexican Institute of Social Security (IMSS), has a structure that favors service integration. Most of its services for the insured population are provided by family physicians in primary care clinics called family health units. Therefore, family planning is integrated with other health services and has been for many years through the predominant role of the family physician. With the new policy framework, attempts are being made to integrate less traditional services, such as cervical cancer prevention and treatment and STD screening, into the family physicians' services. The other major provider of public health services in Mexico is the Ministry of Health, which serves the population not insured through social security. Various new programs have recently been introduced or gained renewed attention in the ministry, including maternal mortality committees in hospitals, postabortion care, and modules for adolescents.

There are several barriers to full implementation of this reproductive health and rights program. The government has expanded the range of family planning method choice somewhat; however, there is still a strong emphasis on physician-controlled, long-term methods. Clients who are using condoms, for example, are not counted as contraceptive users by most health institutions. This attitude toward barrier methods can be problematic in a country where HIV is a growing problem for women in stable unions—the traditional target groups served by family planning programs. The prevalence of STDs among the general population is unknown and, in general, STD programs have been neglected in Mexico. Nonetheless, the Mexican government has taken important steps to promote integration and expansion of reproductive health services in a context of serious economic constraints.

Strengthening Services for Reproductive and
Maternal Health in Uganda[5]

With external assistance, the government of Uganda has begun an effort to strengthen health programs associated with childbirth and sexual behavior in selected districts. Through this new initiative, it expects to increase use of health services and adoption of behaviors to reduce unwanted pregnancies, HIV infection, and maternal and child mortality.

Under Uganda's newly decentralized government structure, the principal responsibility for the provision of primary health care rests with district administrations, although the central Ministry of Health retains policy making, quality control, technical support, and monitoring and evaluation functions and responsibility for all public hospitals. Most districts are ill-equipped to cope with prevailing reproductive health problems. The public health sector is characterized by low salaries, skills, and motivation of staff and insufficiencies in facilities, equipment, supplies, supervision, training and other support systems.

Projected government, donor, and household expenditures on health for 1996-1997 are about $202 million, about $10 per capita. Of this, about $36 million represent recurrent government expenses, another $36 million recurrent donor expenses, with the remaining $130 million being household expenditures. Nongovernmental organizations provide about 60 percent of the health care in Uganda and are often highly dependent on donor funding. There is very limited private-sector provision of modern health care outside urban areas, and few alternatives to public-sector services.

Despite the large proportion of public expenditure currently spent on hospitals, increased emphasis on primary care is an official priority. User fees are charged in most public-sector facilities. Although revenues collected are currently low and financial management procedures and controls are weak, the Ministry of Health now places a priority on local revenue generation, alternative financing mechanisms such as insurance, and increased private-sector provision of care.

The new reproductive/maternal health initiative has four specific objectives. The first is to increase the availability of services by expanding the number of public and private-sector clinical staff capable of providing an integrated package of reproductive/maternal health services. Integrated services will include:

- family planning;
- prenatal care, including screening for pregnancy complications;

---

[5]This section draws heavily on U.S. Agency for International Development (1996).

- maternal nutrition counseling, and tetanus vaccination;
- intrapartum care, including safe deliveries, responses to common obstetric emergencies (along with complications of illegal abortions), and appropriate referral systems;
  - care of the neonate;
  - postnatal care, including the promotion of exclusive breastfeeding, optimal weaning practices, and full childhood immunization;
  - syndromic STD diagnosis and treatment, based on laboratory validation of management algorithms;
  - HIV testing and counseling, with integration of family planning and STD services; and
  - family planning, STD treatment, and counseling for HIV-positive individuals.

This first objective will support the provision of in-service training in the above areas as well as the improvement of preservice training capability at nursing, medical and paramedical schools. Community volunteers, including traditional birth attendants, will be trained to provide education and counseling related to family planning, maternal and infant health and nutrition, including the promotion of breastfeeding and proper weaning practices; and HIV and other STDs and to refer clients to clinics with trained providers. Volunteers will also sell condoms and oral contraceptives that are provided through a social marketing program. Traditional birth attendants are also to be trained to recognize signs of pregnancy complications and supervised by trained midwives. Continued emphasis will be placed on social marketing to increase the number of outlets selling contraceptives and antibiotics for STD treatment, as well as on upgrading the MCH logistics system that distributes such supplies to public facilities.

The second objective is improved quality of services, including improved, routine supervision of clinic and community-based service providers. Trained providers are to be observed during service delivery to assess compliance with formal standards and education and counseling techniques learned during training. The government plans to coordinate with and train district authorities and facility personnel to maintain and accurately report service statistics related to maternal and child health. This will enable monitoring the quantity of various services provided, their provision in an integrated manner, and compliance with service-delivery protocols (including those for STD treatment).

The third objective, enhanced sustainability of services, is to be achieved through several strategies, including standardized financial management systems at health facilities.

The last objective is to increase individuals' desire to use services and adopt behaviors to improve reproductive/maternal health. Service utilization is to be promoted directly by providing accurate information about services and outlet location. Information, education, and communication efforts will concentrate on reducing perceived barriers to service use (such as rumors and misconceptions) and broadening public awareness of the availability and utility of HIV counseling and testing and the link between STDs and HIV. Other desired behavior changes (e.g., correct infant feeding, improved maternal nutrition, condom use, reduction in sexual partners, delayed sexual debut, spousal communication on reproductive health) are to be promoted by encouraging people to assess their risk for unwanted pregnancy, poor pregnancy outcomes, and HIV infection and to obtain care accordingly. Behavior change will also be promoted through mass media campaigns, including talk radio, serial dramas, and music and through similar local activities such as dramas, video shows, and music competitions.

7

Costs, Financing, and Setting Priorities

A verage spending on health care in low-income countries is estimated at only (U.S.) $14 per person, of which less than one-half is from public funds; the corresponding figure in middle-income countries is $62 per person, of which just over one-half is from public funds (World Bank, 1993). Clearly, financial resources are tightly constrained. Our recommendations for improving reproductive health have to be considered in the light of limited financial, as well as managerial and administrative, resources. Funds for new or expanded programs would have to come from a combination of reallocations within the health sector, new resources from public or private sources, and greater efficiency in the use of resources in all types of programs.

In this chapter we set out the parameters within which these decisions will have to be made and discuss the principles that should guide those decisions. In Appendix C we present results from an illustrative model to show how conclusions about the costs of interventions depend on the setting, scale, and design of particular programs. Because of this variability and the lack of research on the cost and effectiveness of program types, we do not attempt to produce a global cost estimate for reproductive health programs. Enough is now known, however, to develop guidelines for setting priorities.

Experimentation and research should proceed in an interactive manner, so that lessons learned from research can be absorbed in new initiatives, which in turn spawn new areas for research. This chapter focuses on interventions to improve reproductive health *within* the health sector, while recognizing that interventions *outside* the health sector, such as investments in the quality and coverage of education for girls, also generate important health benefits.

EXPENDITURES ON REPRODUCTIVE HEALTH

Data on health expenditures, particularly on private out-of-pocket expenditures and on local and provincial public expenditures on health (in contrast to central-level spending) are quite weak in many developing countries. We draw here on World Bank (1993) estimates of the level of spending, activity, and source of finance based on information from government budgets and national accounts, household surveys, and estimates made by international organizations, supplemented by estimates predicted by an imputation model for countries for which direct data are unavailable.

In the world as a whole, an estimated $1.7 trillion was spent on health care from all sources in 1990: about 10 percent, or $170 billion, was spent in developing countries, although about 78 percent of the world's population live in those countries. Two regularities characterize health expenditures across countries. First, as a country's average income level increases, so does the percentage of income spent on health: developing countries spend on average 4.7 percent of their gross national product (GNP) on health; in established market economies, the figure is 9.2 percent. Second, as incomes rise, the share of spending that is public also tends to increase: in developing countries about 50 percent of all spending is public; in established market economies, this share is 60 percent (World Bank, 1993).

Health spending by region varies from as low as $11 per person in China to more than $1,800 per person in established market economies; see Table 7-1. There is also large variation within regions. Tanzania and Ethiopia, for example, spend only about $4 per capita on health, about one-half of which is public ($2 per capita), while spending in South Africa is almost $160 per capita. Such variation among countries in levels of expenditure means that there is no single set of near-term recommendations for reproductive health programs that is realistic in all settings.

No available estimates cover reproductive health as a whole, but some estimates exist for public-sector spending on maternal and child health and family planning; see Table 7-2. These expenditures accounted for about 6 percent of public-sector health expenditures in 1990. The expenditures on family planning varied among the countries shown in Table 7-2 more than ten-fold, from less than (U.S.) $0.10 per person per year in Ghana, Lesotho, and Mauritania to more than $1.00 in El Salvador. No comparable data exist on private spending or on the other types of repro-

TABLE 7-1 Domestic Health Expenditures by Region, 1990

Region	Health Expenditures as a Share of GNP (percent)	Per Capita Spending on Health (Public and Private) (U.S.$)	Per Capita Public Spending (U.S.$)	Public Spending as a Share of the Total (percent)
Sub-Saharan Africa	4.5	24	13	55
India	6.0	21	5	22
China	3.5	11	6	59
Other Asia and Islands	4.5	61	24	39
Latin America and the Caribbean	4.0	105	63	60
Middle East and North Africa	4.1	77	45	58
Formerly Socialist Economies of Europe	3.6	142	101	71
Established Market Economies	9.2	1,860	1,116	60

SOURCE: World Bank (1993:Table A.9).

ductive health programs. Private expenditures are likely to account for a considerably higher proportion of total spending in the middle-income countries than in the lower-income countries, so the differences in total expenditures among countries are likely to be much greater than the public-sector estimates shown in Table 7-2. These estimates are not fully comparable across countries, however, because expenditures are easier to distinguish and assign to family planning in countries where it is centrally funded and operated as a vertical program with its own distinct headings in public budgets. Total expenditures on family planning in developing countries were between $4 and $5 billion in 1990 (Bulatao, 1993), about two-thirds of total health sector expenditures as estimated by the World Bank (1993).

Total external assistance to the health sectors in developing countries was about $4.8 billion in 1990, accounting for less than 3 percent of 1990 spending on health (Michaud and Murray, 1994). Although their share is small, external resources can have a disproportionate effect on new investments and policy.[1]

---

[1]In some countries the share of external aid is considerably larger: for example, aid accounts for more than one-half of all health expenditures in Burkina Faso, Chad, Guinea-Bissau, Mozambique, and Tanzania.

TABLE 7-2 Per Capita Public Sector Expenditures on
Family Planning in Selected Countries, circa 1990

Countries	Family Planning Expenditures, per Capita (U.S.$)
Low-Income Economies	
Bangladesh	0.51
Central African Republic	0.34
Ghana	0.05
India	0.35
Kenya	0.14
Lesotho	0.02
Mauritania	0.07
Nepal	0.20
Sri Lanka	0.18
Middle-Income Economies[a]	
El Salvador	1.22
Malaysia	0.53
Panama	0.13
Turkey	0.49

[a]Middle-income economies are defined as those with GNP per
capita GNP between (U.S.) $600 and $2,500.

SOURCES: Data from Ross, Mauldin, and Miller (1993); World Bank
(1992, 1993).

External assistance is provided though three main channels: official
development assistance, multilateral loans, and through grants to nongovernmental organizations. Over 30 percent of external assistance programs are either directly or closely related to reproductive health
(Michaud and Murray, 1994). Several important conditions are compara-
tively underfinanced in aid programs relative to the disease burden they
impose, including pregnancy-related conditions (Michaud and Murray,
1994). Family planning has traditionally received most of the external
assistance for reproductive health. In 1990 the category of population and
family planning accounted for about 20 percent of all external assistance
to developing countries, and external assistance represented about one-
quarter of the total expenditures on family planning in developing countries (Bulatao, 1993). Maternal and child health accounted for 8 percent,
and prevention and control of sexually transmitted diseases (STDs) and
HIV accounted for 4 percent of external assistance for health in 1990.

There are major problems in the quality of the data on external assistance, and the problems are greater when one tries to estimate flows to

specific health sector activities, such as reproductive health programs.[2] For our purposes, an important drawback is that they underestimate expenditures on reproductive health programs: they do not allocate to reproductive health any expenditures on general health services and hospital projects, even though these expenditures partially support reproductive health.

ROLE OF THE PUBLIC SECTOR

Governments have several approaches to influence reproductive health (Musgrove, 1996):

- inform people and health providers about health risks;
- directly provide health care;
- finance health care;
- mandate that certain activities be carried out; and
- regulate how health activities are carried out.

All of these approaches can be used, and there is no single optimal mix for all situations.

Economic theory and historical experience show that there are some important health-related activities that governments must finance if they are to be provided at all or at socially optimal levels. One set of such activities involve "public goods," activities that the private sector will not undertake, or will undertake at suboptimal levels, because users cannot be charged for them. Many public health interventions—such as spraying for malaria control and health information campaigns—are usually considered public goods. The testing and regulation of contraceptives is an example of a public good in the area of reproductive health. The private sector will not carry out testing and regulation to a socially optimal extent because individuals cannot be effectively charged for the services provided.

Another set of activities that the public sector must help finance involves goods with large positive "externalities," benefits to others than those directly receiving the services. Treatment of STDs is an example of an intervention with large positive externalities. The individual who is

---

[2]The two major data bases on external assistance are the Creditor Reporting System, maintained by the Development Cooperation Directorate, and the Development Assistance Committee of the Organization for Economic Cooperation and Development (OECD) statistics. There are major discrepancies in the numbers reported to these two systems; see Michaud and Murray (1994) for a detailed description of the reporting problems.

treated successfully derives benefits from that treatment, but so does the community at large as the risks of transmission to others are reduced. Therefore, an individual's willingness to pay for these services does not reflect the benefits they generate for society, and public support will be necessary to achieve the optimal level of STD control.

Another type of "market failure" relevant to the health sector occurs when individuals cannot judge the value of a service, at least not without incurring large costs; in these cases, private markets for the service may be impossible to establish and so government financing is needed. Examples might be emergency care of obstetric complications or postabortion care, which occur so rarely in the experience of one person or family that there is no basis to judge whether adequate care is being provided. Governments have a necessary role in accrediting providers or facilities and fostering quality assurance.

Another important rationale for public intervention in health financing relates to poverty. Poor people have the least capacity to pay for health services, and they suffer the largest burden of disease. This is especially true for reproductive health problems, such as maternal mortality. A strong equity rationale therefore supports public subsidies for health services for the poor. This rationale does not lessen the need to provide such services in a cost-effective way.

Health spending patterns around the world indicate that governments typically choose to finance a much larger share of health services than would be narrowly justified by the economic criteria discussed here. At the same time, however, public spending often underfinances particular highly cost-effective public goods and health services with large positive externalities, many of which are reproductive health interventions.

Public spending is inequitable in many countries. Developing countries often attempt to provide free, comprehensive services. But offering free care to all typically leads to some form of rationing, in which better situated populations often have an advantage. Resources may be excessively concentrated in urban facilities serving the middle and upper classes. The poor, particularly the rural poor, especially when referral systems are weak, are left with low-quality public services that are comprehensive in name only.

Rather than achieving little in a vain attempt to provide everything for everyone, developing countries could provide significant health benefits to a large number of people by concentrating public spending on cost-effective public goods and services with large externalities and by subsidizing cost-effective clinical services for the poor. Much of this focus would include public health and clinical services for reproductive health programs.

Public Financing, Private Provision

Even if services are to be financed by government, they need not be provided by government. Rather, combinations of public and private modes of finance and service delivery are possible; see Table 7-3. Governments can finance services and provide them directly, or they can finance care through private providers. Private sources, similarly, can be used to finance public providers or private providers. Most health systems rely on mixed financing and delivery modes. Many countries, especially OECD countries, use a large share of public finance to pay for private provision of services.

The choice of who provides services ideally involves both costs and quality. Is it cheaper for public or private providers to deliver services of equal quality? Which subpopulations are best served by which type of provider? The choice also hinges on governments' abilities to monitor and regulate contracted services. And, in some developing country settings, the private sector may be so poorly developed that contracting out is not a viable option. This is often the case in remote, rural areas. In general, however, most countries are increasingly accepting the view that competition among providers, on the basis of cost and quality, is preferable to the creation of a public monopoly in service provision.

Nongovernmental organizations, financed publicly or privately, play an important role in the delivery of reproductive health services in devel-

TABLE 7-3 Public-Private Modes of Financing and Delivering Reproductive Health Services

Delivery Mode	Financing Mode	
	Public: from general government revenues or publicly mandated insurance	Private: direct, out-of-pocket expenditures and voluntary insurance
Public	Public-sector providers directly supply services.	Governments charge for services they provide, particularly for the wealthy, in order to target public spending on the poor.
Private, for Profit and Not for Profit	Governments subsidize or contract with nongovernmental organizations or private for-profit providers to provide services.	Individuals pay directly for services, which are often delivered through organized networks of private providers.

oping countries, and their role could be strengthened in many countries. Among 22 countries where Demographic and Health Surveys (DHS) were conducted during 1990-1993, for example, the proportion of users of modern contraceptives who obtained clinical services from nongovernment sources ranged from virtually none in a few African countries to well over one-half in several Latin American and Middle Eastern countries (Curtis and Neitzel, 1996:Table 7.2). For methods of modern contraception, at least 10 percent of users relied on sources other than government and pharmacies in one-half of the countries.

In addition to provision of family planning services and supplies, many other tasks in reproductive health are suitable for nongovernmental organizations. For example, providing services to rape victims, providing high-quality abortion services and counseling, and providing information about warning signs of labor complications and what to do about them could all be handled effectively by such organizations. Sometimes, nongovernmental organizations are more efficient and provide services with greater consumer satisfaction than public providers. They are often innovative, testing out new services and delivery modes that are later adopted by other providers. For example, the Bangladesh Women's Health Coalition (BWHC) successfully developed menstrual regulation techniques in Bangladesh. BWHC clinics have also shown that integrated women's reproductive health services and improved care can increase the effective use of services at low cost in comparison with government family planning clinics (Kay, Germain, and Bangser, 1991). Nongovernmental organizations may reach poor women in underserved locations, and they are more accepted there than are government providers. The Aga Khan Development Network, for example, supports safe motherhood activities and other services in remote mountainous areas in rural Pakistan where government services are scarce.

Governments can subsidize nongovernmental organizations or traditional medical practitioners to deliver reproductive health services as appropriate to poor families. For example, about 30 percent of the municipal governments in Brazil provide funding to the Sociedade Civil Bem Estar Familar No Brasil (BEMFAM), a nongovernmental organization that provides services in public-sector health posts and training to public-sector health personnel, as well as operating its own clinics providing a broad array of reproductive health services in state capitals (Gomes, 1994). BEMFAM services are concentrated in the poorest region of the country, the Northeast, where 90 percent of municipal governments have such funding arrangements. Governments can also facilitate such service provision by legalizing nongovernmental organizations, simplifying registration procedures, and offering training, office space, tax relief (import duty exemption), and supplies. In Botswana, government donations of free vaccines and contraceptives to nongovernmental health providers have become a common way to target public subsidies to specific health intervention programs. Subsidies can be provided on a per case, per capita, or a block grant basis.

Public policies can also encourage for-profit providers to deliver high-priority reproductive health services. Incentives range from directly financing for-profit providers to subsidizing in-service training for reproductive health services, such as in STD risk assessment and treatment or the use of new contraceptives. Governments can subsidize inputs for other critical prevention approaches to be bundled with reproductive health services, such as vaccines. However, the development of a private sector for some services, such as family planning, may be delayed by subsidization of public services, especially if subsidies are not targeted to the poor and are continued long after the idea of family planning has become familiar.

Role of Mandates, Regulation, and Information Provision

Public policies to encourage a diversified system of health service delivery, including nongovernmental organizations and for-profit private providers, need to be accompanied by efforts to strengthen the government's capacity to regulate health providers and, through mandates or regulation, to ensure minimum service delivery standards. Governments can mandate the content of educational curriculum to ensure that all graduating physicians have a minimum set of skills in reproductive health or that schools incorporate certain material on reproductive health in their curriculum. Governments can mandate that all insurers include certain high-priority reproductive health services in any insurance package. Governments can accredit hospitals and physicians. They can regulate what medical equipment and drugs and supplies are imported and what types of contraceptives are approved for sale. Such regulatory mechanisms tend to be weak in most developing countries. Providing information—for example, about how to minimize the risks of contracting STDs—is another extremely important role for governments in reproductive health.

USER FEES

Communities, families, and individuals pay some of the cost of publicly provided services in many countries through cash payments, in-kind contributions, and community-based prepayment schemes, as well as illicit fees (for example, tips in order to see a physician). Cost-sharing arrangements have grown in popularity in recent years in many developing countries. A 1995 survey of 37 African countries found that 34 governments impose fees of some kind for government-provided health services (cited in Shaw and Griffin, 1995). This section briefly reviews the main objectives of user fees, the experience from implementation, and implications for women's reproductive health services.

User fees tend to be used in the public sector for three reasons: to mobilize resources, to target public spending to the poor, and to improve efficiency by giving consumers appropriate price signals. For governments in developing countries, revenue generation is usually the main motivation for introducing user fees. Experience indicates that user fees usually contribute a modest amount to government costs—an estimated 4 to 20 percent in sub-Saharan Africa (Shaw and Griffin, 1995)—although in some cases, this is offset by fairly high collection costs. If user fees are largely retained and reinvested at the local facility level, they can improve the quality of services (Foreit and Levine, 1993). Some studies have shown that user fees can actually increase the use of health services by the poor if they are successfully used to improve the quality of services (Litvack and Bodart, 1993). A by-product of user fees is that they may make publicly run facilities more accountable to clients: clients tend to demand more responsive services when they are paying directly for them, especially if local communities are involved in the design and application of user fees.

Some social services in developing countries attempt to target subsidies, either by charging fees on a sliding scale (so that the poorest clients pay less than others), by charging higher fees in locations used mainly by those who can afford to pay, or by charging fees for service at certain hours when waiting times are low (Grosh, 1994). Sliding-scale arrangements can be difficult to administer and are subject to abuse, but if the poorest clients can be readily identified, clinics can charge fees from those better able to afford them without discouraging use of services by the poor. Targeting subsidies by charging fees at some clinics and not others is feasible insofar as the poor live apart from the less poor or use different facilities.

User fees can be used to improve efficiency in a variety of ways. User fees can be used to support a referral system by charging patients who go directly to tertiary facilities for care that should be provided at lower level facilities. User fees at tertiary facilities provide an incentive for patients to seek care at lower levels. User fees can be applied to influence the demand for services: services with high positive externalities (such as STD prevention) can be provided free or almost free of charge so that demand is not curtailed, while services with largely private benefits can carry higher user fees.

Some have argued that user fees should not be imposed for prenatal and delivery care in order to help ensure that babies enter the maternal-child health system and thereby have ready access to immunizations and other preventive services. Children who have been delivered at home tend to be more difficult for the health system to reach. After introduction of user fees in Zambia in 1989, pregnant women appeared to continue to use prenatal services, with modest user fees, but avoided hospital deliveries because of high fees (Booth et al., 1995; see also Prevention of Maternal Mortality Network, 1995). Women expecting complicated deliveries tried to delay hospital admittance until the last possible moment for fear of paying more, and this delay apparently led to higher numbers of infants who did not receive needed services. This in turn probably contributed to the decline in immunization coverage in Zambia from 80 to 50 percent in the early 1990s.

Nongovernmental organizations in some developing countries rely on user fees for much of their revenue. The strategy sometimes has been to charge user fees for services that people are willing to pay for, such as abortions and pregnancy testing, and to use the revenue generated to cross-subsidize other services, such as the supply of contraception (Haaga and Tsui, 1995). This practice may not be appropriate if the services for which high fees are charged should be subsidized, at least for the poor. This might be the case, for example, with provision of safe abortions or prenatal and delivery care. Some of the reproductive health services for which nongovernmental organizations charge high fees—notably pregnancy testing and safe abortions—would be as appropriate or more appropriate to subsidize on public health grounds as the family planning services they are currently subsidizing.

Experience in the 1980s and 1990s has shown that, while user fees for public services have served to mobilize resources, in many cases neither the poor nor certain types of critical services have been adequately protected from the demand-reducing effects of user fees. For reproductive health services, care must be taken to ensure that adequate exemptions are in place so that poor women have access to high-priority services, such as attended deliveries and emergency obstetric services. More data are needed on the practical concerns of how user fees are implemented, whether and how sliding scales for fees operate, and how efficiently fees are collected and whether they augment quality and the total resources available for reproductive health.

SETTING PRIORITIES

Recommendations to redirect public resources to reproductive health activities need to be considered in the context of total resources available for health and comparison with funding requirements for other cost-effective health interventions. A recommendation to increase public spending on reproductive health to $10 per capita when the country's entire public-sector budget for health is only $8 per capita would likely be infeasible, for example, without some plan to mobilize additional resources for the health sector. Arguments to increase spending on reproductive health on the grounds of cost-effectiveness require an examination of the other highly cost-effective interventions that might receive less funding.

Some rationing of health services occurs in all health systems in the world, either implicitly or explicitly. In highly market-oriented health systems, health services are implicitly rationed according to willingness to pay. This approach has both equity and efficiency problems. Equity problems arise because poor people have less access to health services, despite their disproportionately large share of disease burden, because of their lower incomes. Efficiency problems also occur if public goods are left to the market, because they will be undersupplied.

Virtually all governments intervene actively in the health sector. Most governments finance a significant share of health spending (see Table 7-1, above) and in doing so must set priorities and ration the available funds. Developing country governments, with their limited health budgets, face difficult decisions about how to distribute their resources among the enormous needs of their citizens. One common approach is to avoid setting priorities explicitly, but to assume that comprehensive health care can be provided for all with the limited resources available. This strategy has resulted in practice in inefficient spending: tertiary care public hospitals—those that provide the most specialized and sophisticated services and where most clinical research, education, and training takes place—alone may consume 30 to 50 percent of the health budget. Even so, these hospitals often face chronic budget shortages. Health centers (secondary health facilities) typically are short staffed, particularly in rural areas, and face shortages of drugs and supplies. In planning investments in human resources and infrastructure, undue optimism about the future availability of funding has large costs: facilities may be built that are too expensive to run or are run at the cost of reallocating funds from higher priority programs.

One of the most useful instruments for setting priorities for health expenditures is information on the effect of such spending, or value for money, which can be quantified in terms of cost-effectiveness. Cost-effectiveness measures the net gain in health (compared with a benchmark situation) in relation to the incremental cost of an intervention. If costs can be quantified and expressed in a common currency, and if health effects can be summarized in a single metric or index, different interventions can be compared in terms of a single ratio.

As for other health fields, cost-effectiveness estimates for existing reproductive health interventions are imprecise. But even allowing for a wide margin for error, these estimates suggest that several women's reproductive health interventions are among the most cost-effective in the health sector in developing countries (World Bank, 1993). In these estimates, the measured benefits include reductions in mortality, disease, and disability. Under the wider definition of reproductive health of the International Conference on Population and Development (ICPD), which incorporates the benefits of effective fertility control, the benefits of reproductive health programs would be higher. Continuing work is needed to estimate better the costs and effectiveness of health interventions at the country level—both to help set priorities for funding, and to monitor and improve efficiency.

The World Bank has estimated the cost per case or per participant and cost per disability-adjusted life year (DALY), a measure of cost-effectiveness, for several reproductive health interventions.[3] In this exercise costs were measured in terms of dollars and health outcomes were measured in terms of disability-adjusted life years saved; see Table 7-4. For all of these reproductive health interventions, saving a disability-adjusted life year could be achieved with expenditures less than about $110. The cost-effectiveness estimates are presented with a range to emphasize the fact that these are rough estimates. Estimates of cost per case or participant and cost-effectiveness are presented for two settings: low-income countries and middle-income countries. The estimates differ across these two settings because of differences in epidemiologic and demographic characteristics, levels of infrastructure available, and differences in the costs of specific inputs, such as labor. In an analysis of 47 child and adult health interventions in developing countries, cost-effectiveness ranged from as little as $1 per disability-life year saved to over $1,000 per disability-life year saved (Jamison et al., 1993). The reproductive health interventions shown in Table 7-4 are thus among the more cost-effective of those studied by Jamison and his colleagues.

Cost-effectiveness analysis has been criticized on both technical and political grounds, but in our judgment, its advantages in making assumptions explicit outweigh the inevitable limitations of the methods. The criticisms of cost-effectiveness concern data limitations, the assumptions

---

[3]The disability-adjusted life year is a measure that combines healthy life years lost because of premature mortality with those lost from disability. For disability, the number of life years lost was obtained by multiplying the expected duration of the condition (to remission or death) by a severity weight that measured the severity of the disability in comparison with loss of life. After combining death and disability losses, a discount rate is applied. Age weights are also applied so that years of life lost at different ages can be given different relative values. See Murray (1996).

TABLE 7-4 Costs and Cost-Effectiveness of Selected Reproductive Health Interventions in Low-Income and Middle-Income Countries (in U.S.$)

Reproductive Health Intervention	Annual Cost, Per Case or Participant		Cost-Effectiveness (Cost per Disability Adjusted Life Years)	
	Low-Income Countries	Middle-Income Countries	Low-Income Countries	Middle-Income Countries
Public Health				
EPI Plus[a]	15	29	12-17	25-30
Public health information (family planning, nutrition information)	2.4	5	N.A.	N.A.
AIDS prevention program	112	132	3-5	13-18
Clinical Interventions				
Prenatal and delivery care	90	255	30-50	60-110
Family planning	12	20	20-30	100-150
Treatment of STDs	11	18	1-3	10-15

[a]EPI (Expanded Programme on Immigration) Plus includes micronutrient supplementation that is directed at women.

SOURCE: Data from World Bank (1993:106, 117).

used, average versus marginal measurements, political sensitiveness, and exclusion of consumer demand.

Cost-effectiveness analysis requires detailed cost and health impact data. Some countries are investing in these data. In lieu of country-specific estimates, some analysts use data from countries with similar characteristics. Often, differences in cost-effectiveness between one intervention and another are much larger than the variation that can occur from one setting to another or from the range of error in the estimates. When this is the case, even rough estimates may be helpful in setting priorities across interventions.

The disability-adjusted life year (DALY) as a measure of health outcomes incorporates a number of assumptions about valuing the future relative to today, weighing a year of healthy life lost at different ages, and rating the severity of disability (Murray, 1996). These assumptions are necessary to combine both healthy years lost of disability as well as premature mortality into one metric. There are no "correct" assumptions—they could vary by country setting, and they can be estimated through structured interviews with citizens. Sensitivity analysis can be used to illustrate how sensitive conclusions are to the assumptions used. Also, the measure does not incorporate nonhealth effects of interventions; to do so would require either a more inclusive measure of benefits or more complicated models.

The DALY, like other single measures of outcomes such as lives saved, does not include the value of nonhealth outcomes. These can be significant, especially for interventions like family planning, which enhances control over reproduction and frees women's time for activities other than childrearing. These benefits would be valued in a full social cost-benefit analysis, but would not be easy to express in terms commensurate with the reduction of mortality and disability.

Cost-effectiveness changes as interventions are extended throughout the population. Typically, one observes rising marginal costs and decreasing marginal effectiveness as interventions become more universal—but this is difficult to measure or to incorporate in simple models. Sensitivity analysis again can be used to indicate how cost-effectiveness changes as the intervention is extended throughout the population.

Cost-effectiveness is only one element for priority setting in health. Clearly consumer demand must also enter into consideration. For potentially cost-effective services where demand is low, services must be accompanied by demand generation efforts. For less cost-effective services where demand is high, policy makers may wish to try to shift demand through education, user fees, or other measures, or supply the services for reasons of consumer satisfaction.

COST ESTIMATION

Both the potential value and the practical difficulties of estimating costs of reproductive health programs are illustrated by the results of cost models for the Mother-Baby Package of interventions defined by the World Health Organization and other international organizations (see Appendix C). The Mother-Baby Package is a program design for facility-based services, including basic health posts, better-equipped and -staffed clinics, and hospitals equipped for essential care of obstetric complications (see Chapter 5), and it includes clinic-based family planning services. It is not a complete cost model for the programs discussed above, however, because public information campaigns, community-based distribution of contraceptives, and efforts outside the health sector would all have to be accounted for separately. It does include the clinic-based services discussed in Chapters 3, 4, and 5, though (along with more child health interventions than we have discussed), so qualitative results from the model should be relevant to planning reproductive health programs.

The illustrative results show that estimates of the cost of a package of interventions are most sensitive to:

- the salaries of health care providers;
- the methods used to allocate shared costs of multipurpose workers, facilities, and equipment among different functions of health centers; and
- the assumptions about whether fixed facilities are operated at full capacity.

Although we have not performed a similar exercise for programs outside the health sector intended to improve reproductive health, such estimates would likely depend to an even greater extent on how shared costs are allocated, since facilities and staff in education mass media and other sectors are primarily serving other purposes. Cost models like those used for the Mother-Baby Package are valuable mainly in specific applications, for planning and budgeting, and indeed have been adapted for use in several countries, for example, in World Bank sector analyses.

Several qualitative inferences emerge from typical applications. One is that the cost-effectiveness of systems with large fixed-costs of facilities and specialized personnel can be increased when referral systems work, so that the clients with the most serious needs are referred and transported to specialized facilities. Screening and referral are particularly difficult tasks when primary care staff are poorly supervised and motivated, but as we note in Chapter 5, promising examples should be more widely replicated.

The total cost of the package illustrated in Appendix C is greatly influenced by the number of pregnancies in the hypothetical population. This provides some grounds for optimism in countries that have recently seen sharp declines in fertility rates. The task of increasing coverage of attended births and improving the quality of care received should be less daunting. Urban-rural cost comparisons suggest that the increasing urbanization of the populations to be served will significantly reduce costs associated with vehicles and transportation now associated with rural health posts, but whether urbanization will result in any overall cost savings depends on whether salary costs and capital costs for facilities will be greater for expanded services in urban areas. Like our hypothetical rural-urban comparisons, cost estimates prepared using other models for India's Family Welfare Program were highly sensitive to the alternate assumptions about transport needs for rural health centers (Measham and Heaver, 1996:Ch. 6).

Training costs account for much of the total costs of new interventions and for much of the variation between high- and low-cost settings. For example, many of the interventions discussed in previous chapters call for health care and family planning providers to impart knowledge and counsel clients on many subjects about which the providers themselves may not currently know much. The services included in essential care for obstetric complications (Chapter 5) would require a major investment in training in most countries. Moreover, training should not be considered a one-time-only cost incurred in the introduction of reproductive health approaches. Evaluations of health care systems typically recommend proportionally more investment in refresher and in-service training. Training is essential if the reproductive health approach is to be effectively implemented.

Planners should not assume that current programs with staff have no incremental costs. In allocating salary costs of multipurpose workers among functions, analysts typically assume that the workers are in their posts, working the statutory day at their assigned tasks. In countries where workers are poorly paid, poorly motivated, and poorly supervised, the actual output per worker is typically far below what is assumed (Janowitz and Bratt, 1994:46-48; Janowitz et al., 1996:Table III.B.1). The incremental costs of adding services to the job description of currently underemployed workers may appear deceptively low. The true costs of implementing new services would have to include organizational changes required to motivate the increased effort from workers.

CONCLUSIONS

Within the health sector, both the public and private sectors have important roles to play in delivering reproductive health services. Frequently, the focus of government actions is on service delivery. But governments can wield a variety of instruments to influence health—information provision, setting mandates, regulation—in addition to the financing and provision of services. Moreover, even when governments finance services, they do not necessarily have to provide them. In some cases, it may be more efficient to establish contracts with private providers, such as nongovernmental organizations or for-profit institutions, for service delivery.

Users themselves currently bear a large share of the costs of the services they receive in developing countries. Private, out-of-pocket expenditures account for almost one-half of all health expenditures in developing countries. In the past several years, user fees for publicly financed services have become more common. What impact has this trend had on reproductive health? The evidence is mixed. While user fees, properly implemented, can improve resource mobilization, equity, and efficiency, these benefits are often not achieved in practice because of indiscriminate application of user fees. The social benefits of user fees are best achieved if: (1) services with large positive externalities (such as prevention and treatment of sexually transmitted diseases) are fully exempted from fees so as not to deter demand, (2) fees are used to improve quality of care at the point of service, and (3) the poor are either exempted or face only modest fees for high-priority services.

Many investments in women's reproductive health can yield substantial improvements in health in relation to costs. Current global cost-effectiveness estimates, such as those produced for the World Development Report (World Bank, 1993), alternatives prepared for the ICPD Programme of Action, or those we have explored for the Mother-Baby Package, would benefit from a better foundation of empirical studies. But even with wide bands of uncertainty surrounding point estimates, these analyses consistently support the qualitative conclusion that reproductive health programs compare favorably to alternative health-sector investments in both poor and middle-income countries. More external assistance to reproductive health programs, particularly to delivery and neonatal care, would remedy a past imbalance among programs considered for their potential contributions to reducing the burden of disease in developing countries.

Low levels of current spending on the health sector as a whole in the low-income countries affect our recommendations for new expenditures on reproductive health. Our recommendations are designed to help in the planning for more efficient spending of resources that already are devoted to programs like family planning and mother-child health programs. But it is difficult to envision serious reforms and improvement coming with no increment in resources for the sector. Estimates prepared for India's reproductive and child health approach, for example, called for increases in public-sector recurrent spending on the order of 50-60 percent, for a relatively modest package of services (Measham and Heaver, 1996:Ch. 6). The arguments from welfare economics for public funding of health care are persuasive when applied to reproductive health, but even so, private sector funding will also have to be mobilized to achieve these goals in most countries.

Lastly, the rationale for public funding of services is not to be confused with an argument for public provision of services, still less for provision by large centralized public-sector bureaucracies. The most effective organizational forms for delivering services will vary considerably, depending on the existing institutional infrastructure. A good deal of empirical evidence will be needed to test alternative ways to deliver on the promises of the reproductive health approach.

References

CHAPTER 1:
INTRODUCTION

Fathalla, M.
    1988   Research Needs in Human Reproduction. In E. Diczfalusy, P.D. Griffin, and J. Kharlna, eds., *Research in Human Reproduction, Biennial Report (1986-87)*. Geneva, Switzerland: World Health Organization.

Germain, A., and P. Antrobus
    1989   New Partnerships in Reproductive Health Care. *Populi* 16(4):18-30.

National Research Council
    1989   *Contraception and Reproduction: Health Consequences for Women and Children in the Developing World*. Committee on Population, Working Group on Health Consequences of Contraceptive Use and Controlled Fertility. Washington, D.C.: National Academy Press.

United Nations
    1973   *Human Rights: A Compilation of International Instruments of the United Nations*. New York: United Nations.
    1994   *Programme of Action of the 1994 International Conference on Population and Development* (A/CONF.171/13). Reprinted in *Population and Development Review* 21(1):187-213 and 21(2):437-461.
    1995a   *World Population Prospects. The 1994 Revision*. (ST/ESA/SER.A.145) Population Divison. New York: United Nations.
    1995b   *World Urbanization Prospects. The 1994 Revision*. (ST/ESA/SER.A.150) Population Division. New York: United Nations.

CHAPTER 2:
HEALTHY SEXUALITY

Anarfi, J.K.
1993 Sexuality, migration and AIDS in Ghana—a socio-behavioural study. *Health Transition Review* 3(Supplement):45-67.

Awusabo-Asare, K., J.K. Anarfi, and D.K. Agyeman
1993 Women's control over their sexuality and the spread of STDs and HIV/AIDS in Ghana. *Health Transition Review* 3(Supplement):69-84.

Archavanitkul, K., and P. Guest
1994 Migration and the commercial sex sector in Thailand. *Health Transition Review* 4(Supplement):273-295.

Barricklow, D.
1993 Shelter from the storm. *Journal of Family Welfare* 39(1):33-35.

Basnayake, S.
1985 Medical and Sexual Problems: Analysis of a Sample of Letters Addressed to a Newspaper Column. The Family Planning Association of Sri Lanka. Columbo.

Belsey, M.
1996 Health and Psychosocial Dimensions of Commercial Sexual Exploitation of Children. Background paper prepared for World Congress Against Commercial Sexual Exploitation of Children, Stockholm, Sweden, August 27-31, 1996. World Health Organization, Geneva, Switzerland.

Bledsoe, C.H., and N.B. Cohen, eds.
1993 *Social Dynamics of Adolescent Fertility in Sub-Saharan Africa.* Working Group on the Social Dynamics of Adolescent Fertility in Sub-Saharan Africa, Committee on Population, National Research Council. Washington, D.C.: National Academy Press.

Bourqia, R.
1990 The woman's body: Strategy of illness and fertility in Morocco. In Towards More Efficacy in Women's Health and Child Survival Strategies. Report of the Johns Hopkins University-Ford Foundation Workshop, Cairo, Egypt.

Browne, A., and D. Finkelhor
1986 The impact of child sexual abuse: A review of the research. *Psychological Bulletin* 99:66-77.

Bruce, J.
1990 Fundamental elements of the quality of care: A simple framework. *Studies in Family Planning* 21(2):61-91.

Burt, M.R.
1990 Public costs and policy implications of teenage childbearing. *Advances in Adolescent Mental Health* 4:265-280.

Caldwell, P., and J.C. Caldwell
1981 The functions of child-spacing in traditional societies and the direction of change. In H.J. Page and R. Lesthaeghe, eds., *Child Spacing in Tropical Africa: Traditions and Change.* New York: Academic Press.

Caldwell, J.C., P. Caldwell, and P. Quiggin
1989 The social context of AIDS in sub-Saharan Africa. *Population and Development Review* 15(2):185-234.

Caraël, M.
1995 Sexual Behavior. Pp. 75-123 in J. Cleland and B. Ferry, eds., *Sexual Behavior and AIDS in the Developing World.* London: Taylor and Francis.

Cohen, B., and J. Trussell, eds.
1996   *Preventing and Mitigating AIDS in Sub-Saharan Africa: Research and Data Priorities for the Social and Behavioral Sciences.* Panel on Data and Research Priorities for Arresting AIDS in Sub-Saharan Africa, Committee on Population, National Research Council. Washington, D.C.: National Academy Press.
Constantinides, P.
1985   Women heal women: Spirit possession and sexual segregation in a Muslim society. *Social Science and Medicine* 21(6):685-692.
Counts, D.
1987   Female suicide and wife abuse: A cross-cultural perspective. *Suicide and Life Threatening Behavior* 17:194-204.
Counts, D.A., J. Brown, and J. Campbell, eds.
1992   *Sanctions and Sanctuary: Cultural Perspectives of the Beating of Wives.* Boulder, Colo.: Westview Press.
Department of Statistics, Sudan, and Macro International, Inc.
1991   *Sudan Demographic and Health Survey, 1989-90.* Calverton, Md.: Macro International, Inc.
Diawara, Y.
1979   *Sexuality and Education.* Bureau Regional d'Education pour l'Afrique. Dakar, Senegal: UNESCO.
Diaz, M., with K. Moore
1996   The evolution of a sexuality education program: From research to action. Pp. 195-209 in S. Zeidenstein and K. Moore, eds., *Learning about Sexuality: A Practical Beginning.* New York: Population Council and International Women's Health Coalition.
Dixon-Mueller, R.
1993   The sexuality connection in reproductive health. *Studies in Family Planning* 24(5):269-282.
Doniger, W.
1991   *The Laws of Manu.* New Delhi, India: Penguin.
Dualeh, R.H., and M. Fara-Warsame
1982   Female circumcision in Somalia. In T. Baasher, R.H. Bannerman, H. Rushwan, and I. Sharif, eds., *Traditional Practices Affecting the Health of Women and Children.* Alexandria, Egypt: World Health Organization.
Du-Toit, B.M.
1987   Menarche and sexuality among a sample of black South African school-girls. *Social Science and Medicine* 24(7):561-571.
El-Saadawi, N.
1982   Circumcision of girls. In T. Baasher, R.H. Bannerman, H. Rushwan and I. Sharif, eds., *Traditional Practices Affecting the Health of Women and Children.* Alexandria, Egypt: World Health Organization.
El-Zanaty, F., E. Hussein, G.A. Shawky, A.A. Way, and S. Kishor
1996   *Egypt Demographic and Health Survey, 1995.* National Population Council, Cairo, Egypt, and Macro International, Inc. Calverton, Md.: Marcro International, Inc.
Ferguson, A., J. Gitonga, and D. Kabira
1988   Family Planning Needs in Colleges of Education: Report of a Study of Twenty Colleges in Kenya. Ministry of Health, Division of Family Health, Nairobi, Kenya.
Feyisetan, B., and A.R. Pebley
1989   Premarital sexuality in urban Nigeria. *Studies in Family Planning* 20(6):343-354.

Finkelhor, D.
  1995   The victimization of children: A developmental perspective. *American Journal of Orthopsychiatry* 65(2):177-193.
Folch-Lyon, E., L. Macorra, and S.B. Shearer
  1981   Focus group and survey research on family planning in Mexico. *Studies in Family Planning* 12(12):409-432.
Ford Foundation
  1992   Violence against women: Addressing a global problem. Ford Foundation Women's Program Forum (transcript of an international seminar held in New York, February 1991). New York: Ford Foundation.
Fort, A.L.
  1989   Investigation of the social context of family planning: A qualitative study in Peru. *International Family Planning Perspectives* 15(3):88-94.
Gillies, P.A., and R.G. Parker
  1994   Cross-cultural perspectives on sexual behaviour and prostitution. *Health Transition Review* 4(Supplement):257-271.
Gilmore, D.D.
  1990   *Manhood in the Making: Cultural Concepts of Masculinity.* New Haven, Conn.: Yale University Press.
Goddard, V.
  1987   Honor and shame: The control of women's sexuality and group identity in Naples. In P. Caplan, ed., *The Cultural Construction of Sexuality.* London, England: Routledge.
Goparaju, L.
  1994   Discourse and Practice: Rural-Urban Differences in Male Students' Sexual Behaviour in India. Paper presented to seminar (Feb. 28-Mar. 3) "Sexual Cultures and Migration in the Era of AIDS/STDs," organized by the International Union for the Scientific Study of Population, Bangkok, Thailand.
Hathout, H.
  1989   Perspectives of the Middle East. Pp. 222-237 in Z. Bankowski, J. Barzelatto, and A.M. Capron, eds., *Ethics and human values in family planning: Conference highlights, papers, and discussions.* Proceedings of the XXII Conference of the Council for International Organizations of Medical Sciences, Bangkok, Thailand, 19-24 June 1988. Geneva, Switzerland: Conference of the Council for International Organizations of Medical Sciences.
Heise, L.
  1994   Gender-based violence and women's reproductive health. *International Journal of Gynecology and Obstetrics* 46:221-229.
Heise, L., K. Moore, and N. Toubia
  1995   *Sexual Coercion and Reproductive Health: A Focus on Research.* New York: Population Council.
Heise, L., with J. Pitanguy and A. Germain
  1994   *Violence Against Women: The Hidden Health Burden.* World Bank Discussion Paper No. 255. Washington, D.C.: World Bank.
Howson, C.P., P.F. Harrison, D. Hotra, and M. Law, eds.
  1996   *In Her Lifetime: Female Morbidity and Mortality in Sub-Saharan Africa.* Institute of Medicine. Washington, D.C.: National Academy Press.
IMIFAP (Instituto Mexicano de Investigacion de Familia y Poblacion) and Gallup Corporation
  1993   Mexico National Sex Education and Abortion Opinion Survey. Final report presented to the Moriah Fund, Prospect Hill Foundation, and John Merck Fund. IMIFAP, Mexico City, D.F., Mexico.

International Planned Parenthood Federation
   1995   *Challenges: Women's Health, Women's Rights.* London, England: International Planned Parenthood Federation.
Jenny, C., T.M. Hooten, A. Bowers, M.K. Compass, J.N. Krieger, S.L. Hiller, N. Kiviat, and L. Cory
   1990   Sexually transmitted diseases in victims of rape. *New England Journal of Medicine* 322:713-716.
Kapur, P.
   1973   *Love, Marriage and Sex.* New Delhi, India: Vikas Publishing House.
Khattab, M.
   1992   *The Silent Endurance: Social Conditions of Women's Reproductive Health in Rural Egypt.* Amman, Jordon: UNICEF Regional Office; Cairo, Egypt: The Population Council.
   1996   *Women's Perceptions of Sexuality in Rural Giza.* Monographs in Reproductive Health. Cairo, Egypt: The Population Council.
Kiragu, K.
   1995   Female genital mutilation: A reproductive health concern. Supplement to A.P. McCauley and C. Slater, *Meeting the Needs of Young Adults.* Population Reports No. 47. Baltimore, Md.: Johns Hopkins University.
Kirby, D.
   1994   *Sex Education in the Schools.* Menlo Park, Calif.: Henry J. Kaiser Family Foundation.
Kirby, D., L. Short, J. Collins, D. Rugg, L. Kolbe, M. Howard, B. Miller, F. Sonenstein, and L. Zabin
   1994   School-based programs to reduce sexual risk behaviors: A review of effectiveness. *Public Health Reports* 109:339-360.
Koenig, M.A., and R. Simmons
   1992   Constraints on supply and demand for family planning: Evidence from rural Bangladesh. Pp. 259-275 in J.F. Phillips and J.A. Ross, eds., *Family Planning Programmes and Fertility.* Oxford, England: Oxford University Press.
Koss, M. P., L. Heise, and N.F. Russo
   1994   The global health burden of rape. *Psychology of Women Quarterly* 18:499-527.
Laumann, E.O., J.H. Gagnon, R.T. Michael, and S. Michaels
   1995   *The Social Organization of Sexuality: Sexual Practices in the United States.* Chicago: University of Chicago Press.
Levinson, D.
   1989   *Violence in Cross-Cultural Perspective.* Newbury Park, Calif.: Sage.
Martin, S.L., A.O. Tsui, K. Maitra, and R. Marinshaw
   1997   Wife Abuse in Northern India. Unpublished paper, Carolina Population Center, University of North Carolina.
Mashaly, A.Y. P.L. Graicer, and Z.M. Youssef
   1993   Injury in Egypt: Injury as a Public Health Problem. Ministry of Health, Cairo, Egypt.
Mauldon, J., and K. Luker
   1996   The effects of contraceptive education on method use at first intercourse. *Studies in Family Planning* 28(1):19-24.
Meekers, Dominique.
   1990   Marriage and Premarital Childbearing in Cote d'Ivoire. Unpublished doctoral dissertation, Department of Demography, University of Pennsylvania.
   1992   The process of marriage in African societies: A multiple indicator approach. *Population and Development Review* 18(1):61-78.

Mernissi, F.
1977   View from the Near East/North Africa. In D.J. Bogue, K. Oettinger, M. Thompson, and P. Morse, eds., *Adolescent Fertility*. Chicago: University of Chicago Press.

Murray, C.J.L., G. Yang, and X. Qiao
1992   Adult mortality: Levels, patterns, and causes. Pp. 23-112 in Richard G.A. Feachem et al., eds., *The Health of Adults in the Developing World*. New York: Oxford University Press.

Nguelebe, E.
1995   L'Excision. Pp. 201-206 in R. Ndamossi, G. Mboup, and E. Nguelebe, *Enquete Demographique et de Sante, Republique Centrafricaine, 1994-95*. Bangui, Central African Republic: Direction des Statistiques Demographiques et Sociales, Bangui, Central African Republic, and Macro International, Inc.

Orubuloye, I.O., J.C. Caldwell, and P. Caldwell
1993   African women's control over their sexuality in an era of AIDS: A study of the Yoruba in Nigeria. *Social Science and Medicine* 37(7):859-872.

Orubuloye, I.O, J.C. Caldwell, and P. Caldwell
1994   Commercial sex workers in Nigeria in the shadow of AIDS. Pp. 101-116 in I.O. Orubuloye, J.C. Caldwell, P. Caldwell, and G. Santow, eds., *Sexual Networking and AIDS in Sub-Saharan Africa: Behavioural Research and the Social Context*. Canberra, Australia: Health Transition Centre, Australian National University.

Oyeneye, O.Y., and S. Kawonise
1993   Sexual networking in Ijebu-Ode, Nigeria: An exploratory study. *Health Transition Review* 3(Supplement):171-183.

Paltiel, F.
1987   Women and mental health: A post-Nairobi perspective. *World Health Statistics* 40:233-266.

Pick, S., J.C. Hernandez, M. Alvarez, and R. Vernon
1992   *An Operational Test to Institutionalize Life Education in Secondary Schools in Mexico*. Mexico City: IMIFAP (Instituto Mexicano de Investigacion de Familia y Población) and the Population Council.

Pick, S., M. Givaudan, and E. Aldaz
1996   *Conducta sexual y prevención del SIDA en hombres y mujeres de la Ciudad de Mexico*. Mexico City: Instituto Mexicano de Investigacion de Familia y Población (IMIFAP).

Pickering, H., and H.A. Wilkins
1993   Do unmarried women in African towns have to sell sex, or is it a matter of choice? *Health Transition Review* 3(Supplement):17-27.

Rajani, R., and M. Kudrati.
1996   The varieties of sexual experience of the street children of Mwanza, Tanzania. Pp. 301-323 in S. Zeidenstein and K. Moore, eds., *Learning about Sexuality: A Practical Beginning*. New York: The Population Council and International Center for Research on Women.

Renne, E.P.
1993   Changes in adolescent sexuality and the perception of virginity in a southwestern Nigerian village. *Health Transition Review* 3(Supplement):121-133.

Rogow, D.
1990   Meeting male reproductive health care needs in Latin America. *Quality/Calidad/Qualite* 2. New York: Population Council.

Sanday, P.R.
1981   The socio-cultural context of rape: A cross-cultural study. *Journal of Social Issues* 37(4):5-27.

Savara, M., and C.R. Sridhar
  1994   Sexual behavior among different occupational groups in Maharashtra, India, and
          the implications for AIDS education. *The Indian Journal of Social Work* 14(4):617-
          632.
Shamim, I., and Q.A. Chowdhury
  1993   *Homeless and Powerless: Child Victims of Sexual Exploitation.* Dhaka, Bangladesh:
          Bangladesh Sociology Association.
Stewart, S.
  1996   Changing attitudes toward violence against women: The Musasa project. Pp.
          343-362 in S. Zeidenstein and K. Moore, eds., *Learning about Sexuality: A Practical
          Beginning.* New York: The Population Council and International Center for Re-
          search on Women.
Taylor, A.P.
  1984   Reproduction and the family: The role of family planning. In *The 1984 Interna-
          tional Conference on Population: The Liberian Experience.* Liberia: Ministry of Plan-
          ning and Economic Affairs.
Thongkrajai, E., J. Stoeckel, M. Kievying, C. Leelakraiwan, S. Anusornteerakul, K. Keitisut,
          P. Thingkrajai, N. Winiyakul, P. Leelaphanmetha, and C. Elias
  1993   *AIDS Prevention Among Adolescents: An Intervention Study in Northeast Thailand.*
          Women and AIDS Research Program, Report-in-Brief. Washington, D.C.: Inter-
          national Center for Research on Women.
Udry, J.R.
  1993   Coitus as demographic behavior. In R. Gray, H. Leridon, and A. Spira, eds.,
          Biomedical and Demographic Determinants of Reproduction. Oxford, England:
          Clarendon Press.
United Nations
  1989   *Violence Against Women in the Family.* New York: United Nations.
van der Kwaak, A.
  1992   Female circumcision and gender identity: A questionable alliance? *Social Science
          and Medicine* 35(6):777-787.
van de Walle, E.
  1990   The social impact of AIDS in sub-Saharan Africa. *Milbank Quarterly* 68(1):10-32.
Whiting, J.W., V.K. Burbank, and M.S. Ratner
  1986   The duration of maidenhood across cultures. In J.B. Lancaster and B.A. Ham-
          burg, eds., *School Age Pregnancy and Parenthood: Biosocial Dimensions.* New York:
          Aldine de Gruyter.
World Health Organization
  1994   WHO leads action against female genital mutilation. *World Health Forum*
          15:416.111.

CHAPTER 3:
INFECTION-FREE SEX AND REPRODUCTION

Alan Guttmacher Institute
  1994   *Clandestine Abortion: A Latin American Reality.* New York: Alan Guttmacher Insti-
          tute.
Alary, M., J.R. Joly, and C. Poulin
  1989   Incidence of four sexually transmitted diseases in a rural community: A prospec-
          tive study. *American Journal of Epidemiology* 130:547-556.

Anderson, R.M.
   1989   Editorial review: Mathematical and statistical studies of the epidemiology of
          HIV. *AIDS* 3:333-346.
Andrus, J.K., D.W. Fleming, D.R. Harger, M.Y. Chin, D.V. Bennett, J.M. Horan, G. Oxman,
B. Olson, and L.R. Foster
   1990   Partner notification: Can it control epidemic syphilis? *Annals of Internal Medicine*
          112:539-543.
Apao, M., and C. Darden
   1993   Integrating HIV/AIDS Education Into NGO Family Planning Clinics Nationwide
          via Social Marketing Techniques. DKT-UNFPA Social Marketing Project, DKT
          International, Philipines.
Aral, S.O., and K.K. Holmes
   1990   Epidemiology of sexual behavior and sexually transmitted diseases. Pp. 19-36 in
          Holmes, K.K., P. Mardh, P.F. Sparling, P.J. Wiesner, et al., *Sexually Transmitted
          Diseases, Second Edition*. New York: McGraw-Hill.
Aral, S.O., and T.A. Peterman
   1993   Defining behavioral methods to prevent sexually transmitted diseases through
          intervention research. Pp. 861-873 in M.S. Cohen, E.W. Hook III, and
          P.J. Hitchcock, eds., *Infectious Disease Clinics of North America: Sexually Transmit-
          ted Diseases in AIDS Era: Part I*. Philadelphia, Pa.: W.B. Saunders Company.
Asamoah-Adu, A., S. Weir, M. Pappoe, N. Kanlisi, A. Neequaye, and P. Lamptey
   1994   Evaluation of a targeted AIDS prevention intervention to increase condom use
          among prostitutes in Ghana. *AIDS* 8:239-246.
Asuzu, M.C., N.A. Rotowa, and I.O. Ajayi
   1990   The use of mail reminders in STD contact tracing in Ibadan, Nigeria. *East African
          Medical Journal* 67:75-78.
AVSC International and Program for Appropriate Technology in Health (Access to Volun-
          tary and Safe Contraception)
   1994   Proceedings from a working meeting (September 25) "Cervical Cancer Preven-
          tion, Screening, and Treatment." Montreal, Canada.
Bang, R.A, A.T. Bang, M. Baitule, Y. Choudhary, S. Sarmukaddam, and O. Tale
   1989   High prevalence of gynaecological diseases in rural Indian women. *Lancet* 1:85-
          87.
Basch, C., E.M. Sliepcevich, R.S. Gold, D.F. Duncan, and L.J. Kolbe
   1985   Avoiding type III errors in health education program evaluations: A case study.
          Health Education Quarterly 12(4):315-331.
Baylis, M.G., and A.M. Myers
   1990   Combatting sexual assault: An evaluation of prevention programs. *Canadian
          Journal of Public Health* 81(5):341-344.
Begley, C., L. McGill, and P. Smith
   1989   The incremental cost of screening, diagnosis, and treatment of gonorrhea and
          chlamydia in a family planning clinic. *Sexually Transmitted Diseases* 16(2):63-67.
Behets, F.M.T., Y. Williams, A. Briathwaite, T. Hylton-Kong, I.F. Hoffman, G. Dallabetta, E.
Ward, M.S. Cohen, and J.P. Figueroa
   1995   Management of vaginal discharge in women treated at a Jamaican sexually trans-
          mitted disease clinic: Use of diagnostic algorithms compared with laboratory
          testing. *Clinical Infectious Diseases* 21(6):1450-1455.
Berg, A.O.
   1990   The primary care physician and sexually transmitted diseases control. Pp. 1095-
          1098 in K.K. Holmes et al., eds., *Sexually Transmitted Diseases*. New York: McGraw
          Hill.

Berkely, S.
  1994   Diagnostic tests for sexually transmitted diseases: A challenge. *Lancet* 343:685-686.
Blumenthal, P.D., L. Gaffikin, N.M. Maier, and P. Riseborough, eds.
  1994   Issues in cervical cancer: Seeking alternatives to cytology. *Proceedings from the Cervical Cancer Screening Workshop.* Baltimore, Md.: Johns Hopkins Program for International Education in Reproductive Health.
Bosch, F.X., M.M. Manos, M. Munoz, M. Sherman, A.M. Jansen, J. Peto, M.H. Schiffman, V. Moreno, R. Kurman, and K.V. Shah
  1995   Prevalence of human papilloma virus in cervical cancer: A worldwide perspective. *Journal of the National Cancer Institute* 87:796-802.
Brabin, L., J. Kemp, O.K. Obunge, J. Ikamalo, N. Dollimore, N.N. Odu, C.A. Hart, and N.D. Briggs
  1995   Reproductive tract infections and abortion among adolescent girls in rural Nigeria. *Lancet* 345:300-304.
Brinton, L.A., C. Schairer, W. Haenszel, P. Stolley, H.F. Lehman, R. Levine, and D. Savitz
  1986   Cigarette smoking and invasive cervical cancer. *Journal of the American Medical Association* 255:3265-3269.
Brown, Z.A., J. Benedetti, R. Ashley, S. Burchett, S. Selke, S. Berry, L.A. Vontver, and L. Corey
  1991   Neonatal herpes simplex virus infection in relation to asymptomatic maternal infection at the time of labor. *New England Journal of Medicine* 324:1247-1252.
Brunham, R.C., and J.E. Embree
  1992   Sexually transmitted diseases: Current and future dimensions of the problem in the third world. Pp. 35-58 in A. Germain, K.K. Holmes, P. Piot, and J.N. Wasserheit, eds., *Reproductive Tract Infections Global Impact and Priorities for Women's Reproductive Health.* New York: Plenum Press.
Brunham, R.C., and A. Ronald
  1991   Epidemiology of sexually transmitted diseases in developing countries. Pp. 61-80 in J.N. Wasserheit, S.O. Aral, and K.K. Holmes, eds., *Research Issues in Human Behavior and Sexually Transmitted Diseases in the AIDS Era.* Washington, D.C.: American Society of Microbiology.
Brunham, R.C., K.K. Holmes, and J.E. Embree
  1990   Sexually transmitted diseases in pregnancy. Pp. 771-802 in K.K. Holmes, P. Mardh, P.F. Sparling, P.J. Wiesner, et al., eds., *Sexually Transmitted Diseases, Second Edition.* New York: McGraw-Hill.
Buckley, J.D., R.W. Harris, R. Doll, M.P. Vessey, and P.T. Williams
  1981   Case-control study of the husbands of women with dysplasia or carcinoma of the cervix uteri. *Lancet* 2(8254):1010-1015.
Caldwell, J.C., I.O. Orubuloye, and P. Caldwell
  1991   The destabilization of the traditional Yoruba sexual system. *Population and Development Review* 17(2):229-262,373-375.
Caraël, M., J. Cleland, J-C. Deheneffe, B. Ferry, and R. Ingham
  1995   Sexual behavior in developing countries: Implications for HIV control. *AIDS* 9:1171-1175.
Cates, W., Jr.
  1995   Sexually transmitted diseases. Pp. 57-84 in B.P. Sachs, R. Beard, E. Papiernik, C. Russell, eds., *Reproductive Health Care for Women and Babies: Analysis of Medical, Economic, Ethical and Political Issues.* New York: Oxford University Press.

Cates, W., Jr., and K.K. Holmes
  1992   Sexually transmitted diseases. Pp. 99-114 in J. Last, R.B. Wallace, eds., *Maxcy-Rosenau's Public Health and Preventive Medicine*. (13th Edition). Norwalk, Conn.: Appleton and Lange.
Cates, W., Jr., and K.M. Stone
  1992   Family planning, sexually transmitted diseases, and contraceptive choice: A literature update (part I and part II). *Family Planning Perspectives* 24:75-84,122-128.
Cates, W., Jr., and J.N. Wasserheit
  1991   Genital chlamydial infections: Epidemiology and reproductive sequelae. *American Journal of Obstetrics and Gynecology* 164:1771-1781.
Cates, W., Jr., T.M.M. Farley, P.J. Rowe, and the WHO Task Force on the Diagnosis and Treatment of Infertility.
  1985   Worldwide patterns of infertility: Is Africa different? *Lancet* 2:596-598.
Cates, W., Jr., R.T. Rolfs, Jr., and S.O. Aral
  1990   Sexually transmitted diseases, pelvic inflammatroy disease, and infertility: An epidemiological update. *Epidemiological Review* 12:199-220.
Cates, W., Jr., M.R. Joesoef, and M.B. Goldman
  1993   Atypical pelvic inflammatory disease: Can we identify clinical predictors? *American Journal of Obstetrics and Gynecology* 169:341-346.
Cates, W., Jr., R.B. Rothenberg, and J.W. Blount
  1996   Syphilis control: The historical context and epidemiologic basis for interrupting sexual transmission of *Treponema pallidum*. *Sexually Transmitted Diseases* 23(1):68-75.
Centers for Disease Control and Prevention
  1988a   Condoms for prevention of sexually transmitted diseases. *Morbidity and Mortality Weekly Report* 37:133-137.
  1988b   Guidelines for the prevention and control of congenital syphilis. *Morbidity and Mortality Weekly Report* 37(S1):1-13
  1993a   Sexually transmitted diseases treatment guidelines. Division of STD/HIV Prevention. *Morbidity and Mortality Weekly Report* 42(RR-14):1-102.
  1993b   Update: Barrier protection against HIV infection and other sexually transmitted diseases. *Morbidity and Mortality Weekly Report* 42(30):589-91,597.
  1994   *1993 Annual Report*. Division of STD/HIV Prevention. Atlanta, Ga.: Centers for Disease Control and Prevention.
  1995   First 500,000 AIDS cases, United States. *Mortality and Morbidity Weekly Report* (44):849-853.
Chen, H.T., and H.R. Rossi
  1983   Evaluating with sense The theory-driven approach. *Evaluation Review* 7:283-302.
Choi, K.H., and T.J. Coates
  1994   Prevention of HIV infection. *AIDS* 8:1371-1389.
Chow, W-H., J.R. Daling, W. Cates, Jr., and R.S. Greenberg
  1987   Epidemiology of ectopic pregnancy. *Epidemiologic Reviews* 9:70-94.
Cleary, J.
  1994   Female Condom Efficacy, Acceptability and Relationship to the Women's Hierarchy of Risk Reduction. AIDS Research Coordinating Unit, Division of HIV Prevention, State Department of Health, Albany, N.Y.
Cleland, J., and B. Ferry
  1995   *Sexual Behavior and AIDS in the Developing World*. London, England: Taylor and Francis.

Clottey, C., and G. Dallabetta
    1993   Sexually transmitted diseases and human immunodeficiency virus: Epidemio-
            logical synergy? *Infectious Disease Clinics of North America Sexually Transmitted
            Diseases in the AIDS Era* 7(4):753-770.
Coates, T.J., and H.J. Makadon
    1995   Does sex education work? In *HIV Prevention Looking Back, Looking Ahead*. UCSF
            Center for AIDS Prevention Studies and Harvard AIDS Institute. San Francisco:
            University of California.
Cohen, I., J.C. Veille, and B.M. Calkins
    1990   Improved pregnancy outcome following successful treatment of chlamydial in-
            fection. *Journal of the American Medical Association* 263:3160-3163.
Corey, L.
    1994   The current trend in genital herpes: Progress in prevention. *Sexually Transmitted
            Diseases* 21(suppl 2):S38-S44.
Dating Violence Intervention Project
    1988   Three Session Curriculum on Teen Dating Violence Prevention and Peer leader
            Training Manual. Dating Violence Intervention Project, Cambridge, Mass.
de Vincenzi, I.
    1994   A longitudinal study of human immunodeficiency virus transmission by hetero-
            sexual partners. *New England Journal of Medicine* 331:341-346.
DiClemente, R.J., M. Durbin, D. Siegel, F. Krasnovsky, N. Lazarus, and T. Comacho
    1992   Determinants of condom use among junior high school students in a minority,
            inner-city school district. *Pediatrics* 89(2):197-202.
Dorfman, L.E., P.A. Derish, and J.B. Cohen
    1992   Hey girlfriend: An evaluation of AIDS prevention among women in the sex
            industry. *Health Education Quarterly* 19(1):25-40.
Dwyer, J., and T. Jezowski
    1995   *Quality Management for Family Planning Services: Practical Experience from Africa.*
            AVSC Working Paper No. 7. New York: Association for Voluntary Safe Contra-
            ception.
Ehrhardt, A.A., and J.N. Wasserheit
    1991   Age, gender, and sexual risk behaviors for sexually transmitted diseases in the
            United States. Pp. 97-121 in J.N. Wasserheit, S.O. Aral, and K.K. Holmes, eds.,
            Research Issues in Human Behavior and Sexually Transmitted Diseases in the AIDS Era.
            Washington, D.C.: American Society of Microbiology.
Elias, C.
    1991   *Sexual Transmitted Disease and the Reproductive Health of Women in Developing Coun-
            tries.* Programs Division Working Paper No. 5. New York: The Population
            Council.
Elias, C., and L. Heise
    1994   Challenges for the development of female-controlled vaginal microbicides. *AIDS*
            8:1-9.
Elias, C.J., and A. Leonard
    1995   Family planning and sexually transmitted diseases: The need to enhance contra-
            ceptive choice. *Current Issues in Public Health* 1:191-199.
Ellertson, C., B. Winikoff, E. Armstrong, S. Camp, and P. Senanayake
    1995   Expanding Access to Emergency Contraception in Developing Countries. Un-
            published paper. The Populaton Council, New York.
Feldblum, P., and C. Joanis
    1994   *Modern Barrier Methods Effective Contraception and Disease Prevention.* Chapel Hill,
            N.C.: Family Health International.

Ferry, B.
  1995   Risk factors related to HIV transmission: Sexually transmitted disease, alcohol
         consumption, and medically related injection. Pp. 193-207 in J. Cleland and B.
         Ferry, eds., *Sexual Behaviour and AIDS in the Developing World*. London, England:
         Taylor and Francis.
Finger, W.
  1994   Should family planning include STD services? *Network* 144-147. Family Health
         International, Research Triangle Park, N.C.
Flisher, A.J., M.M. Roberts, and R.J. Blignaut
  1992   Youth attending Cape Peninsula day hospitals. *South African Medical Journal*
         82:104-106.
Frerichs, R.R., N. Silarug, N. Eskes, P. Pagcharoenpol, A. Rodklai, S. Thangsupachai, C.
         Wongba
  1994   Saliva-based HIV antibody testing in Thailand. *AIDS* 8(7):885-894.
Funk, R.E.
  1993   *Stopping Rape: A Challenge for Men*. Philadelphia, Pa.: New Society Publishers.
Gershman, K.A., and R.T. Rolfs
  1991   Diverging gonorrhea and syphilis trends in the 1980s: Are they real? *American
         Journal of Public Health* 81(10):1263-1267.
Gotardi, G., P. Gritti, M. Marzi, and M. Sideri
  1984   Colposcopic finding in virgin and sexually active teenagers. *Obstetrics and Gyne-
         cology* 63(5):613-615.
Gravett, M.G., H.P. Nelson, T. DeRouen, C. Critchlow, D.A. Eschenbach, and K.K. Holmes
  1986   Independent associations of bacterial vaginosis and *Chlamydia trachomatis* infec-
         tion with adverse pregnancy outcome. *Journal of the American Medical Association*
         256(14):1899-1903.
Grosskurth, H., P. Mayaud, G. ka-Gina, F. Mosha, and J. Todd
  1994   Risk assessment for the diagnosis of sexually transmitted diseases. *Prevention and
         Management of Sexually Transmitted Diseases in Eastern and Southern Africa*. Mono-
         graph No. 3. Nairobi, Kenya: NARESA, Network of AIDS Researchers of East-
         ern and Southern Africa.
Grosskurth, H., F. Mosha, J. Todd, E. Mwijarubi, A. Klokke, K. Senkoro, P. Mayaud, J.
         Changalucha, A. Nicoll, G. ka-Gina, et al.
  1995   Impact of improved treatment of sexually transmitted diseases on HIV infection
         in rural Tanzania: Randomized controlled trial. *Lancet* 346(8974):530-536.
Handsfield, H.H., L.L. Jasmin, P.L. Roberts, V.W. Hanson, R.L. Kothenbeutel, and W.E.
         Stamm
  1986   Criteria for selective screening for *Chlamydia trachomatis* infection in women at-
         tending family planning clinics. *Journal of the American Medical Association*
         255:1735-1738.
Hanenberg, R.S., W. Rojanapithayakorn, P. Kunasol, and D.C. Sokal
  1994   Impact of Thailand's HIV-control program as indicated by the decline of sexually
         transmitted diseases. *Lancet* 344:243-245.
Hanson, K., and C. Gidycz
  1993   Evaluation of a sexual assault prevention program. *Journal of Consulting and Clini-
         cal Psychology* 61(6):1046-1052.
Harris, R.W., L.A. Brinton, R.H. Cowdell, D.C. Skegg, P.G. Smith, M.P. Vessey, and R. Doll
  1980   Characteristics of women with dysplasia or carcinoma in situ of the cervix uteri.
         British Journal of Cancer 42(3):359-369.
Heise, L., and C. Elias
  1995   Transforming AIDS prevention to meet women's needs A focus on developing
         countries. *Social Science and Medicine* 40(7):931-943.

Higgins, D.L., C. Galavotti, K.R. O'Reilly, et al.
1991   Evidence for the effects of HIV-antibody and testing on risk behaviors. *Journal of the American Medical Association* 266:2419-2429.

Hildesheim, A., L.A. Brinton, K. Mallin, et al.
1990   Barrier and spermicidal contraceptive methods and risk of invasive cervical cancer. *Epidemiology* 1:266-272.

Hillier, S.L., M.A. Krohn, S.J. Klebanoff, and D.A. Eschenbach
1992   The relationship of hydrogen peroxide producing lactobacilli to bacterial vaginosis and genital microflora in pregnant women. *Obstetrics and Gynecology* 79:369-373.

Hira, S.K., G.J. Bhat, and D.M. Chikamata
1990   Syphilis intervention in pregnancy: Zambian demonstration project. *Genitourinary Medicine* 66:159-164.

Holcomb, D.R., P.D. Sarvela, K.A. Sondag, and L.C. Holcomb
1993   An evaluation of a mixed gender date rape prevention workshop. *Journal of American College Health* 41(4):159-164.

Holmes, K.K.
1994   Human ecology and behavior and sexually transmitted bacterial infections. *Proceedings of the National Academy of Sciences, USA* 91:2448-2455.

Holmes, K.K., P. Mardh, P.F. Sparling, P.J. Wiesner, et al.
1990   *Sexually Transmitted Diseases, Second Edition.* New York: McGraw-Hill.

Holmes, K.K, D.W. Johnson, P.A. Kvale, C.W. Halverson, T.F. Keys, and D.H. Martin
1996   Impact of a gonorrhea control program, including selective mass treatment, in female sex workers. *Journal of Infectious Diseases* 174(supp.2):S230-S239.

Holtzman, D., R. Lowry, L. Kann, J.L. Collins, and L.J. Kolbe
1994   Changes in HIV-related information sources, instruction, knowledge behaviors among US high-school students, 1989 and 1990. *American Journal of Public Health* 84:388-393.

Howard, M., and J. McCabe
1990   Helping teenagers postpone sexual involvement. *Family Planning Perspectives* 22:21-26.

Hulka, B.S.
1982   Risk factors for cervical cancer. *Journal of Chronic Diseases* 35:3-11.

Jain, A., and J. Bruce
1993   A reproductive health approach to the objectives and assessment of family planning programs. Pp. 193-209 in G. Sen, A. Germain, and L. Chen, eds., *Population Policies Reconsidered: Health, Empowerment, and Rights.* Cambridge, Mass.: Harvard Center for Population and Development Studies.

Johnson, R.E., F. Lee, A. Hadgu, G. McQuillan, S.O. Aral, S. Keesling, and A. Nahmias
1994   U.S. genital herpes trends during first decade of AIDS Prevalences increased in young whites and elevated in blacks. *Sexually Transmitted Diseases* 21(2)(Supplement):S109

Judson, F.N., and F.C. Wolf
1978   Tracing and treating contacts of gonorrhea patients in clinic for sexually transmitted diseases. *Public Health Reports* 93:460-463.

Kahn, J.G., C.K. Walker, A.E. Washington, D.V. Landers, and R.L. Sweet
1991   Diagnosing pelvic inflammatory disease. *Journal of the American Medical Association* 266:2594-2604.

Karim, Q. Abdool, E. Preston-Whyte, and S.S. Abdool Karim
1992   Teenagers seeking condoms at family planning services. *South African Medical Journal* 82:356-359.

Kegeles, S.M., R.B. Hayes, and T.J. Coates
1995   The Mpowerment project: A community-level HIV prevention intervention for young gay men. *American Journal of Public Health* 86(8)1:1075-1076.
Kelly, J.A., J.S. St. Lawrence, L.Y. Stevenson, A.C. Hauth, S.C. Kalichman, Y.E. Diaz, T.L. Brasfield, J.J. Koob, and M.G. Morgan
1992   Community AIDS/HIV risk reduction: The effects of endorsements by popular people in three cities. *American Journal of Public Health* 82(11):1483-1489.
Kirby, D., R. Barth, N. Leland, and J.V. Fetro
1991   Reducing the risk: Impact of a new curriculum on sexual risk-taking. *Family Planning Perspectives* 23(6):253-263.
Kirby, D., L. Short, J. Collins, D. Rugg, L. Kolbe, M. Howard, B. Miller, F. Sonenstein, and L.S. Zabin
1994   School-based programs to reduce sexual risk behaviors: A review of effectiveness. *Public Health Reports* 109(3):339-360.
Kost, K., and J.D. Forrest
1992   American women's sexual behavior and exposure to risk of sexually transmitted diseases. *Family Planning Perspectives* 24:244-254.
Kreiss, J., E. Ngugi, K. Holmes, J. Ndinya-Achola, P. Waiyaki, et al.
1992   Efficacy of nonoxynol 9 contraceptive sponge use in preventing heterosexual acquisition of HIV in Nairobi prostitutes. *Journal of the American Medical Association* 268(4):477-482.
Krieger, L., and J. Stryker
1995   What is the role of testing at home? In *HIV Prevention Looking Back, Looking Ahead*. San Francisco, Calif.: San Francisco Center for AIDS Prevention Studies.
Ladipo, O.A., G. Farr, E. Otolorin, J.C. Konje, K. Sturgen, P. Cox, and C.B. Champion
1991   Prevention of IUD-related pelvic infection: The efficacy of prophylactic doxcycline at IUD insertion. *Advances in Contraception* 7(1):43-54.
Laga, M.
1994   Epidemiology and control of sexually transmitted diseases in developing countries. *Sexually Transmitted Diseases* 21:S45-S50.
Laga, M., A. Meheus, and P. Piot
1989   Epidemiology and control of gonococcal ophthalmia neonatorum. *Bulletin of the World Health Organization* 57(5):471-478.
Lamptey, P., D. Rugg, D. Zewdie, and C. Kendall
1995   Primary Prevention Strategies for Sub-Saharan Africa, Unpublished paper. AIDSCAP Project, John Snow International, Arlington, Va.
Larsen, S., E. Hunter, and E. Creighton
1990   Syphilis. Pp. 927-934 in Holmes, K.K., P. Mardh, P.F. Sparling, and P.J. Wiesner, *Sexually Transmitted Diseases, Second Edition*. New York: McGraw-Hill.
Lemon, S., and J. Newbold
1990   Viral hepatitis. Pp. 449-466 in K.K. Holmes, P. Mardh, P.F. Sparling, and P.J. Wiesner, *Sexually Transmitted Diseases, Second Edition*. New York: McGraw-Hill.
Marrazzo, J.M., C.L. Celum, D. Fine, S. Leslie, D.J. Mosure, and H.H. Handsfield
1997   Performance and cost-effectiveness of selective screening criteria for Chlamydia trachomatis infection in women. Implications for a national Chlamydia control strategy. *Sexually Transmitted Diseases* 24(3):131-141.
Mayaud, P., J. Changalucha, H. Grosskurth, G. ka-Gina, J. Rugemalila, J. Nduba, J. Newell, R. Hayes, and D. Mabey
1992   The value of urine specimens in screening for male urethritis and its microbial aetiologies in Tanzania. *Genitourinary Medicine* 68(6):361-365.

McGrath, J.W., C. Rwabukwali, D. Schumann, J. Pearson-Marks, S. Nakayiwa, B. Namande, L. Nakyobe, and R. Mukasa
  1993   Anthropology and AIDS: The cultural context of sexual risk behavior among urban Baganda women in Kampala, Uganda. *Social Science and Medicine* 36(4):429-439.
McLaurin, K.E., C.E. Hord, and M. Wolf
  1990   Health systems' role in abortion care: The need for a pro-active approach. *Issues in Abortion Care*. No. 1. Carrboro, N.C.: International Projects Assistance Services.
Meheus, A., K.F. Schulz, and W. Cates, Jr.
  1990   Development of prevention and control program for sexually transmitted diseases in developing countries. Pp. 1041-1046 in K.K. Holmes, P.-A. Mårdh, P.F. Sparling, P.J. Wiesner, W. Cates, Jr., S.M. Lemon, and W.E. Stamm, eds., *Sexually Transmitted Diseases, Second Edition*. New York: McGraw-Hill.
Miller, B.
  1988   Date rape: Time for a new look at prevention. *Journal of College Student Development* 29:553-555.
Moore, P., and Y. Chang
  1995   Detection of herpes virus-like DNA sequences in Kaposi's sarcoma in patients with and those without HIV infection. *New England Journal of Medicine* 332(18): 1181-1185.
Moses, S., F.A. Plummer, E.N. Ngugi, N.J.D. Nagelkerke, A.O. Anzala, and J.O. Ndinya-Achola
  1991   Controlling HIV in Africa: Effectiveness and cost of an intervention in a high-frequency STD transmitter core group. *AIDS* 5:407-411.
Moses, S., F.A. Plummer, J.E. Bradley, J.O. Endinya-Achola, N.J.D. Nagelkerke, and A.R. Ronald
  1994   The association between lack of male circumcision and risk for HIV infection: A review of the epidemiological data. *Sexually Transmitted Diseases* 21:201-210.
Mosley, W.H., J.L. Bobadilla, and D.T. Jamison
  1993   The health transition: Implications for health policy in developing countries. Pp. 673-682 in D.T. Jamison, et al., eds., *Disease Control Priorities in Developing Countries*. New York: Oxford University Press.
Niruthisard, S., R. Roddy, and S. Chutivongse
  1992   Use of nonoxynol-9 and reduction in rate of gonococcal and chlamydial cervical infections. *Lancet* 339:1371-1375.
Oakley, A., D. Fullerton, and J. Holland
  1995   Behavioral interventions for HIV/AIDs prevention. *AIDS* 9:479-486.
Olukoya, A., and C. Elias
  1994   *Perceptions of Reproductive Morbidity among Nigerian Men and Women: Implications for Family Planning Services*. Final Report. Africa Operations Research and Technical Assistance Project. New York: The Population Council.
O'Reilly, K., and M. Islam
  1995   Interventions for STD/HIV Prevention and Treatment. Global Programme on AIDS. Geneva, Switzerland: The World Health Organization.
Over, M., and P. Piot
  1993   HIV infection and sexually transmitted diseases. Pp. 455-527 in D.T. Jamison, W.H. Mosley, A.R. Measham, and J.L. Bobadilla, eds., *Disease Control Priorities in Developing Countries*. New York: Oxford University Press.
Padian, N.S., E. Vittinghoff, and S. Shiboski
  1994   Letter. *New England Journal of Medicine* 331:341-346.

Pan American Health Organization
  1983   *Acute Respiratory Infections in Children.* RD 21/1. Washington, D.C.: Pan American Health Organization.
Patton, D.L., D.E. Moore, L.R. Spadoni, M.R. Soules, S.A. Halbert, and S.P. Wang
  1989   A comparison of the fallopian tube's response to overt and silent salpingitis. *Obstetrics and Gynecology* 74:622-630.
Piot, P., and M.Q. Islam
  1994   Sexually transmitted diseases in the 1990s: Global epidemiology and challenges for control. *Sexually Transmitted Diseases* 21:S7-S13.
Population Services International
  1994   1993/1994 Annual Report. Washington, D.C.: Population Services International.
Quinn, T.
  1994   Recent advances in diagnosis of sexually transmitted diseases. *Sexually Transmitted Diseases* 21(suppl 2):S19-S27.
Randolph, A.G., A.E. Washington, and C.G. Prober
  1993   Ceasarean delivery women presenting with genital herpes lesions: Efficacy, risks, and costs. *Journal of the American Medical Association* 270:77-82.
Rees, M.
  1993   Menarche: When and why? *Lancet* 342:1375-1376.
Rojanapithayakorn, W.
  1992   One Hundred Percent Condom Programme. VIII International Conference on AIDS. Abstract PoD-5654. Amsterdam, The Netherlands.
Rolfs, R.T., and A.K. Nakashima
  1990   Epidemiology of primary/secondary syphilis in the United States, 1981-1988. *Journal of the American Medical Association* 264:1432-1437.
Rooks, J., and B. Winikoff
  1990   *A Reassessment of the Concept of Reproductive Risk in Maternity Care and Family Planning Services.* Robert H. Ebert Program on Critical Issues in Reproductive Health and Population, February 12-13. New York: The Population Council.
Roper, W.L., H.B. Peterson, and J.W. Curran
  1993   Commentary: Condoms and HIV/STD prevention—clarifying the message. *American Journal of Public Health* 83:501-503.
Rosenberg, M.J., and E.L. Gollub
  1992   Commentary: Methods women can use that may prevent sexually transmitted disease, including HIV. *American Journal of Public Health* 82(11):1473-1478.
Rothenberg, R.B.
  1983   The geography of gonorrhea: Empirical demonstration of core group transmission. *American Journal of Epidemiology* 117:688-694.
  1990   Analytic approaches to the epidemiology of sexually transmitted diseases. Pp. 37-42 in K.K. Holmes, P.-A. Mårdh, P.F. Sparling, P.J. Wiesner, W. Cates, Jr., S.M. Lemon, and W.E. Stamm, eds., *Sexually Transmitted Diseases, Second Edition.* New York: McGraw-Hill.
Rowe, P.J., P.C. Comhaire, T.B. Hargreave, and H.J. Mellows
  1993   *WHO Manual for the Standardized Investigation and Diagnosis of the Infertile Couple.* Cambridge, U.K.: Cambridge University Press.
Schulz, K.F., J.M. Schulte, and S.M. Berman
  1992   Maternal health and child survival: Opportunities to protect both women and children from the adverse consequences of reproductive tract infections. In A. Germain et al., eds., *Reproductive Tract Infections.* New York: Plenum Press.
Science
  1995   Testing AIDS interventions: When is the price too high? Staging ethical trials in Africa. *Science* 269:1332-1335.

Shafer, M.A., and R.L. Sweet
   1989   Pelvic inflammatory disease in adolescent females epidemiology, pathogenesis,
            diagnosis, treatment and sequelae. *Pediatric Clinics of North America* 36:513-533.
Shafer, M.A., J. Schachter, A.B. Moscicki, A. Weiss, J. Shalwitz, E. Vaughan, S.G. Millstein
   1989   Urinary leukocyte esterase screening test for asymptomatic chlamydial and gono-
            coccal infections in males. *Journal of the American Medical Association* 262(18):2562-
            2566.
Simmons, R., and C. Elias
   1993   The study of client-provider interactions: A review of methodological issues.
            The Population Council Working Papers. No. 7. New York: The Population Coun-
            cil.
Sinei, S.K.A., K.F. Schulz, P.R. Lamptey, D.A. Grimes, J.K. Mati, S.M. Rosenthal, M.J.
Rosenberg, G. Riara, P.N. Njage, V.B. Bhullar, et al.
   1990   Preventing IUD-related pelvic infection: The efficacy of prophylactic doxycy-
            cline at insertion. *British Journal of Obstetrics and Gynecology* 97(5):412-419.
Singh, V., M.M. Gupta, L. Satyanarayana, A. Parashari, A. Sehgal, D. Chattopadhya, and P.
Sodhani
   1995   Association between reproductive tract infections and cervical inflammatory epi-
            thelial changes. *Sexually Transmitted Diseases* 22:25-30.
Soper, D.E., E. Shoupe, G.A. Shangold, M.M. Shangold, J. Gutmann, and L. Mercer
   1993   Prevention of vaginal trichomoniasis by compliant use of the female condom.
            Sexually Transmitted Diseases 20(3):137-139.
Stein, Z.
   1992   Editorial: The double bind in science policy and the protection of women from
            HIV infection. *American Journal of Public Health* 82(11):1471-1472.
Stoeckel, J.
   1992   *Intervention Research on Child Survival*. The Population Council. New York:
            McGraw-Hill Book Company.
Stover, J.
   1988   The Impact of AIDS on the Use of Condoms for Family Planning in Mexico, a
            SOMARC Special Study. Unpublished paper. The Futures Group, Washington,
            D.C.
Stray-Pederson, B.
   1983   Economic evaluation of maternal screening to prevent congenital syphilis. *Sexu-
            ally Transmitted Diseases* 10(4):167-172
Sweat, M.D., and J.A. Denison
   1995   Reducing HIV incidence in developing countries with structural and environ-
            mental interventions. *AIDS* 9(suppl A):S251-S257.
Tawil, O., K.R. O'Reilly, and A. Verster
   1995   Enabling approaches in HIV/AIDs prevention: Influencing the social and envi-
            ronmental determinants of risk (editorial review); unpublished.
Temmerman, M., F. Mohamedali, and L. Fransen
   1993   Syphilis prevention in pregnancy An opportunity to improve reproductive and
            child health in Kenya. *Health Policy and Planning* (Oxford University Press)
            8(2):122-127.
Temmerman, M., J. Ndinya-Achola, J. Ambani, and P. Piot
   1995   The right not to know HIV-test results. *Lancet* 345:969-970.
Temmerman, M., S. Moses, D. Kiragu, S. Fusallah, I.A. Wamola, and P. Piot
   1990   Impact of single session post-partum counselling of HIV infected women on their
            subsequent reproductive behavior. *AIDS Care* 2(3):247-252.

Toomey, K.E., J.S. Moran, M.P. Rafferty, and G.A. Beckett
   1993   Epidemiological considerations of sexually transmitted diseases in underserved
             populations. *Infectious Disease Clinics of North America* 7:739-752.
Trachtenberg, A.I., A.E. Washington, and S. Halldorson
   1988   A cost-based decision analysis for chlamydia screening in California family plan-
             ning clinics. *American Journal of Obstetrics and Gynecology* 71:101-108.
UNAIDS and World Health Organization
   1996   *HIV/AIDS: The Global Epidemic.* Geneva, Switzerland: UNAIDS.
Van Landingham, M., C. Saengtienchai, J. Knodel, and A. Pramualratana
   1995   *Friends, Wives and Extramarital Sex in Thailand: A Qualitative Study of Peer and
             Spousal Influence on Thai Male Extramarital Sexual Behavior and Attitudes.* Bangkok,
             Thailand: Mahidol University, Institute for Population Studies.
Vernon, R., G. Ojeda, and R. Murad
   1990   Incorporating AIDS Prevention Activities into a Family Planning Organization in
             Colombia. *Studies in Family Planning* 21(6):335-343.
Vuylsteke, B., M. Laga, M. Alary, M.M. Gerniers, J. Lebughe, N. Nzila, F. Behets, E. Van
Dyck, and P. Piot
   1993   Clinical algorithms for the screening of women for gonococcal and chlamydia
             infection: Evaluation of pregnant women and prostitutes in Zaire. *Clinical Infec-
             tious Diseases* 17(1):82-88.
Wallace, R.
   1988   A synergism of plagues: "Planned shrinkage," contagious housing destruction,
             and AIDS in the Bronx. *Environmental Research* 47(1):1-33.
Walter, H.J., and R.D. Vaugh
   1993   AIDS risk reduction among a multi-ethnic sample of urban high-school students.
             Journal of American Medical Association 270:725-730.
Wasserheit, J.N.
   1989   The significance and scope of reproductive tract infections among third world
             women. *International Journal of Gynaecology and Obstetrics* 27(suppl 3):145-168.
   1992   Epidemiological synergy: Interrelationships between human immunodeficiency
             virus infection and other sexually transmitted diseases. *Sexually Transmitted Dis-
             eases* 19:61-77.
   1994   Effect of changes in human ecology and behavior on patterns of sexually trans-
             mitted diseases, including human immunodeficiency virus infection. *Proceedings
             of the National Academy of Sciences, USA* 9(1):2430-2435.
Wasserheit, J.N., J.R. Harris, J. Chakraborty, B.A. Kay, and K.J. Mason
   1989   Reproductive tract infections in a family planning population in rural Bangladesh:
             A neglected opportunity to promote MCH-FP programs. *Studies in Family Plan-
             ning* 20(2):69-80.
Wawer, M.J.
   1995   STD Control for AIDS Preventions: Design and feasibility of a community-based
             mass treatment trial. 11 Meeting, 27-29 August 1995, International Society for
             STD Research, New Orleans, La.
Wawer, M.J., R.H. Gray, T.C. Quinn, N.K. Sewankambo, F. Wabwire-Mangen, D. Serwadda,
and L. Paxton
   1995   Design and feasibility of population-based mass STD treatment, rural Rakai dis-
             trict, Uganda. Abstract 079. XIth Meeting of the International Society for STD
             Research, August 27-30, 1995, New Orleans, La.
Way, P.O., and K.A. Stanecki
   1994   *The Impact of HIV/AIDS on World Population.* Bureau of the Census. Washington,
             D.C.: U.S. Department of Commerce.

Webster, L.A., S.M. Berman, and J.R. Greenspan
  1993   Surveillance for gonorrhea and primary and secondary syphilis among adoles-
          cents, United States—1981-1991. *CDC Surveillance Summaries, Morbidity and Mor-
          tality Weekly Report* 42(SS3):1-11.
Webster, L.A., and R.T. Rolfs
  1993   Surveillance for primary and secondary syphilis—United States, 1991. *CDC Sur-
          veillance Summaries, Morbidity and Mortality Weekly Report* 42(SS3):13-19.
Wenger, N.S., L.S. Linn, M. Epstein, and M.F. Shapira
  1991   Reduction of high-risk sexual behavior among heterosexuals undergoing HIV-
          antibody testing A randomized clinical trial. *American Journal of Public Health*
          81:1580-1585.
Williams, E., N. Lamson, S. Efem, S. Weir, and P. Lamptey
  1992   Implementation of an AIDS prevention program among prostitutes in the Cross
          River State of Nigeria. *AIDS* 6:229-230.
Wilson, D., B. Myathi, and M. Whariwa
  1992   A community-level AIDS prevention program among sexually vulnerable groups
          and the general population in Bulawayo, Zimbabwe. In *Effective Approaches to
          AIDS Prevention.* Report of a meeting, 26-29 May 1992.
          Geneva, Switzerland: World Health Organization.
Winifield, J., and A.S. Latif
  1985   Tracing contacts of persons with sexually transmitted diseases in a developing
          country. *Sexually Transmitted Diseases* 12:5-7.
Wölner-Hansen, P.D. Eschenbach, J. Paavonen, C. Stevens, N. Kiviat, C. Critchlow, et al.
  1990   Association between vaginal douching and acute pelvic inflammatory disease.
          Journal of the American Medical Association 263:1936-1941.
World Health Organization
  1986   *WHO Expert Report on Venereal Diseases and Treponematoses, Sixth Report.* Techni-
          cal Series 736. Geneva, Switzerland: World Health Organization.
  1991   *Management of Patients with Sexually Transmitted Diseases.* Report from a Technical
          Meeting, July 3-6, 1990. Technical Report Series 810. Geneva, Switzerland: World
          Health Organization.
  1994   STD Case Management Workbook Module Two: Using Flow Charts for
          Syndromic Management. Field Test Version. World Health Organization,
          Geneva, Switzerland.
World Health Organization, Global Programme on AIDS
  1995a   WHO Estimate of HIV Infection Tops 19 Million. Press release WHO/30. World
          Health Organization, Global Programme on AIDS, Geneva, Switzerland.
  1995b   An Overview of Selected Curable Sexually Transmitted Diseases. Unpublished
          paper. World Health Organization, Global Programme on AIDS, Geneva, Swit-
          zerland.
Younis, N., H. Khattab, H. Zurayk, M. El-Mouelhy, M.F. Amin, and A.M. Farag
  1993   A community study of gynecological and related morbidities in rural Egypt. *Stud-
          ies in Family Planning* 24:175-186.
Zekeng, L., P.J. Feldblum, R.M. Oliver, and L. Kaptue
  1993   Barrier contraceptive use and HIV infection among high-risk women in
          Cameroon. *AIDS* 7:725-731.
Zurayk, H., H. Khattab, N. Younis, O. Kamal, and M. El-Helw
  1995   Comparing women's reports with medical diagnoses of reproductive morbidity
          conditions in rural Egypt. *Studies in Family Planning* 26(1):14-21.

CHAPTER 4:
INTENDED BIRTHS

Alexander, N.J.
  1995   Future contraceptives. *Scientific American* (September):136-141.
Asif, R., S.N. Sinha, M. Yunus, M. Zaheer, and S. Mohsin
  1994   Contraceptive behaviour in women carrying an unwanted pregnancy. *Journal of Family Welfare* 40(2):26-30.
Baker, J., and S. Khasiani
  1991   Induced abortion in Kenya: Case histories. *Studies in Family Planning* 23(1):34-44.
Bledsoe, C.H., and B. Cohen, eds.
  1993   *Social Dynamics of Adolescent Fertility in Sub-Saharan Africa.* Working Group on the Social Dynamics of Adolescent Fertility in Sub-Saharan Africa, Committee on Population, National Research Council. Washington, D.C.: National Academy Press.
Bongaarts, J.
  1990   The measurement of unwanted fertility. *Population and Development Review* 16(3):487-506.
  1991   Do reproductive intentions matter? *Demographic and Health Surveys World Conference* 1:223-248.
Bongaarts, J., and J. Bruce
  1995   The causes of unmet need for contraception and the social content of services. *Studies in Family Planning* 26(2):57-76.
Brown, S.S., and L. Eisenberg, eds.
  1995   *The Best Intentions: Unintended Pregnancy and the Well-Being of Children and Families.* Committee on Unintended Pregnancy, Institute of Medicine. Washington, D.C.: National Academy Press.
Bruce, J.
  1990   Fundamental elements of the quality of care: A simple framework. *Studies in Family Planning* 21(2):61-91.
Buckner, B.C., A.O. Tsui, A.I. Hermalin, and C. McKaig, eds.
  1995   *A Guide to Methods of Family Planning Program Evaluation, 1965-1990.* Chapel Hill, N.C.: Carolina Population Center.
Caldwell, J.C.
  1986   Routes to low mortality in poor countries. *Population and Development Review* 12(2):171-220.
Casterline, J., A.E. Perez, and A.E. Biddlecom
  1996   Factors Underlying Unmet Need for Family Planning in the Philippines. Research Division working paper no. 84. New York: Population Council.
Cleland, J., and C. Wilson
  1987   Demand theories of the fertility transition: An iconoclastic view. *Population Studies* 41:5-30.
Cleland, J., J.F. Phillips, S. Amin, and G.M. Kamal
  1994   *The Determinants of Reproductive Change in Bangladesh: Success in a Challenging Environment.* World Bank regional and sector studies. Washington, D.C.: World Bank.
Cochrane, S., and F. Sai
  1993   Excess fertility. Pp. 333-362 in D.T. Jamison, et al., eds., *Disease Control Priorities in Developing Countries.* New York: Oxford University Press.
Coeytaux, F.
  1988   Induced abortion in sub-Saharan Africa: What we do and do not know. *Studies in Family Planning* 19(3):186-190.

Cook, R.
   1989   Abortion laws and policies: Challenges and opportunities. *International Journal of Obstetrics and Gynecology* Supp. 3:61-87.
Costa, S., and M. Vessey
   1993   Misoprostol and illegal abortion in Rio de Janeiro, Brazil. *Lancet* 341(8855):1258-1261.
Curtis, S.L., and K. Neitzel
   1996   *Contraceptive Knowledge, Use, and Sources.* DHS Comparative Studies No. 19. Columbia, Md.: Institute for Resource Development.
Davis, K.
   1967   Population policy: Will current programs succeed? *Science* 158(3802):730-739.
Desai, S.
   1995   When are children from large families disadvantaged? Evidence from cross-national analyses. *Population Studies* 49:195-210.
Dixon-Mueller, R.
   1989   Psychosocial consequences to women of contraceptive use and controlled fertility. Pp. 140-160 in A.M. Parnell, ed., *Contraceptive Use and Controlled Fertility: Health Issues for Women and Children.* Committee on Population, National Research Council. Washington, D.C.: National Academy Press.
Dixon-Mueller, R., and A. Germain
   1992   Stalking the elusive "unmet need" for family planning. *Studies in Family Planning* 23(5):330-335.
Ezeh, A.C., M. Seroussi, and H. Raggers
   1996   *Men's Fertility, Contraceptive Use, and Reproductive Preferences.* DHS Comparative Studies No. 18. Columbia, Md.: Institute for Resource Development.
Foster, A., and N. Roy
   1996   The dynamics of education and fertility: Evidence from a family planning experiment. Working paper, Department of Economics. University of Pennsylvania.
Frenzen, P.D., and D.P. Hogan
   1982   The impact of class, education, and health care on infant mortality in a developing society: The case of rural Thailand. *Demography* 19:391-408.
Haaga, J.
   1989   Mechanisms for the association of maternal age, parity, and birth spacing with infant health. Pp. 96-139 in A.M. Parnell, ed., *Contraceptive Use and Controlled Fertility: Health Issues for Women and Children.* Committee on Population, National Research Council. Washington, D.C.: National Academy Press.
Harrison, P.F., and A. Rosenfield, eds.
   1996   *Contraceptive Research and Development: Looking to the Future.* Committee on Contraceptive Research and Development, Institute of Medicine. Washington, D.C.: National Academy Press.
Henshaw, S., and E. Morrow
   1990   *Induced Abortion: A World Review. 1990 Supplement.* New York: Alan Guttmacher Institute.
Hirschman, C.
   1986   The recent rise in Malay fertility: A new trend or a temporary lull in a fertility transition? *Demography* 23(2):161-184.
Huntington, D., and S.R. Schuler
   1993   The simulated client method: Evaluating client-provider interactions in family planning clinics. *Studies in Family Planning* 24(3):187-193.

Huntington, D., B. Mensch, and V.C. Miller
    1996   Survey questions for the measurement of induced abortion. *Studies in Family Planning* 27(3):155-161.
International Planned Parenthood Federation
    1995   *Consensus Statement on Emergency Contraception.* London: International Planned Parenthood Federation.
Jain, A., and J. Bruce
    1994   A reproductive health approach to the objectives and assessment of family planning programs. Pp. 193-209 in G. Sen, A. Germain, and L. Chen, eds., *Population Policies Reconsidered: Health, Empowerment, and Rights.* Cambridge, Mass.: Harvard Center for Population and Development Studies.
Kenney, G.M.
    1993   Assessing Legal and Regulatory Reform in Family Planning: Manual on Legal and Regulatory Reform. OPTIONS Projects Policy Paper No. 1. The Futures Group, Washington, D.C.
Knodel, J., A. Chamratrithirong, and N. Debavalya
    1987   *Thailand's Reproductive Revolution: Rapid Fertility Decline in a Third World Setting.* Chapter 7:117-142, "Societal Change and the Demand for Children." Madison: University of Wisconsin Press.
Koenig, M.A., and R. Simmons
    1992   Constraints on supply and demand for family planning: Evidence from rural Bangladesh. Pp. 259-275 in J.F. Phillips and J.A. Ross, eds., *Family Planning Programmes and Fertility.* New York: Oxford University Press.
Koenig, M.A., V. Fauveau, A.I. Chowdhury, J. Chakraborty, and M.A. Khan
    1988   Maternal Mortality in Matlab, Bangladesh, 1976-1985. *Studies in Family Planning* 19(2):69-80.
Kost, K., and J.D. Forrest
    1995   Intention status of U.S. births in 1988: Differences by mother's socioeconomic and demographic characteristics. *Family Planning Perspectives* 27(1):11-17.
Larsen, U.
    1994   Sterility in Sub-Saharan Africa. *Population Studies* 48(3):459-474.
Larsen, U., and J. Menken
    1989   Measuring sterility from incomplete birth histories. *Demography* 26:185-202.
Laumann, E.O., J.H. Gagnon, R.T. Michael, and S. Michaels
    1994   *The Social Organization of Sexuality: Sexual Practices in the United States.* Chicago: University of Chicago Press.
Lincoln, R., and L. Kaeser
    1988   Whatever happened to the contraceptive revolution? *Family Planning Perspectives* 20(1):20-24.
Lissance, D.M., and W.P. Schellstede
    1993   *Evaluating the Effectiveness of a Family Planning IE&C Program in Bangladesh.* Washington, D.C.: Population Services International.
Lloyd, C.
    1994   Investing in the next generation: The implications of high fertility at the level of the family. Pp. in 181-202 in Robert Cassen, ed., *Population and Development: Old Debates, New Conclusions.* New Brunswick, N.J.: Transaction Publishers.
Lloyd, C., and A. Gage-Brandon
    1994   High fertility and children's schooling in Ghana: Sex differences in parental contributions and educational outcomes. *Population Studies* 48(2):293-306.

MacDonald, P., with S. Soekir, A. Gunadi, and M. Yadnya
  1995 *Assessing Performance, Improving Quality: The Peer Review Program of the Indonesian Midwives Association.* Bethesda, Md.: Quality Assurance Project, Center for Human Services.
Mashalaba, N.N.
  1989 Commentary on the causes and consequences of unwanted pregnancy from an African perspective. *International Journal of Gynecology and Obstetrics* Supp. 3:15-19.
Mason, K.O., and A.M. Taj
  1987 Differences between women's and men's reproductive goals in developing countries. *Population and Development Review* 13:611-638.
McLaurin, K.E., C.E. Hord, and M. Wolf
  1990 *Health Systems' Role in Abortion Care: The Need for a Pro-active Approach.* Issues in Abortion Care no. 1. Carrboro, N.C.: International Projects Assistance Services.
Mensch, B., M. Arends-Kuenning, and A. Jain
  1994 Assessing the Impact of the Quality of Family Planning Services on Contraceptive Use in Peru: A Case Study Linking Situation Analysis Data to the DHS. Research Division working paper no. 67. Population Council, N.Y.
Muhuri, P., and S. Preston
  1991 Effects of family composition on mortality differentials by sex among children in Matlab, Bangladesh. *Population and Development Review* 17(1):415-434.
Nag, M.
  1983 The Equity-Fertility Hypothesis as an Explanation of the Fertility Differential Between Kerala and West Bengal. Center for Policy Studies working paper no. 96. Population Council, N.Y.
Phillips, J., and J.A. Ross, eds.
  1992 *Family Planning Programmes and Fertility.* Oxford, England: Clarendon Press.
Piotrow, P.T., K.A. Treiman, J.G. Rimon, Sung Yee Hun, and B.V. Lozare
  1994 Strategies for Family Planning Promotion. World Bank technical paper no. 223. World Bank, Washington, D.C.
Population Reference Bureau
  1995 *Reproductive risk: A worldwide assessment of women's sexual and maternal health.* Washington, D.C.: Population Reference Bureau.
Pritchett, L.H.
  1994 Desired fertility and the impact of population policies. *Population and Development Review* 20(1):1-55.
Robey, B.K., S.O. Rutstein, and L. Morris
  1992 The reproductive revolution: New survey findings. *Population Reports* Series M, no. 11.
Rosenzweig, M., and K. Wolpin
  1993 Maternal expectations and ex post rationalizations. *Journal of Human Resources* 28(2):205-229.
Ross, J.A., and W.P. Mauldin
  1996 Family planning programs: Efforts and results, 1972-94. *Studies in Family Planning* 27(3):137-147.
Rutstein, S.O.
  1995 Do Family Planning Programs Decrease Fertility? Paper presented at annual meeting of the Population Association of America, San Francisco. Macro International, Inc., Calverton, Md.
Senanayake, P.
  1996 Emergency contraception: The International Planned Parenthood Federation's experience. *International Family Planning Perspectives* 22:69-70.

Sheon, A., W. Schellstede, and B. Derr
   1987   Contraceptive social marketing. Pp. 367-390 in R.J. Lapham and G.B. Simmons, eds., *Organizing for Effective Family Planning Programs*. Committee on Population, National Research Council. Washington, D.C.: National Academy Press.

Sherris, J.D., B. Ravenholt, and R. Blackburn
   1985   *Contraceptive Social Marketing: Lessons from Experience*. Population Reports, J-30. Baltimore, Md.: Johns Hopkins University.

Simmons, G.B., and R. Lapham
   1987   The determinants of family planning program effectiveness. Pp. 683-706 in R.J. Lapham and G.B. Simmons, eds., *Organizing for Effective Family Planning Programs*. Committee on Population, National Research Council. Washington, D.C.: National Academy Press.

Sinding, S., J. Ross, and A. Rosenfield
   1994   Seeking common ground: Unmet need and demographic goals. *International Family Planning Perspectives* 20(1):23-27.

Trottier, D.A., L.S. Potter, B. Taylor, and L.H. Glover
   1994   User characteristics and oral contraceptive compliance in Egypt. *Studies in Family Planning* 25(4):284-292.

Trussell, J., and C. Ellertson
   1995   The efficacy of emergency contraception. *Fertility Control Reviews* 4(2):8-11.

Trussell, J., C. Ellertson, and F. Stewart
   1996   The effectiveness of the Yuzpe regimen of emergency contraception. *Family Planning Perspectives* 28(2):58-87.

United Nations
   1994   *Programme of Action of the 1994 International Conference on Population and Development*. (A/CONF.171/13) Reprinted in *Population and Development Review* 21(1): 187-213 and 21(2):437-461.

Weller, R.H., D. Sly, A. Sukamdi, and R. Ekawati
   1991   The wantedness status of births in Indonesia. *Demographic and Health Surveys World Conference* 1:275-290. Calverton, Md.: Macro International, Inc.

Westley, S.B.
   1995   Evidence mounts for sex-selective abortion in Asia. *Asia-Pacific Population and Policy*, No. 34. Honolulu, Hawaii: East-West Population Center.

Westoff, C.F.
   1990   Reproductive intentions and fertility rates. *International Family Planning Perspectives* 16(3):84-89.

Westoff, C.F., and A. Bankole
   1995   *Unmet Need: 1990-1994*. DHS Comparative Studies No. 16. Calverton, Md.: Macro International, Inc.

Winikoff, B., C. Elias, and K. Beattie
   1994   Special issues of IUD use in resource-poor settings. Pp. 230-238 in C.W. Bardin and D.R. Mishell, Jr., eds., *Proceedings of the Fourth International Conference on IUDs*. New York: Population Council.

Working Group on the Health Consequences of Contraceptive Use and Controlled Fertility
   1989   *Contraception and Reproduction: Health Consequences for Women and Children in the Developing World*. Committee on Population, National Research Council. Washington, D.C.: National Academy Press.

World Health Organization
   1986   *Essential Obstetric Functions at First Referral Level*. Report of a Technical Working Group, 23-27 June. Geneva, Switzerland: World Health Organization.

1994   *Abortion: A Tabulation of Available Data on the Frequency and Mortality of Unsafe Abortion.* 2nd ed., WHO Division of Family Health. (Doc. WHO/FHE/MSM/93.13) Geneva, Switzerland: World Health Organization.

Zimicki, S.
1989   The relationship between maternal mortality and fertility. Pp. 1-47 in A.M. Parnell, ed., *Contraceptive Use and Controlled Fertility: Health Issues for Women and Children.* Committee on Population, National Research Council. Washington, D.C.: National Academy Press.

CHAPTER 5:
HEALTHY PREGNANCY AND CHILDBEARING

Achadi, E., K. Winnard, W.M. Brody, and M. Marshall
1994   Trip Report: Indonesia Assessment, September 19-October 5, 1994. Report prepared for U.S. Agency for International Development. MotherCare Project #5966-C-00-3038-00. John Snow, Inc., Arlington, Va.

Alisjahbana, A., C. Williams, R. Dharmayanti, D. Hermawan, B.E. Kwast, and M. Koblinsky
1995   An integrated village maternity service to improve referral patterns in a rural area in West Java. *International Journal of Gynecology and Obstetrics* 48(Suppl):s83-s94.

Ambaretnani, N.P., C. Hessler-Radelet, and L.E. Carlin
1993   *Qualitative Research for the Social Marketing Component of the Perinatal Regionalization Project, Tanjungsari, Java.* MotherCare Working Paper #19 prepared for the U.S. Agency for International Development. Project #936-5966. Arlington, Va.: John Snow, Inc.

Bailey, P.E., J.A. Szaszdi, and B. Schieber
1994   *Analysis of the Vital Events Reporting System of the Maternal and Neonatal Health Project: Quetzaltenango, Guatemala.* MotherCare Working Paper #3 prepared for the U.S. Agency for International Development. Project #DPE-5966-Z-00-8083-00. Arlington, Va.: John Snow, Inc.

Bailey, P.E., R.C. Dominik, B. Janowitz, and L. Araujo
1991   Obstetrica e Mortalidade Perinatal em uma Area Rural do Nordeste Brasileiro. *Boletin de la Oficina Sanitaria Panamericana* 111(4):306-318.

Bartlett, A.
1991   Inquisivi, Bolivia Technical Report #2. Report prepared for the U.S. Agency for International Development. MotherCare Project #936-5966. John Snow, Inc., Arlington, Va., and Institute of Nutrition of Central America and Panama, Johns Hopkins University.

Bhaskaram, C., and V. Reddy
1975   Cell-mediated immunity in iron and vitamin-deficient children. *British Medical Journal* 3:522.

Bhatt, R.V.
1989   Professional responsibility in maternity care: Role of medical audit. *International Journal of Gynecology and Obstetrics* 30:47-50.

Bothwell, T.H., and R. Charlton
1981   *Iron Deficiency in Women.* Washington, D.C.: International Nutrition Anemia Consultative Group.

Bower, B., and A. Perez
1993   Final Project Report: Cochabamba Reproductive Health Project. Report prepared for the U.S. Agency for International Development. MotherCare Project #5966-C-00-3038-00. John Snow, Inc., Arlington, Va.

Bruce, J.
  1990   Fundamental elements of the quality of care: A simple framework. *Studies in Family Planning* 21(2):61-91.
The Center for Health Research, Consultation and Education, and MotherCare/John Snow, Inc.
  1991   *Qualitative Research on Knowledge, Attitudes, and Practices Related to Women's Reproductive Health.* MotherCare Working Paper #9 prepared for the U.S. Agency for International Development. MotherCare Project #936-5966. Arlington, Va.: John Snow, Inc.
Chandramohan, D., F. Cutts, and P. Millard
  1995   The effects of stay in a maternity waiting home on perinatal mortality in rural Zimbabwe. *Journal of Tropical Medicine and Hygiene* 98:261-267.
Colgate-Goldman, S., C. Conroy, P. Daunas, and C. Godinez
  1994   Guatemala Assessment Report, July 18-August 4, 1994. Prepared for the U.S. Agency for International Development. MotherCare Project #5966-C-00-3038-00. John Snow, Inc., Arlington, Va.
Coria-Soto, I.L., J.L. Bobadilla, and F. Notzon
  1996   The effectiveness of antenatal care in preventing intrauterine growth retardation and low birth weight due to preterm delivery. *International Journal for Quality in Health Care* 8(1):13-20.
Dallman, P.R.
  1989   Changing characteristics of childhood anemia. *Journal of Pediatrics* 114:161-164.
  1993   Iron deficiency anemia: A synopsis of current scientific knowledge and U.S. recommendations for prevention and treatment. In R. Earl and C.E. Woteki, eds., *Iron Deficiency Anemia: Recommended Guidelines for the Prevention, Detection and Management Among U.S. Children and Women of Childbearing Age.* Committee on the Prevention, Detection, Management of Iron Deficiency Anemia Among U.S. Children and Women of Childbearing Age. Food and Nutrition Board, Institute of Medicine. Washington, D.C.: National Academy Press.
Danell, I., L. Grummer-Strawn, M. Caceres, and P. Stupp
  1994   *Maternal Mortality and Morbidity in El Salvador: FESAL-93.* Atlanta, Ga.: Centers for Disease Control and Prevention and National Center for Health Statistics.
Das, R.K.
  1971   Genital prolapse in pregnancy and labor. *International Surgery* 56(4):260-265.
De Graft-Johnson, J.
  1994   Maternal Morbidity in Ghana. Paper presented at the Annual Meeting of the Population Association of America, Miami, Fla., May 5-7. Carolina Population Center, University of North Carolina.
Eades, C., C. Brace, L. Osei, and K. LaGuardia
  1993   Traditional birth attendants and maternal mortality in Ghana. *Social Science and Medicine* 36(11):1503-1507.
The Eclampsia Trial Collaborative Group
  1995   Which anticonvulsant for women with eclampsia? Evidence from the collaborative eclampsia trial. *Lancet* 345:1455-1463.
Enwonu, C., ed.
  1990   *Functional Significance of Iron Deficiency.* Nashville, Tenn.: Meharry Medical College.
Family Health Services Project, MotherCare/John Snow, Inc., and the Johns Hopkins University/Population Communication Services
  1993   *Interpersonal Communication and Counseling Curriculum for Midwives.* MotherCare Project. John Snow, Inc., Arlington, Va.

Fauveau, V., M. Koenig, J. Chakraborty, and A. Chowdhury
  1988   Causes of maternal mortality in rural Bangladesh, 1976-1985. *Bulletin of the World Health Organization* 66(5):643-651.
Fauveau, V., B. Wojtyniak, G. Mostafa, A.M. Sarder, and J. Chakraborty
  1990   Perinatal mortality in Matlab, Bangladesh: A community-based study. *International Journal of Epidemiology* 19:606-612.
Fauveau, V., K. Stewart, S.A. Khan, and J. Chakraborty
  1991   Effect on mortality of community-based maternity-care programme in rural Bangladesh. *Lancet* 338:1183-1186.
Fauveau, V., M. Mamdani, R. Steinglass, and M. Koblinsky
  1993   Maternal tetanus: Magnitude, epidemiology and potential control measures. *International Journal of Gynecology and Obstetrics* 40:3-12.
Fortney, J.A.
  1995   Antenatal risk screening and scoring: A new look. *International Journal of Gynecology and Obstetrics* 2(suppl.):s53-s58.
Galloway, R., and J. McGuire
  1994   Determinants of compliance with iron supplementation: Supplies, side effects, or psychology? *Social Science and Medicine* 39(3):381-390.
Garn, S.M., S.A. Ridella, A.S. Petzold, and F. Falkner
  1981   Maternal hematologic levels and pregnancy outcomes. *Seminars in Perinatology* 5:55-62.
Golding, J., T. Shenton, and I. MacGillivray
  1988   Could oedema and proteinuria in pregnancy be used to screen for high risk? *Pediatric and Perinatal Epidemiology* 2:25-42.
Govindasamy, P., K. Stewart, S. Rutstein, J. Boerma, and A. Sommerfelt
  1993   *High-Risk Births and Maternity Care.* Demographic and Health Surveys Comparative Studies No. 8. Columbia, Md.: Macro International, Inc.
Hall, M.H., P.K. Chng, and I. MacGillivray
  1980   Is routine antenatal care worthwhile? *Lancet* 2:78-80.
Harrison, K.A.
  1985   Child-bearing, health and social priorities: A survey of 22,774 consecutive hospital births in Zaria, Northern Nigeria. *British Journal of Obstetrics and Gynecology* 5(suppl.):1-119.
Hessler-Radelet, C.
  1993   Lessons Learned about the Impact of the Regionalization of Perinatal Care Project. Field report prepared for MotherCare Project. John Snow, Inc., Arlington, Va.
Hetzel, B.
  1993   The control of iodine deficiency. *American Journal of Public Health* 33(4):494-495.
Hogberg, U., and S. Wall
  1986   Secular trends in maternal mortality in Sweden from 1750 to 1980. *Bulletin of the World Health Organization* 64(1):79-84.
Hogberg, U., S. Wall, and G. Brostroin
  1986   The impact of early medical technology on maternal mortality in the late 19th century Sweden. *International Journal of Gynecology and Obstetrics* 24:251-261.
Howard-Grabman, L., G. Seoane, and C.A. Davenport
  1994   *The Warmi Project: A Participatory Approach to Improve Maternal and Neonatal Health: An Implementor's Manual.* MotherCare Project. John Snow, Inc., Arlington, Va.
Hughes, A.
  1991   Anemia in Pregnancy. Background discussion paper of the meeting of the Technical Working Group on Prevention and Treatment of Severe Anemia in Pregnancy, Geneva, 20-22 May 1991. Maternal Health and Safe Motherhood, Division of Family Health, World Health Organization.

Janowitz, B., P.E. Bailey, R.C. Dominik, and L. Araujo
    1988   TBAs in rural northeast Brazil: Referral patterns and perinatal mortality. *Health Policy and Planning* 3(1):48-58.
Kitay, D., and R. Harbort
    1975   Iron and folic acid deficiency in pregnancy. *Clinical Perinatology* 2:255-273.
Koblinsky, M.A.
    1995   Beyond maternal mortality—magnitude, interrelationship, and consequences of women's health, pregnancy-related complications and nutritional status on pregnancy outcomes. *International Journal of Gynecology and Obstetrics* 48(suppl.):21-32.
Koblinsky, M.A., O. Campbell, and S. Harlow
    1993   Mother and more: A broader perspective on women's health. In M.A. Koblinsky, J. Timyan, and J. Gay, eds., *The Health of Women: A Global Perspective*. Boulder, Colo.: Westview Press.
Kramer, M.S.
    1987   Determinants of low birth weight: Methodological assessment and meta-analysis. *Bulletin of the World Health Organization* 65(5):663-737.
Kutzin, J.
    1993   Obstacles to women's access: Issues and options for more effective interventions to improve women's health. *Human Resources Development and Operations Policy*. Human Resources working paper no. 13. Washington, D.C.: World Bank.
Lawson, J.
    1992   Vaginal fistulae. *Journal of the Royal Society of Medicine* 85:254-256.
Leslie, J., and G.R. Gupta
    1989   *Utilization of Formal Services for Maternal Nutrition and Health Care in the Third World*. Paper prepared for the U.S. Agency for International Development. Project #DAN-1010-A-00-7061-00. Washington, D.C.: International Center for Research on Women.
Levin, H., E. Pollitt, R. Galloway, and J. McGuire
    1993   Micronutrient deficiency disorders. In D. Jamison, H. Mosley, A. Measham and J.L. Bobadilla, eds., *Disease Control Priorities in Developing Countries*. New York: Oxford University Press.
Loudon, I.
    1991   On maternal and infant mortality 1900-1960. *The Society for the Social History of Medicine* 4:29-73.
Macro International, Inc.
    1994   Selected statistics from DHS. *Demographic and Health Surveys Newsletter* (6)2.
Mahomed, K., and F. Hytten
    1989   Iron and folate supplementation in pregnancy. In T. Chalmers, M. Enkin, and M.J.N.C. Keirse, eds., *Effective Care in Pregnancy and Childbirth*. London: Oxford University Press.
Maine, D.
    1991   *Safe Motherhood Programs: Options and Issues*. Center for Population and Family Health, School of Public Health. New York: Columbia University.
Maine, D., M.Z. Akalin, J. Chakraborty, A. de Francisco, and M. Strong
    1996   Why did maternal mortality decline in Matlab? *Studies in Family Planning* 27:179-187.
Mantz, M.L., and P. Okong
    1994   *Evaluation Report: Uganda Life Saving Skills Program for Midwives, October-November, 1994*. Report prepared for the U.S. Agency for International Development. MotherCare Project #5966-C-00-3038-00. John Snow, Inc., Arlington, Va.

Marshall, M.A., and S.T. Buffington
  1991   *Life-Saving Skills Manual for Midwives.* 2nd ed. Washington, D.C.: American College of Nurse-Midwives.
Ministry of Health
  1994   *National Maternal Mortality Study: Egypt, 1992-1993.* Alexandria, Egypt: Ministry of Health, Child Survival Project.
Murphy, M.
  1981   Social consequences of vesico-vaginal fistula in northern Nigeria. *Journal of Biosocial Sciences* 13:139-150.
Murphy, J.F., J. O'Riordan, R.G. Newcombe, E.C. Coles, and J.F. Pearson
  1986   Relation of haemoglobin levels in first and second trimesters to outcome of pregnancy. *Lancet* 1:992-995.
Mustapha, A., and H. Rushwan
  1971   Acquired genito-urinary fistulae in the Sudan. *Journal of Obstetrics and Gynecology of the British Commonwealth* 78:1039-1043.
National Statistics Office [Philippines] and Macro International, Inc.
  1994   *Philippines National Safe Motherhood Survey 1993.* Calverton, Md.: National Statistics Office and Macro International, Inc.
Omran, A.R., and C.C. Standley, eds.
  1981   *Further Studies on Family Formation Patterns and Health: An international collaborative study in Colombia, Egypt, Pakistan, and the Syrian Arab Republic.* Geneva, Switzerland: World Health Organization.
O'Rourke, K.
  1995   The effect of hospital staff training on management of obstetrical patients referred by traditional birth attendants. *International Journal of Gynecology and Obstetrics* 48(Suppl.):s95-s102.
Otubu, J.A., and B.U. Ezem
  1982   Genital prolapse in the Hausa/Fulani of northern Nigeria. *East African Medical Journal* 59(9):605-609.
Payne, L., C. Hooks, and M. Marshall
  1993   Trip Report MotherCare Project Nigeria: Needs Assessment, December 4-18, 1994. Report prepared for the U.S. Agency for International Development. MotherCare Project #5966-C-00-3038-00. John Snow, Inc., Arlington, Va.
Pinotti, J.A., H.B. Brenelli, and J.D. Moragues
  1993   Preventive obstetrics and gynecological program: Pilot plan for integrated medical care. *Bulletin of Pan American Health Organization* 15(2):104-112.
Poedje, R., L. Setjalilakusuma, A. Abadi, B. Soegianto, S. Rihadi, A. Djaeli, and W. Budiarto
  1993   Final Project Report: East Java Safe Motherhood Study. Report prepared for the U.S. Agency for International Development. MotherCare Project #936-5966. John Snow, Inc., Arlington, Va.
Poovan, P., F. Kifle, and B. Kwast
  1990   A maternity waiting home reduces obstetric catastrophes. *World Health Forum* 11:440-445.
Prevention of Maternal Mortality Network (PMM)
  1995   Situational analyses of emergency obstetric care: Examples from eleven operations research projects in West Africa. *Social Science and Medicine* 40(Suppl.):657-667.
Public Opinion Polls
  1993   *MotherCare Nigeria Maternal Healthcare Project Qualitative Research.* MotherCare Working Paper #17B prepared for the U.S. Agency for International Development. Project #936-5966. Arlington, Va.: John Snow, Inc.

Rooney, C.
1992   *Antenatal Care and Maternal Health: How Effective is it? A Review of the Evidence.*
        WHO/MSM/92.4. Geneva, Switzerland: World Health Organization.
Rosenfield, A., and D. Maine
1985   Maternal mortality—A neglected tragedy: Where is the M in MCH? *Lancet*
        8446(2):83-85.
Schieber, B.
1993   *MotherCare—Guatemala: Final Report.* Prepared for the U.S. Agency for International Development. MotherCare Project #936-5966. John Snow, Inc., Arlington, Va.
Schieber, B.A., M. Mejia, S. Koritz, C. Gonsalez, and B. Kwast
1995   *Medical Audit of Early Neonatal Deaths: INCAP: Quetzaltenango Maternal and Neonatal Health Project.* Technical Working Paper #1 prepared for the U.S. Agency for International Development. MotherCare Project #936-5966. John Snow, Inc., Arlington, Va.
Seoane, G., and M. Castrillo
1995   Analysis Situacional de Cinco Districtos de Salud de La Paz y Cochabamba. Report prepared for the U.S. Agency for International Development. MotherCare Project #5966-C-00-3038-00. John Snow, Inc., Arlington, Va.
Shah, U., A.K. Pratinidhi, and P.V. Bhatlawande
1984a   Perinatal mortality in rural India: A strategy for reduction through primary care. I. Stillbirths. *Journal of Epidemiology and Community Health* 38:134-137.
1984b   Perinatal mortality in rural India: Intervention through primary health care. II. Neonatal mortality. *Journal of Epidemiology and Community Health* 38:138-142.
Sloan, N.L., E.A. Jordan, and B. Winikoff
1992   *Does Iron Supplementation Make a Difference?* MotherCare Working Paper #15 prepared for the U.S. Agency for International Development. MotherCare Project #936-5966. John Snow, Inc., Arlington, Va.
Sood, S.K., K. Ramachandran, M. Mathur, K. Gupta, V. Ramalingaswamy, C. Swarnabai, J. Ponniah, V.I. Mathan, and S.J. Baker
1975   WHO-sponsored collaborative studies on nutritional anemia in India. Part I: The effects of supplemental oral iron administration to pregnant women. *Quarterly Journal of Medicine* 174:241-258.
Srikantia, S.G., C. Bhaskaram, J.S. Prasad, and K. Krishnamachari
1976   Anemia and immune response. *Lancet* 1:1307-1309.
Stewart, M.K., and M. Festin
1995   Validation study of women's reporting and recall of major obstetric complications treated at the Philippine general hospital. *International Journal of Gynecology and Obstetrics* 48(Suppl.):s53-s66.
Stinnett, J.D.
1983   *Nutrition and the Immune Response.* Boca Raton, Fla.: CRC Press.
Stone, J.L., C.J. Lockwood, G. Berkowitz, M. Alvarez, R. Lapinski, and R. Berkowitz
1994   Risk factors for severe preeclampsia. *Obstetrics and Gynecology* 83:357-361.
Sundari, T.K
1992   The untold story: How the health care systems in developing countries contribute to maternal mortality. *International Journal of Health Service* 22(3):513-528.
Tahzib, F.
1983   Epidemiological determinants of vesicovaginal fistulae. *British Journal of Obstetric Gynaecology* 90:387-391.

Tahzib, F.
1985   Vesicovaginal fistula in Nigerian children. *Lancet* 2(8467):1291-1293.
Task Force on Validation of Women's Reporting of Obstetric Complications
1997   Statement on Validity of Self-Report Data (September 16-17). MotherCare Project, John Snow, Inc., Arlington, Va., and Demographic and Health Surveys, Macro International, Inc., Calverton, Md.
Thaddeus, S., and D. Maine
1994   Too far to walk: Maternal mortality in context. *Social Science and Medicine* 38(8):1091-1110.
United Nations
1991   *Controlling Iron Deficiency.* A report based on an Administrative Committee on Coordination/Subcommittee on Nutrition workshop, Nutrition State-of-the-Art Series, Nutrition Policy Discussion Paper No. 9. Geneva, Switzerland: United Nations.
1996   *World Population Prospects: The 1996 Revision.* Department for Economic and Social Information and Policy Analysis. New York: United Nations.
Villar, J., U. Farnot, F. Barros, C. Victora, A. Langer, and J. Belizan
1992   A randomized trial of psychosocial support during high-risk pregnancies. *New England Journal of Medicine* 327:1266-1271.
Villar, J., and P. Bergsjo
1996   Scientific Basis for the Content of Routine Antenatal Care: With Emphasis in Primary Care Settings. Unpublished manuscript, Institute of Nutrition of Central America and Panama, Guatemala City, Guatemala.
Wedderburn, M., and M. Moore
1990   *Qualitative Assessment of Attitudes Affecting Childbirth Choices of Jamaican Women.* Working Paper No. 5 prepared for the U.S. Agency for International Development. MotherCare Project #936-5966. MotherCare Project and Manoff Group. Arlington, Va.: John Snow, Inc.
Women's Global Network for Reproductive Rights
1991   Maternal mortality and morbidity: Obstetric fistula. *Newsletter* 37.
World Bank
1993   *World Development Report 1993: Investing In Health.* New York: Oxford University Press.
World Health Organization
1991   *Maternal Mortality: A Global Factbook.* Geneva, Switzerland: World Health Organization.
1993a   *Coverage of Maternity Care: A Tabulation of Available Information.* WHO/FHE/MSM/93.7. Geneva, Switzerland: World Health Organization.
1993b   Making Maternity Care More Accessible. Press Release No. 59. Geneva, Switzerland: World Health Organization.
1993c   The Global Burden of Disease. Background paper prepared for the *World Development Report*, Geneva, Switzerland.
1994a   *Maternal Health and Safe Motherhood Programme: Research Progress Report 1987-1992.* WHO/FHE/MSM94.18. Geneva, Switzerland: World Health Organization.
1994b   *The Mother-Baby Package: Implementing Safe Motherhood in Countries.* Document FRH/MSM/94.11. Geneva, Switzerland: World Health Organization.
1995   Essential or Emergency Obstetric Care. *Safe Motherhood Newsletter* 18(2):1-2.
1996   *Perinatal Mortality.* Document FRH/MSM/96.7. Geneva, Switzerland: World Health Organization.

World Health Organization and UNICEF

1996   *Revised Estimates of Maternal Mortality: A New Approach by WHO and UNICEF.* Geneva, Switzerland: World Health Organization.

Younis, N., H. Khattab, H. Zurayk, M., el-Mouelhy, M. Fadle Amin, and A.M. Farag

1993   A community study of gynecological and related morbidities in rural Egypt. *Studies in Family Planning* 24(3):175-186.

Younis, N., K. Khalil, H. Zurayk, and H. Khattab

1994   *Learning about the Gynecological Health of Women.* Policy Series in Reproductive Health, No. 2. Giza, Egypt: The Population Council.

Zurayk, H., N. Younis, and H. Khattab

1995   Rethinking family planning policy in light of reproductive health research. In C. Makhlouf Obermeyer, ed., *Family, Gender and Population in the Middle East: Policies in Context.* Cairo, Egypt: American University Cairo Press.

CHAPTER 6:
PROGRAM DESIGN AND IMPLEMENTATION

Bulatao, R.A.

1993   *Effective Family Planning Programs.* Washington, D.C.: World Bank.

Cates, W., Jr., and K. Stone

1992   Family planning: The responsibility to prevent both pregnancy and reproductive tract infections. Pp. 93-129 in A. Germain, K. Holmes, P. Piot, and J. Wasserheit, eds., *Reproductive Tract Infections: Global Impact and Priorities for Women's Reproductive Health.* New York: Plenum Press.

Cleland, J., and C. Wilson

1987   Demand theories of the fertility transition: An iconoclastic view. *Population Studies* 41:5-30.

Cleland, J., J.F. Phillips, S. Amin, and G.M. Kamal

1994   *Determinants of Reproductive Change in Bangladesh.* Washington, D.C.: World Bank.

Daley, D.

1994   Reproductive health and AIDS-related services for women: How well are they integrated? *Family Planning Perspectives* 26(6):264-269.

Fisher, A., R. Miller, I. Askew,, B. Mensch, A. Jain, and D. Huntington

1994   The Situation Analysis Approach to Assessing the Supply Side of Family Planning Programs. The Population Council, New York.

Germain, A., and R. Dixon-Mueller

1992   Stalking the elusive 'unmet need' for family planning. *Studies in Family Planning* 23(5):330-335.

Gish, O.

1992   Malaria eradication and the selective approach to health care: Some lessons from Ethiopia. *International Journal of Health Services* 22(1):179-192.

Grupo Interinstitucional de Salud Reproductiva

1995   *Programa de salud reproductiva y planificación familiar: 1995-2000.* Mexico City: Poder Ejecutivo Federal.

Haaga, J., and R. Maru

1996   The effect of operations research on program changes in Bangladesh. *Studies in Family Planning* 27(2):76-87.

Hardee, K., and K. Yount

1995   From Rhetoric to Reality: Delivering Reproductive Health Promises through Integrated Services. Working Paper. Family Health International, Research Triangle Park, N.C.

Heaver, R.
1995   Managing primary health care: Implications of the health transition. *World Bank Discussion Papers* No. 276. Washington, D.C.: World Bank.

Khattab, M.
1992   *The Silent Endurance: Social Conditions of Women's Reproductive Health in Rural Egypt.* Amman, Jordan and Cairo, Egypt: UNICEF Regional Office and The Population Council.

Liese, B.
1995   Intercountry comparative analysis of vertical and integrated programmes. Pp. 347-360 in H. Rashad, R. Gray and T. Boerma, eds., *Evaluation of the Impact of Health Interventions.* Liege, Belgium: Ordina Editions, International Union for the Scientific Study of Population.

Martínez Manatou, J.
1994   *Sucedió en México: Del nacimiento de la pildora a la reducción de la tasa de crecimiento poblacional.* Mexico City: Instituto Mexicano de Seguridad Social.

McGinn, T., D. Maine, J. McCarthy, and A. Rosenfield.
1996   *Setting Priorities in International Reproductive Health Programs: A Practical Framework.* New York: Center for Population and Family Health, Columbia University.

Measham, A.R., and R.A. Heaver
1996   *India's Family Welfare Program: Moving to a Reproductive and Child Health Approach.* Washington, D.C.: World Bank.

Mercenier, P., and M. Prevot
1983   Guidelines for a Research Protocol on Integration of a Tuberculosis Programme and Primary Health Care. WHO/TB/83.142. World Health Organization, Geneva, Switzerland.

Mosley, W.H.
1988   Is there a middle way? Categorical programs for primary health care. *Social Science and Medicine* 26(9):907-908.

Nowak, R.
1995   New push to reduce maternal mortality in poor countries. *Science* 269(August 11):780-782.

Pachauri, S.
1995   Defining a Reproductive Health Package for India: A Proposed Framework. South and East Asia working paper no. 4. The Population Council, Delhi, India.

Pathfinder International
1995   *Service Delivery Expansion Support (SDES) Baseline.* Working paper no. 1. Mexico City, D.F.: Pathfinder International.

Riquer Fernandez, M.F.
1995   *Aspectos Sociodemográficos de la Población Rural y Urbana.* Mexico City, D.F.: Consejo Nacional de Población.

Rosero-Bixby, L.
1986   Infant mortality in Costa Rica: Explaining the recent decline. *Studies in Family Planning* 17(2):57-65.

Simmons, G.B., and R.J. Lapham
1987   The determinants of family planning program effectiveness. Pp. 683-706 in R.J. Lapham and G.B. Simmons, eds., *Organizing for Effective Family Planning Programs.* Committee on Population, National Research Council. Washington, D.C.: National Academy Press.

Simmons, R., and J.F. Phillips
1987   The integration of family planning with health and development. Pp. 185-211 in Robert J. Lapham and George B. Simmons, eds. *Organizing for Effective Family Planning Programs* Washington, D.C.: National Academy Press.

Simmons, R., and J. Phillips
  1992   The proximate operational determinants of fertility regulation behavior. Pp. 181-
          201 in J. Phillips and J. Ross, eds., *Family Planning Programmes and Fertility*. Ox-
          ford, England: Clarendon Press.
Smith, D., and J. Bryant
  1988   Building the infrastructure for primary health care: An overview of vertical and
          integrated approaches. *Social Science and Medicine* 26(9):909-917.
Toubia, N.
  1995   *Doing More with Less: The Marie Stopes Clinics in Sierra Leone*. *Quality/Calidad/
          Qualité 7*. New York: The Population Council.
Townsend, J., and M.E. Khan
  1996   Indicators and a management information and evaluation system for a reproduc-
          tive and child health program. Pp. 72-82 in A.R. Measham and R.A. Heaver, eds.,
          *Supplement to India's Family Welfare Program: Moving to a Reproductive and Child
          Welfare Approach*. Washington, D.C.: World Bank.
UNICEF
  1995   Monitoring Progress Toward the Goals of the World Summit for Children: A
          Practical Handbook for Multiple-Indicator Surveys. United Nations Children's
          Fund, Programme Division, New York.
United Nations
  1994   *Report of the International Conference on Population and Development*. Document No.
          A/CONF.171/13. New York: United Nations.
U.S. Agency for International Development
  1996   Strategic Objective 4: Increased Utilization and Changed Behaviors Related to
          Reproductive/Maternal/Child Health in Selected Districts. U.S. Agency for In-
          ternational Development, Kampala, Uganda.
Wilkinson, M.I., W. Njogu, and N. Abderrahim
  1993   *The Availability of Family Planning and Maternal and Child Health Services*. Demo-
          graphic and Health Surveys Comparative Studies No. 7. Columbia, Md.: Macro
          International Inc.
World Bank
  1985   *World Development Report 1985: International Capital and Economic Development*.
          New York: Oxford University Press.
  1993   *World Development Report 1993: Investing in Health*. New York: Oxford University
          Press.
World Health Organization
  1994   *The Mother-Baby Package: Implementing Safe Motherhood in Countries*. Document
          FRH/MSM/94.11. Geneva, Switzerland: World Health Organization.
World Health Organization and UNICEF
  1996   *Revised Estimates of Maternal Mortality: A New Approach by WHO and UNICEF*.
          Geneva, Switzerland: World Health Organization.

CHAPTER 7:
COSTS, FINANCING, AND SETTING PRIORITIES

Booth, D., J. Milimo, G. Bond, et al.
  1995   *Coping with Cost Recover: A Study of the Social Impact and Responses to Cost Recovery
          in Basic Services (Health and Education) in Poor Communities in Zambia*. Task Force
          on Povery Reduction. Working paper no. 3. Stockholm, Sweden: Swedish Inter-
          national Development Agency.

Bulatao, R.
1993   *Effective Family Planning Programs.* Washington, D.C.: World Bank.
Curtis, S., and K. Neitzel.
1996   *Contraceptive Knowledge, Use, and Sources.* DHS comparative study no. 19. Calverton, Md.: Macro International.
Foreit, K.G., and R.E. Levine
1993   *Cost Recovery and User Fees in Family Planning.* Policy papers no. 5, OPTIONS Project. Washington, D.C.: The Futures Group.
Gomes, C.
1994   Strengthening the collaboration between private and public sector for family planning expansion: A case study of Brazil. Pp. 75-87 in Jay Satia, Carl Schonmeyr, and Sharifah Tahir, eds., *Managing a New Generation of Population Programmes for: Challenges of the Nineties.* Kuala Lumpur, Malaysia: International Council on Management of Population Programmes.
Grosh, M.
1994   *Administering Targeted Social Programs in Latin America: From Platitudes to Practice.* Washington, D.C.: World Bank.
Haaga, J., and A.O. Tsui, eds.
1995   *Resource Allocation for Family Planning in Developing Countries: Report of a Meeting.* Committee on Population, National Research Council. Washington, D.C.: National Academy Press.
Jamison, D.W., H. Mosley, A. Measham, and J.L. Bobadilla, eds.
1993   *Disease Control Priorities in Developing Countries.* New York: Oxford University Press.
Janowitz, B., and J. Bratt
1994   *Methods for Costing Family Planning Services.* Research Triangle Park, N.C.: United Nations Population Fund and Family Health International.
Janowitz, B., K. Jamil, J. Chowdhury, B. Rahman, and D. Hubacher
1996   *Productivity and Costs for Family Planning Service Delivery in Bangladesh: The Government Program.* Research Triangle Park, N.C.: Family Health International.
Kay, B., A. Germain, and M. Bangser
1991   The Bangladesh Women's Health Coalition. *Quality/Calidad/Qualité* 3. New York: Population Council.
Litvack, J.I., and C. Bodart
1993   User fees plus quality equals improved access to health care: Results of a field experiment in Cameroon. *Social Science and Medicine* 37(3):369-383.
Measham, A.R., and R. Heaver
1996   *India's Family Welfare Program: Moving to a Reproductive and Child Health Approach.* Washington, D.C.: World Bank.
Michaud, C., and C.J.L. Murray
1994   External assistance to the health sector in developing countries: A detailed analysis, 1972-1990. *Bulletin of the World Health Organization* 72(4):639-651.
Murray, C.
1996   Rethinking DALYs. Pp. 1-98 in Christopher J.L. Murray and Alan D. Lopez, eds. *The Global Burden of Disease.* Cambridge, Mass.: Harvard University Press.
Musgrove, P.
1996   Public and Private Roles in Health: Theory and Expenditure Patterns. Discussion paper. World Bank, Washington, D.C.
Prevention of Maternal Mortality Network (PMM)
1995   Situational analysis of emergency obstetric care: Examples from eleven operations research projects in West Africa. *Social Science and Medicine* 40(Suppl.):657-667.

Ross, J., W.P. Mauldin, and V. Miller
    1993   *Family Planning and Population: A Compendium of International Statistics.* New York: The Population Council.
Shaw, R.P., and C. Griffin
    1995   *Financing Health Care in Sub-Saharan Africa Through User Fees and Insurance.* Washington, D.C.: World Bank.
World Bank
    1992   *World Development Report 1992: Development and the Environment.* Washington, D.C.: World Bank.
    1993   *World Development Report 1993: Investing in Health.* Washington, D.C.: World Bank.

Appendices

APPENDIX

A

WHO Recommendations for Treatment of STD-Associated Syndromes

In 1991, the World Health Organization (WHO) (1991) published recommendations for the comprehensive management of patients with sexually transmitted diseases (STDs) within the broader context of control, prevention and care programmes for STD and human immunodeficiency virus (HIV) infection. A WHO Advisory Group Meeting on Sexually Transmitted Diseases Treatment subsequently reviewed and updated treatment recommendations in the light of recent developments (World Health Organization/UNAIDS, 1997). This appendix presents the revised recommendations for a syndromic approach to the management of patients with STD symptoms. It discusses the management of the most common clinical syndromes caused by sexually transmitted agents and provides flow charts (algorithms) for the management of each syndrome.

The use of appropriate standardized protocols is strongly recommended in order to ensure adequate treatment at all levels of health service. Such standardized treatment also facilitates the training and supervision of health providers, delays the development of antimicrobial resistance in sexually transmitted agents, such as *Neisseria gonorrhoeae* and *Haemophilus ducreyi*, and is an important factor in rational drug procurement.

For all these conditions (except vaginitis) the sexual partner(s) of patients should also be examined for STDs and promptly treated for the same condition(s) as the index case. Partner notification and management are considered in the full report of the WHO Advisory Group (World Health Organization/UNAIDS, 1997).

Note. The therapies for uncomplicated gonorrhea, syphilis, chancroid, and granuloma inguinale are all described in Section 3 (World Health Organization/UNAIDS, 1997).

URETHRAL DISCHARGE

Male patients complaining of urethral discharge and/or dysuria should be examined for evidence of discharge. If none is seen, the urethra should be gently massaged from the ventral part of the penis towards the meatus. If microscopy is available, a urethral specimen should be collected; a Gram-stained urethral smear showing more than 5 polymorphonuclear leukocytes per field (x1000) in areas of maximal cellular concentration is indicative of urethritis.

The major pathogens causing urethral discharge are *N. gonorrhoeae* and *C. trachomatis*. Unless a diagnosis of gonorrhoea can be definitively excluded by laboratory tests, the treatment of the patient with urethral discharge should provide adequate coverage of these two organisms.

Recommended Regimens (see Figures A-1 and A-2)

> therapy for uncomplicated gonorrhoea
> *plus either*
> doxycycline, 100mg orally, twice daily for 7 days
> *or*
> tetracycline, 500mg orally, 4 times daily for 7 days.

Alternative regimen when tetracyclines are contraindicated or not tolerated

> therapy for uncomplicated gonorrhoea
> *plus*
> erythromycin, 500mg orally, 4 times daily for 7 days.

Alterative regimen where single-dose therapy for gonorrhoea is not available

> trimethoprim (80mg) / sulfamethoxazole (400mg), 10 tablets orally, daily for 3 days
> *plus either*
> doxycycline, 100mg orally, twice daily for 7 days
> *or*
> tetracycline, 500mg orally, 4 times daily for 7 days.

Urethral discharge

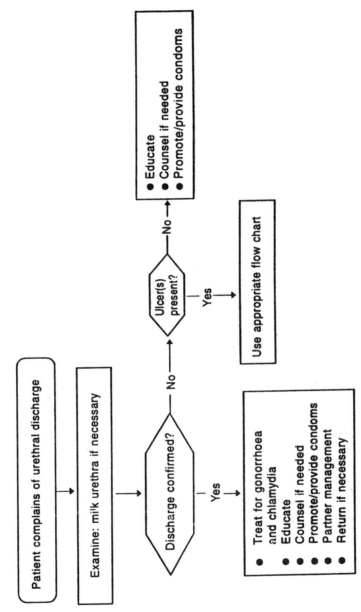

FIGURE A-1 Algorithm for the management of urethral discharge. SOURCE: World Health Organization/UNAIDS (1997).

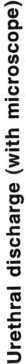
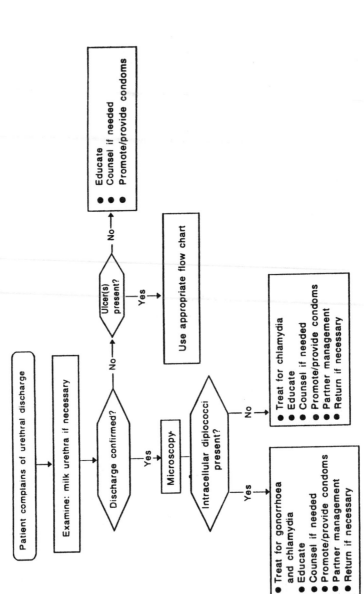

Urethral discharge (with microscope)

Patient complains of urethral discharge

↓

Examine: milk urethra if necessary

↓

Discharge confirmed?

— No → Ulcer(s) present?

Ulcer(s) present? — No →
- Educate
- Counsel if needed
- Promote/provide condoms

Ulcer(s) present? — Yes → Use appropriate flow chart

Discharge confirmed? — Yes → Microscopy

↓

Intracellular diplococci present?

— Yes →
- Treat for gonorrhoea and chlamydia
- Educate
- Counsel if needed
- Promote/provide condoms
- Partner management
- Return if necessary

— No →
- Treat for chlamydia
- Educate
- Counsel if needed
- Promote/provide condoms
- Partner management
- Return if necessary

FIGURE A-2 Algorithm for the management of urethral discharge (with microscope). SOURCE: World Health Organization/UNAIDS (1997).

Note. This regimen should only be used in areas where trimethoprim/sulfamethoxazole has been shown to be effective against uncomplicated gonorrhoea.

Follow-up

Patients should be advised to return if symptoms persist 7 days after start of therapy.

Persistent or recurrent symptoms may be due to poor compliance, reinfection, infection with a resistant strain of *N. gonorrhoeae* or infection with *T. vaginalis*. Where symptoms persist or recur after adequate treatment of the index patient and partner(s), both (or all) should be referred for laboratory investigation. The investigation should include a Gram stain to confirm the presence of urethritis and to look for *N. gonorrhoeae*. *T. vaginalis* may be identified by microscopic examination of a first-voided urine sample, although this test has a fairly low sensitivity in comparison with a culture. If the presence of *T. vaginalis* is confirmed, metronidazole, 2g, should be given as a single oral dose.

Note. Patients taking metronidazole should be cautioned to avoid alcohol.

GENITAL ULCERS

The frequency with which genital ulcers are caused by specific organisms varies dramatically in different parts of the world. Clinical differential diagnosis of genital ulcers is inaccurate, particularly in settings where several etiologies are common. Clinical manifestations may be further altered in the presence of HIV infection.

After examination to confirm the presence of genital ulceration, treatment appropriate to local etiologies and antibiotic sensitivity patterns should be given. For example, in areas where both syphilis and chancroid are prevalent, patients with genital ulcers should be treated for both conditions at the time of their initial presentation to ensure adequate therapy in case of loss to follow-up. In areas where granuloma inguinale is also prevalent, treatment for this condition should be included.

Laboratory-assisted differential diagnosis is rarely helpful at the initial visit, and mixed infections are common. For instance, in areas of high syphilis incidence, a reactive serological test may reflect a previous infection and give a misleading picture of the patient's present condition.

Recommended regimens (see Figure A-3)

> therapy for syphilis
> *plus either*
> therapy for chancroid
> *or*
> therapy for granuloma inguinale

Genital ulcer and HIV infection

In HIV-infected patients, prolonged courses of treatment may be necessary for chancroid. Moreover, where HIV infection is prevalent, an increasing proportion of cases of genital ulcers are likely to harbor herpes simplex virus. Herpetic ulcers may be atypical and persist for long periods in HIV-infected patients.

Follow-up

Patients with genital ulcers should be followed up weekly until the ulceration shows signs of healing.

INGUINAL BUBO

Inguinal bubo, an enlargement of the lymph nodes in the groin area, is rarely the sole manifestation of an STD and is usually found together with other genital ulcer diseases. Nonsexually transmitted local and systemic infections (e.g., infections of the lower limb) can also cause swelling of inguinal lymph nodes.

Recommended regimens (see Figure A-4)

> doxycycline, 100mg orally, twice daily for 14 days
> *or*
> tetracycline, 500mg orally, 4 times daily for 14 days.

Alternative regimen:

> erythromycin, 500mg orally, 4 times daily for 14 days
> *or*
> sulfadiazine, 1g orally, 4 times daily for 14 days.

Some cases may require longer treatment than the 14 days recommended above. Fluctuant lymph nodes should be aspirated through

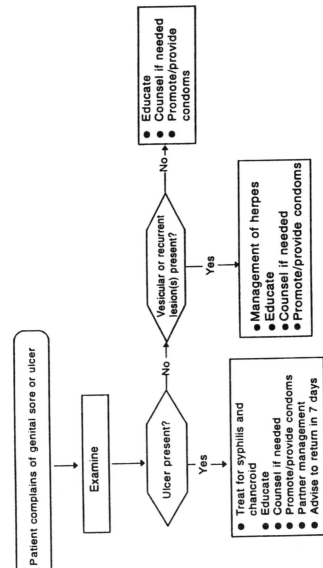

FIGURE A-3 Algorithm for the management of genital ulcers. SOURCE: World Health Organization/UNAIDS (1997).

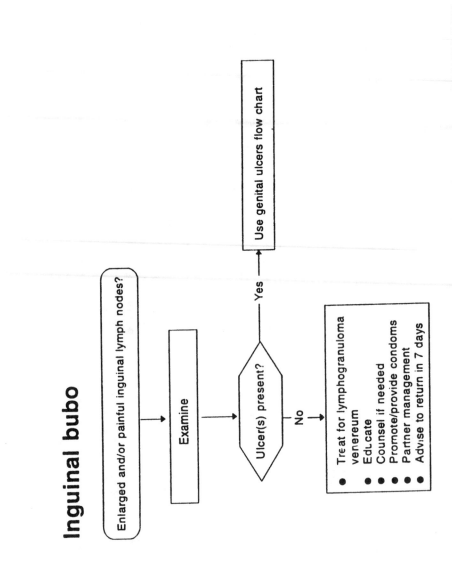

FIGURE A-4 Algorithm for the management of inguinal bubo. SOURCE: World Health Organization/UNAIDS (1997).

healthy skin. Incision and drainage or excision of nodes will delay healing and is contraindicated.

SCROTAL SWELLING

Scrotal swelling can be caused by trauma, a tumor, torsion of the testis or epididymitis. Inflammation of the epididymis is usually accompanied by pain, oedema and erythema and sometimes by urethral discharge, dysuria and/or frequency. The adjacent testis is often also inflamed (orchitis), producing epididymo-orchitis. Sudden onset of unilateral swollen scrotum may be due to trauma or testicular torsion and requires immediate referral. When not effectively treated, STD-related epididymitis may lead to infertility. The most important causative organisms are *N. gonorrhoeae* and *C. trachomatis*.

Recommended regimen (see Figure A-5)

> therapy for uncomplicated gonorrhoea
> *plus either*
> doxycycline, 100mg orally, twice daily for 7 days
> *or*
> tetracycline, 500mg orally, 4 times daily for 7 days.

Alternative regimen when tetracyclines are contraindicated or not tolerated

> therapy for uncomplicated gonorrhoea
> *plus*
> erythromycin, 500mg orally, 4 times daily for 7 days.

Alternative regimen where single-dose therapy for gonorrhoea is not available

> trimethoprim (80mg) / sulfamethoxazole (400mg), 10 tablets orally, once daily for 3 days
> *plus*
> doxycycline, 100mg orally, twice daily for 7 days
> *or*
> tetracycline, 500mg orally, 4 times daily for 7 days.

Note. This regimen should only be used in areas where trimethoprim/sulfamethoxazole has been shown to be effective against uncomplicated gonorrhoea.

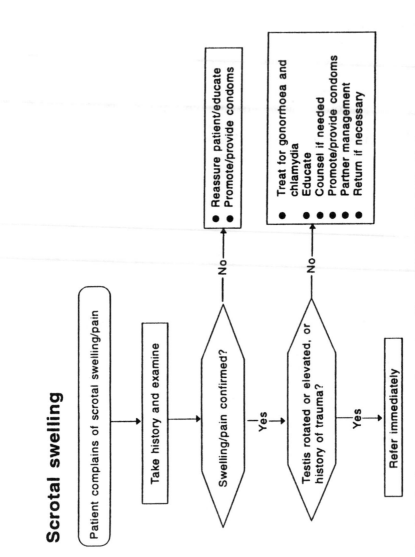

Scrotal swelling

Patient complains of scrotal swelling/pain

Take history and examine

Swelling/pain confirmed?

No → • Reassure patient/educate
    • Promote/provide condoms

Yes

Testis rotated or elevated, or history of trauma?

No → • Treat for gonorrhoea and chlamydia
    • Educate
    • Counsel if needed
    • Promote/provide condoms
    • Partner management
    • Return if necessary

Yes

Refer immediately

FIGURE A-5 Algorithm for the management of scrotal swelling. SOURCE: World Health Organization/UNAIDS (1997).

Adjuncts to therapy

Bed rest and scrotal elevation until local inflammation and fever subside.

VAGINAL DISCHARGE

Vaginal discharge is most commonly caused by vaginitis, but it may also be the result of cervicitis. *N. gonorrhoeae* and *C. trachomatis* infection cause cervicitis, and *Trichomonas vaginalis, Candida albicans* and a synergistic combination of *Gardnerella sp.* and anaerobic bacterial infection (bacterial vaginosis) cause vaginitis. Effective management of cervicitis is more important from a public health point of view, as cervicitis may have serious sequelae. However, clinical differentiation between the two conditions is difficult. The symptom of vaginal discharge is neither sensitive nor specific for either condition. Recent studies suggest that an assessment of the woman's risk status helps greatly in making a diagnosis of cervicitis, but further evaluation using the flow charts below is needed, particularly with regard to risk factors, which vary from country to country. Where it is not possible to differentiate between cervicitis and vaginitis, and risk assessment is positive, patients should be treated for both conditions.

Cervicitis

Recommended regimen (see Figures A-6, A-7, and A-8)

therapy for uncomplicated gonorrhoea
  plus either
doxycycline, 100mg orally, twice daily for 7 days
  or
tetracycline, 500mg orally, 4 times daily for 7 days.

Note. Tetracyclines are contraindicated in pregnancy.

Alterative regimen when tetracyclines are contraindicated or not tolerated

therapy for uncomplicated gonorrhoea
  plus
erythromycin, 500mg orally, 4 times daily for 7 days.

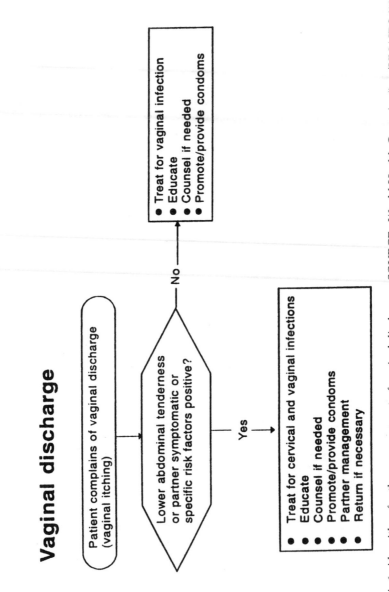

FIGURE A-6 Algorithm for the management of vaginal discharge. SOURCE: World Health Organization/UNAIDS (1997).

Vaginal discharge (with speculum)

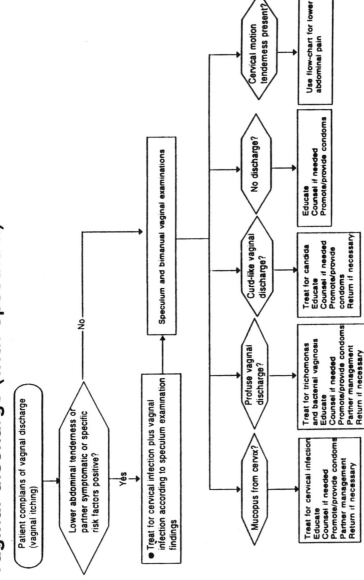

FIGURE A-7 Algorithm for the management of vaginal discharge (with speculum). SOURCE: World Health Organization/UNAIDS (1997).

248

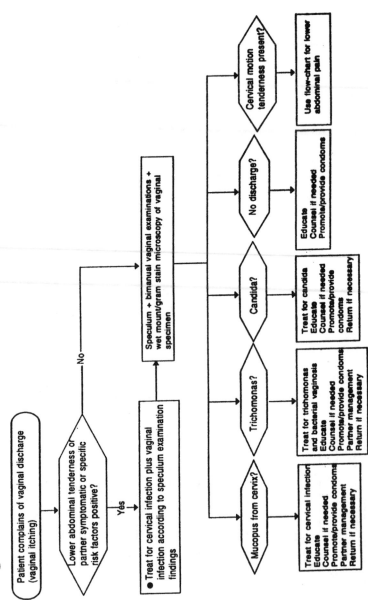

Vaginal discharge (with speculum and microscope)

Patient complains of vaginal discharge (vaginal itching)

Lower abdominal tenderness or partner symptomatic or specific risk factors positive?

Yes

- Treat for cervical infection plus vaginal infection according to speculum examination findings

No

Speculum + bimanual vaginal examinations + wet mount/gram stain microscopy of vaginal specimen

Mucopus from cervix?

Treat for cervical infection
Educate
Counsel if needed
Promote/provide condoms
Partner management
Return if necessary

Trichomonas?

Treat for trichomonas and bacterial vaginosis
Educate
Counsel if needed
Promote/provide condoms
Partner management
Return if necessary

Candida?

Treat for candida
Educate
Counsel if needed
Promote/provide condoms
Return if necessary

No discharge?

Educate
Counsel if needed
Promote/provide condoms

Cervical motion tenderness present?

Use flow-chart for lower abdominal pain

FIGURE A-8 Algorithm for the management of vaginal discharge (with speculum and microscope). SOURCE: World Health Organization/UNAIDS (1997).

Alterative regimen where single dose therapy for gonorrhoea is not available

> trimethoprim (80mg) / sulfamethoxazole (400mg), 10 tablets orally, once daily for 3 days
> *plus either*
> doxycycline, 100mg orally, twice daily for 7 days
> *or*
> tetracycline, 500mg orally, 4 times daily for 7 days.

Note. This regimen should only be used in areas where trimethoprim/sulfamethoxazole has been shown to be effective against uncomplicated gonorrhoea. Tetracyclines are contraindicated in pregnancy.

Vaginitis

Recommended regimen (see Figures A-6, A-7, and A-8)

> metronidazole, 2g orally as a single dose,
> *or*
> metronidazole, 400-500mg orally, twice daily for 7 days
> *plus either*
> nystatin, 100 000 IU intravaginally, once daily for 14 days
> *or*
> miconazole or clotrimazole, 200mg intravaginally, once daily for 3 days
> *or*
> clotrimazole, 500mg intravaginally, as a single dose.

Note. Patients taking metronidazole should be cautioned to avoid alcohol.

LOWER ABDOMINAL PAIN

All sexually active women presenting with lower abdominal pain should be carefully evaluated for the presence of salpingitis and/or endometritis—pelvic inflammatory disease (PID). In addition, routine bimanual and abdominal examinations should be carried out on all women with a presumptive STD since some women with PID or endometritis will not complain of lower abdominal pain. Women with endometritis may present with complaints of vaginal discharge and/or bleeding and/or uterine tenderness on pelvic examination. Symptoms suggestive of PID include abdominal pain, dyspareunia, vaginal discharge, menometrorrhagia, dysuria, pain associated with menses, fever, and sometimes nausea and vomiting.

PID is difficult to diagnose because clinical manifestations are varied. PID becomes highly probable when one or more of the above symptoms are seen in a woman with adnexal tenderness, evidence of lower genital tract infection, and cervical motion tenderness. Enlargement or induration of one or both fallopian tubes, tender pelvic mass, and direct or rebound tenderness may also be present. The patient's temperature may be elevated but is normal in many cases. In general, clinicians should err on the side of overdiagnosing and treating milder cases.

Hospitalization of patients with acute pelvic inflammatory disease should be seriously considered when: (a) the diagnosis is uncertain; (b) surgical emergencies such as appendicitis and ectopic pregnancy need to be excluded; (c) a pelvic abscess is suspected; (d) severe illness precludes management on an outpatient basis; (e) the patient is pregnant; (f) the patient is unable to follow or tolerate an outpatient regimen; (g) the patient has failed to respond to outpatient therapy; or (h) clinical follow-up 72 hours after the start of antibiotic treatment cannot be guaranteed. Many experts recommend that all patients with PID should be admitted to hospital for treatment.

Etiological agents include *N. gonorrhoeae, C. trachomatis,* anaerobic bacteria (*Bacteroides* spp. and Gram-positive cocci). Facultative Gram-negative rods and *Mycoplasma hominis* have also been implicated. As it is impossible to differentiate between these clinically, and a precise microbiological diagnosis is difficult, the treatment regimens must be effective against this broad range of pathogens. The regimens recommended below are based on this principle.

Inpatient Therapy

Recommended regimens (see Figure A-9)

1. ceftriaxone, 500mg by intramuscular injection, once daily
     plus
   doxycycline, 100 mg orally or by intravenous injection, twice daily, or tetracycline, 500mg orally 4 times daily
     plus
   metronidazole, 400-500mg orally or by intravenous injection, twice daily, or chloramphenicol, 500mg orally or by intravenous injection, 4 times daily.

2. clindamycin, 900mg by intravenous injection, every 8 hours
     plus

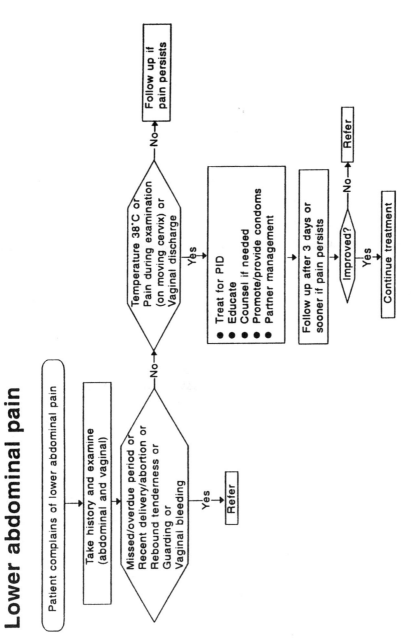

FIGURE A-9 Algorithm for the management of lower abdominal pain. SOURCE: World Health Organization/UNAIDS (1997).

gentamicin, 1.5 mg/kg by intravenous injection every 8 hours.

3. ciprofloxacin, 500mg orally, twice daily, or spectinomycin 1g by intramuscular injection, 4 times daily
     plus
    doxycycline, 100mg orally or by intravenous injection, twice daily, or tetracycline, 500mg orally, 4 times daily
     plus
    metronidazole 400-500mg orally or by intravenous injection, twice daily, or chloramphenicol, 500mg orally or by intravenous injection, 4 times daily.

Note. For all three regimens, therapy should be continued until at least 2 days after the patient has improved and should then be followed by either doxycycline, 100mg orally, twice daily for 14 days, or tetracycline, 500mg orally, 4 times daily, for 14 days. Patients taking metronidazole should be cautioned to avoid alcohol. Tetracyclines are contraindicated in pregnancy.

Outpatient Therapy

Recommended regimen

single-dose therapy for uncomplicated gonorrhoea (single-dose ceftriaxone has been shown to be effective; other single dose regimens have not been formally evaluated as treatments for PID)
 plus
doxycycline, 100mg orally twice daily, or tetracycline, 500mg orally, 4 times daily for 14 days
 plus
metronidazole, 400-500mg orally, twice daily for 14 days.

Note. Patients taking metronidazole should be cautioned to avoid alcohol. Tetracyclines are contraindicated in pregnancy.

Alternative regimen where single dose therapy for gonorrhoea is not available

trimethoprim (80mg) / sulfamethoxazole (400mg), 10 tablets orally once daily for 3 days, and then 2 tablets orally, twice daily for 10 days
 plus

doxycycline, 100mg orally, twice daily, or tetracycline, 500mg orally, 4 times daily for 14 days
  plus
metronidazole, 400-500mg orally, twice daily for 14 days.

Note. This regimen should only be used in areas where trimethoprim/sulfamethoxazole has been shown to be effective in the treatment of uncomplicated gonorrhoea. Patients taking metronidazole should be cautioned to avoid alcohol.

Adjuncts to therapy: removal of an intrauterine device (IUD)

The IUD is a risk factor for the development of PID. Although the exact effect of removing an IUD on the response of acute salpingitis to antimicrobial therapy and on the risk of recurrent salpingitis is unknown, removal of the IUD is recommended soon after antimicrobial therapy has been initiated. When an IUD is removed, contraceptive counselling is necessary.

Follow-up

Outpatients with PID should be followed up at 72 hours and admitted if their condition has not improved.

NEONATAL CONJUNCTIVITIS

Neonatal conjunctivitis (ophthalmia neonatorum) can lead to blindness when caused by *N. gonorrhoeae*. The most important sexually transmitted causes of ophthalmia neonatorum are *N. gonorrhoeae and C. trachomatis.* In developing countries, *N. gonorrhoeae* accounts for 20-75 percent and *C. trachomatis for* 15-35 percent of cases brought to medical attention. Other common causes are *Staphylococcus aureus, Streptococcus pneumoniae, Haemophilus spp. and Pseudomonas spp.* Newborn babies are generally presented because of redness and swelling of the eyelids or "sticky eyes," or because of discharge from the eye(s).

Recommended regimen (see Figures A-10 and A-11)

Neonatal conjunctivitis

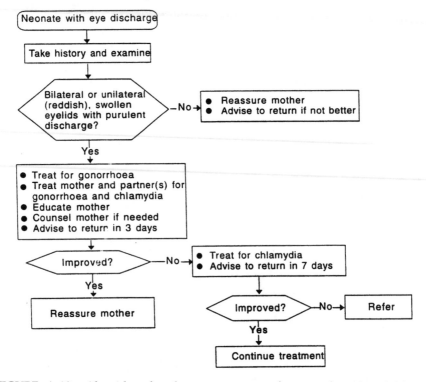

FIGURE A-10   Algorithm for the management of neonatal conjunctivitis.
SOURCE: World Health Organization/UNAIDS (1997).

Neonatal conjunctivitis (with microscope)

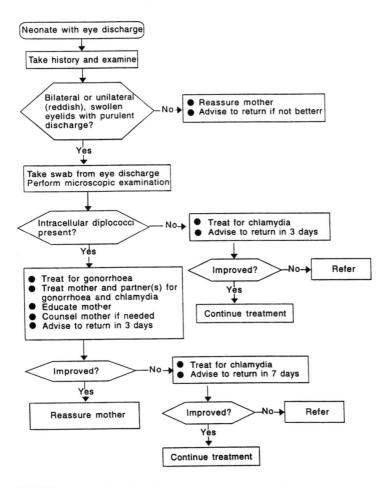

FIGURE A-11 Algorithm for the management of neonatal conjunctivitis (with microscope). SOURCE: World Health Organization/UNAIDS (1997).

REFERENCES

World Health Organization
   1991   *Management of patients with sexually transmitted diseases: Report of a WHO Study Group* WHO Technical Report Series, No. 810. Geneva, Switzerland: World Health Organization.
   1997   *Management of Sexually Transmitted Diseases*. World Health Organization, Joint United Nations Programme on HIV/AIDS Publication, Document GPA/TEM/ 94.1 Rev. 1., Sections 2.1-2.7:3-17. Geneva, Switzerland: World Health Organization.

APPENDIX

B

Examples of Programs to Promote Safe Pregnancy and Delivery

This appendix describes several projects that involve interventions at each step of the process of care for obstetric complications outlined in Chapter 5. We present these descriptions because they illustrate concretely some of the principles discussed in the chapter, because many of the reports are not widely available, and because the published literature still contains few evaluations of outcomes.

STEP 1: RECOGNITION OF THE PROBLEM

Can behaviors be changed by making families aware of the signs of complications and where to go in response to them? In one project, women's groups and community strategy meetings were organized in rural areas of Bolivia. Two other examples focus on information, education, and communication efforts in urban areas in Latin America where women are already more familiar with the available services.

Women's Groups in Inquisivi, Bolivia, 1989-1993

A population of 15,000 people, primarily of Aymara heritage, and living in a remote and difficult area, separated by high plains, high Andean valleys and subtropical valleys, is served by three health posts that lack basic equipment, supplies, and skills to manage obstetrical or newborn complications. The maternal mortality ratio (over 1,000 maternal deaths per 100,000 live births) and perinatal mortality ratios (103 perinatal deaths per 1,000 live births) reflect the isolation and poverty of these people (Howard-Grabman, Seoane, and Davenport, 1993). Women with complications would have to be referred to La Paz or Oruro, the two closest cities, which takes 4 to 6 hours over difficult roads. Traditional birth attendants do not exist, although traditional healers are sometimes consulted when complications arise. Husbands are the main providers of assistance in labor and delivery.

A simple model for community-level problem solving was implemented, consisting of four steps:

(1) identification and prioritization of maternal and neonatal health problems ("auto-diagnosis") by 50 women's groups;

(2) development of strategies and actions to solve the problems by the women's groups and members of their communities and local authorities;

(3) implementation of the groups' plans which involved: training 45 *parteras* (empirical midwives); educating both women and men in management of hemorrhage; providing family planning services in seven communities in collaboration with a local nongovernmental organization; developing and distributing a home-based women's health card, a manual for *parteras*, four booklets for women on reproductive health and five radio programs with a local nongovernmental organization;

(4) participatory evaluation.

Over one-half of women in the 52 communities participated in this process between 1991 and 1993. As they and their families became more involved, health practices and service utilization changed: tetanus toxoid immunization coverage, iron tablet distribution, immediate breastfeeding, consumption of iodized salt, prenatal and postnatal care visits, and the number of women attended by a trained birth attendant increased.

The intervention was evaluated using a pre- and postintervention treatment and comparison-area design, with data collected from a village-based information system. The most striking result was a reduction in the number of perinatal deaths, from 75 to 31 deaths over a 2-year period. This decrease was likely due to more immediate neonatal care. For each delivery, a person was designated to take responsibility for drying and warming the child before the placenta was delivered and placing the baby on the mother's breast within the first hour of life. (Previously, the newborn baby was set aside until after delivery of the placenta.) Use of modern contraceptives rose from 0 to 27 percent, reflecting that several of the groups had identified "too many children" as their main health concern (Howard-Grabman, Seoane, and Davenport, 1993).

Cochabamba Reproductive Health Project, Bolivia, 1990-1993

Just over one-half the population of Cochabamba, the third most populous department of Bolivia, is urban. Rapid growth of the urban population is due to the migration of Quechua and Aymara people from both rural parts of the department and the rest of the country. The maternal mortality ratio is very high (480 deaths/100,000), as are the infant mortality rates (126/1,000) and perinatal mortality rates (110/1,000) (Bower and Perez, 1993). The major causes of maternal mortality are complications of induced abortions and the poor conditions under which women have home births and even institutional deliveries.

Traditional health beliefs are dominant: only 13 percent of the urban population exclusively use the Western medical system. In 1991, only 34 percent of pregnant women ever received prenatal care during their pregnancies, and only 13 percent had four prenatal visits, the number stipulated by national norms.

Working with the local public health authority and several local nongovernmental organizations offering health services, the MotherCare program sought to increase demand for reproductive health services, improve the quality of those services and, consequently, contribute to an eventual decline in maternal and neonatal mortality in an area of approximately 500,000 people. A formative study of women's reproductive health knowledge, attitudes, and practices was conducted. The findings of the study were used to develop intervention strategies to improve home practices, increase the appropriate use of formal health services, and train health care providers to offer services more respectful of women's needs and wishes.

A health communication plan was initiated in three phases: (1) sensitization, aimed at creating awareness among policy makers and health providers of the problems of maternal and neonatal health and the differences in perspectives on health care between Quechua-Aymara peoples and the formal health system; (2) prenatal care, to create an awareness of the importance of routine and emergency prenatal care; and (3) safer/cleaner home delivery, promoting the use of sterile materials to cut and tie the umbilical cord, the recognition of and response to obstetrical complications, the avoidance of labor augmenters, and safe delivery of the placenta.

Each phase lasted 3 months and used educational video and radio programs covering the general theme, with television and radio spots for each major subtheme and one flip-chart per subtheme (with instructional guides) that was provided to families. Representatives of each participating agency attended workshops in health communications skills to institutionalize capability to develop and implement the various phases.

Training was conducted with providers to upgrade their skills and to adapt case management procedures to the needs of clients.

According to a household survey, in participating clinics prenatal care attendance rose by 17 percent to more than 100 percent, compared with a baseline period 2 years earlier, although there was no significant increase in the Cochabamba department as a whole (Bower and Perez, 1993). Women who could identify one of the danger signs increased from 26 percent to 43 percent. The percentage of women who could identify edema (traditionally thought to be a positive sign promising an easy birth) as a danger sign rose from 2 percent to 64 percent.

By various means (mass media, group participation, interpersonal communication), pregnant women were empowered to go to their prenatal care providers knowing specifically why they were there and what questions to ask about their own babies' health. This approach was developed in response to the need for information that many pregnant women complained about when interviewed in the qualitative and baseline studies. Women had pointed out that during prenatal care they did not receive all of the information that they wanted in order to leave confident that their pregnancy was progressing normally.

Psychosocial Support for High-Risk Pregnancies, 1989-1991

A highly structured home visit program in four Latin American cities—Rosario, Argentina; Pelotas, Brazil; Havana, Cuba; and Mexico City, Mexico—evaluated the effect of psychological and social support and health education for women at high risk for poor pregnancy outcomes (Villar et al., 1992). A total of 2,235 women at higher-than-average risk for poor pregnancy outcomes were recruited before their 20th week of pregnancy. All women planned to and did have an institutional delivery.

Through random assignment to an intervention or control group, women received either (1) four to six home visits from a nurse or social worker in addition to routine prenatal care or (2) only routine prenatal care (with a mean of eight prenatal visits). The main objective of the home visits was the strengthening of a pregnant woman's social network. Beginning with the first visit, a support person (husband or partner, mother, sister, friend, or neighbor) was selected by the patient to share all intervention activities. The support person was strongly encouraged to remain involved with the woman throughout the pregnancy, to participate in the decision-making process, to help the woman resolve personal problems, to promote healthful behavior, and to encourage attendance at visits for prenatal care. A second objective of the study was to provide health education during the home visits, including education on nutrition, reducing smoking, alcohol, or drug use, and complications during pregnancy, labor, and delivery; preparation for delivery and the postpartum experiences; and what to do in case of emergencies. A third objective was to reinforce adequate health services utilization for the pregnant woman and her support person. Complementing these activities were efforts to make the hospital more accessible to women—a hot-line to respond to questions, no appointment required for visits, and a guided tour of the obstetric facility to familiarize the client with labor, delivery, and emergency services.

The result of the program was virtually no change in behavior or outcomes. The women who received the home visits as well as routine prenatal care had outcomes that differed little from those of the women who received only routine care. The risks of low birth weight, preterm delivery, and intrauterine growth retardation were similar in the two groups (Villar et al., 1992). There was significant improvement in the knowledge of seven of nine danger signs considered and in two of three labor onset signs. But there was no evidence that the intervention had any significant effect on specific behaviors—the type of delivery, length of hospital stay, or use of health services. There was no protective effect of the psychosocial support program, even among the mothers at highest risk.

That improvements in knowledge did not translate into changes in health-related behaviors, such as improved use of health services, may have been due to the short duration of the intervention—3 months—and to continued barriers to access (Belizan et al., 1995). Women's behaviors during pregnancy and delivery may not be easy to change with short interventions.

STEP 2: MAKING THE DECISION TO SEEK CARE

The Perinatal Regionalization Project, Tanjungsari, West Java, Indonesia, 1989-1993

The Perinatal Regionalization Project aimed to develop a comprehensive maternal health program to improve maternal and perinatal health outcomes. Located in a rural subdistrict of West Java, Tanjungsari has a population of 90,000; it is served by three government health centers with midwives (one of which has delivery beds for normal births) and a district hospital 40 kilometers away in an adjacent subdistrict. Villages in this mountainous area are connected by roads, but some are impassable even for a four-wheel-drive ambulance regardless of season. While the health infrastructure is well utilized by women for prenatal care and children's health, traditional birth attendants are the primary providers during the intrapartum and postpartum periods.

The program consisted of three interventions:

- The first part was to train traditional birth attendants in the recognition and referral of maternal and newborn complications.
- The second part was to establish community birthing homes (*polindes*) at the village level in 10 of 27 villages in the intervention subdistrict. Each birthing home was to serve as the practice base for a community nurse-midwife and as residence for her if at all possible. (The Indonesian government has mandated the training of one midwife, a *bidan di desa*, to be available per village throughout the country.) Equipped with beds, scales, instruments and medical supplies, prenatal and delivery services for normal births were available in the *polindes*; on a monthly basis, child health, immunization, and family planning services were also provided. A two-way radio was installed in each of the ten *polindes*, the three health centers in the subdistrict and the district hospital. In case of a delivery, the traditional birth attendant and a community worker might manage the woman together at the birthing home unless a midwife was available or needed by the traditional birth attendant. The radios could be operated by the traditional birth attendants, community workers, or village headman and his wife to call for assistance from a doctor or midwife or for an ambulance.
- The third part was to train for maternal providers at all levels of the system, informal and formal. The traditional birth attendants had been previously trained, but their knowledge and skills were reinforced through practice with the midwives and monthly discussions at the health centers with doctors and midwives. Once maternal and perinatal death audits began, a physician visiting the families in the village would also discuss cases with the traditional birth attendants. Both the health center doctors and midwives had continuing education courses provided by consultants and senior midwives in the district hospital. The specialist obstetric staff of the nearby medical school collaborated with the consultant obstetrician and pediatrician of the district hospital in the formulation of management protocols for hospital, health center, and the midwives in the *polindes*.

Following the establishment of the birthing homes, an information, education, and communication strategy was implemented in the last 6 months of the project to improve the awareness and responsiveness of women, their husbands, community leaders, and traditional birth attendants concerning the purpose and use of the birthing huts (for routine care) and timely recognition of danger signs and referral. Parades, contests of knowledge among traditional birth attendants, and "open house" days at the *polindes*, where the ambulance and two-way radio services were demonstrated, brought messages directly into villages. Promotional leaflets for pregnant women, husbands, and traditional birth attendants addressed several issues:

- the importance of attending prenatal care, especially when feeling sick or experiencing one of the pictured conditions (bleeding, swollen face, feet, and hands, fever with chills, headache, and breech or transverse lie);
- where to get prenatal care;
- why to use a birthing hut for prenatal and delivery care; and
- when to take the first step to a place where a pregnant woman has decided to deliver.

The program was evaluated through interviews with all 2,275 women who had a singleton birth during the 15-month project period in 1992-1993 in the intervention area and all 1,000 new mothers in the control subdistrict of Cisalak where public services continued as usual.

Approximately 32 percent of women reported complications during the antepartum and intrapartum periods, while 29 percent suffered problems during the puerperium. The vast majority of deliveries in both the study and control areas were attended by traditional birth attendants (86 and 87 percent, respectively). The site of delivery was, however, different: in Tanjungsari, 85 percent delivered at home, compared with 96 percent in Cisalak. Much of this difference had to do with where women with complications sought care: in Tanjungsari, 31 percent (120 of 390 women) with delivery complications delivered in a health facility; in Cisalak, 11 percent did so.

How much of this use of health facilities for delivery because of complications was due to the recognition and referral of traditional birth attendants, the primary care providers? Unfortunately, the overall rate of intrapartum referral of women with complications during either the prenatal or intrapartum periods was low—13 percent in Tanjungsari and 6 percent in Cisalak. For those who suffered in the intrapartum period, 18 percent were referred in Tanjungsari and 9 percent in Cisalak. More women with "no complications" as perceived by themselves, or with only prenatal complications, were referred in Tanjungsari as well, possibly a precautionary measure made by traditional birth attendants trained in recognizing danger signs of complications.

Compliance with referral in these areas was relatively high, with the rate of compliance for intrapartum referral higher in Tanjungsari (87 percent) than in Cisalak (69 percent). Approximately 65 percent (98 cases) of complicated cases that were delivered in facilities in Tanjungsari had been recognized and referred by a traditional birth attendant, compared with only 14 complicated cases delivered in facilities in Cisalak. The traditional birth attendants' initial enthusiasm for making referrals dissipated over time. In focus groups, some of them expressed concern about undermining their status by referring cases to higher levels of care. They were afraid that women or other traditional birth attendants would say that they were unable to handle complications on their own. Several said they would refer only if they felt the family would comply.

How much did the program change the birthing pattern? The evaluation showed that women's knowledge of complications during pregnancy, labor, and delivery was higher in the intervention area than in the control area and that knowledge was more complete following the communications campaign. Use of birthing huts for prenatal care also increased following the campaign, from 9 to 26 percent (Hessler-Radelet, 1993). But use of delivery care proved more resistant to change. Focus group discussions and observations revealed that:

- Women did not care for take-home materials that depicted danger signs and complications, as they believed these illustrations would be prophetic.
- Women also felt that knowing about danger signs was important, but thought, if the danger sign (e.g., edema) didn't hurt or was a common occurrence during pregnancy and disappeared after delivery or didn't inhibit everyday chores, it could not be very dangerous.
- Traditional birth attendants felt uncomfortable referring more than the "usual" number of clients to a birthing hut; they felt it undermined their authority in the eyes of the community. However, the community generally respected their decisions in terms of referral for danger signs and complications (Winnard, 1993).

Indonesian women do not like to think about negative events or plan ahead for them. They believe that planning for a negative event will disrupt their sense of inner calm and may cause that negative event to occur. Cost, distance, and the desire to remain privately at home near family members are the reasons most cited by women for not accepting referral for a delivery place outside the home. Changing time-tried patterns of birthing will require more than 6 months of information and education, although use of prenatal services appears fairly easy to increase.

In villages in Tanjungsari with *polindes*, 19 percent of all pregnant women (and 37 percent of those with complications) delivered in health facilities, compared with 12 percent (and 26 percent of those with complications) in villages without them. Women do not appear to use the birthing huts for delivery; rather, the effect of the huts may have been to familiarize women with formal health sector personnel and to provide the means to better access other health facilities during labor and delivery (Kwast, 1995).

In summary, women with complications in Tanjungsari were more likely to be referred and to deliver in a health facility with a doctor than their counterparts in Cisalak, although most women in both sites, with or without complications, still delivered at home with a traditional birth attendant. Perinatal death rates were not significantly different between the two sites, though the numbers of births were small enough that this statistical test had very low power (99 perinatal deaths and 2,275 births in Tanjungsari; 37 perinatal deaths and 1,000 births in Cisalak). More women with intrapartum complications (especially prolonged labor) in Tanjungsari than in Cisalak gave birth in the hospital with a doctor. Yet deaths in the hospital actually increased, which suggests either that cases arrived too late for care or that the care was not adequate.

The Quetzaltenango Project, Guatemala, 1989-1993

In rural Guatemala, traditional birth attendants deliver 70-90 percent of infants. Obstetric skills are only available at hospitals at the department level, although prenatal and child care are available at health posts and centers. Midwifery training was abolished 20 years ago in Guatemala, so delivery care is primarily in the hands of traditional birth attendants.

In the intervention area of rural Quetzaltenango, the Institute of Nutrition of Central America and Panama (INCAP) trained government nursing staff to train over 400 traditional birth attendants in 3-day sessions in the recognition and timely referral of maternal and newborn complications, including bleeding, swelling of hands and face during pregnancy, malpresentation, prolonged labor, retained placenta, depressed newborn, postpartum bleeding, and maternal and neonatal infections. Working with doctors at the referral hospital and health personnel at health centers and posts, protocols for recognition and referral or management of complications were developed and implemented. A strong emphasis was placed on fostering good working relationships between the different levels of health care and improving humane treatment of both women and traditional birth attendants by health staff. Posters were also placed in all health facilities reminding health care providers that everyone in the community is trying to save the lives of women and their newborns on the difficult road from home to the formal health care facilities.

The outcome of this interaction was mixed. One year after the traditional birth attendant training, community-level behaviors had not

changed significantly. Through interviews with a sample of recently delivered women in target communities, levels of complications and use of
health services were determined retrospectively in both intervention and
control areas (total population 165,000) and before and after the interventions. Levels of complications were the same before and after the interventions, except for postpartum complications, which decreased from 6
percent to 2 percent. Approximately 20 percent of all women reported
they suffered complications during the prenatal, labor and delivery, and
puerperium, and one in ten newborns was said to have a complication.
Nearly one-half of the women with maternal complications used health
services even before the interventions, and this percentage did not significantly increase after the interventions (49 percent vs. 52 percent) (Bailey,
Szaszdi, and Schieber, 1994). Approximately one-fifth of the women with
complications who used health facilities did so after referral by traditional birth attendants. After the interventions, this proportion decreased
to 13 percent (Bailey, Szaszdi, and Schieber, 1994), but more women were
going to health facilities directly after the interventions. Traditional birth
attendants did not recognize complications (recognition declined from 81
percent to 68 percent), did not refer the women, or the woman stated she
did not accept her referral but went to a health facility anyway.

More than four out of five women saw a traditional birth attendant
for prenatal care, regardless of whether they experienced a complication.
Intrapartum and postpartum complications seemed to signal more danger to families: 52 percent and 65 percent of women with such complications, respectively, who used services did so directly without consulting a
traditional birth attendant. Fetal and newborn complications caused
women to go directly to health facilities (Bailey, Szaszdi, and Schieber,
1994).

The effect of the community-based interventions appears negligible
because traditional birth attendants were already referring a significant
proportion of complicated cases they saw before the interventions and
because women with complications were already going to health facilities
without consulting a traditional birth attendant. These data suggest an
independence on the part of the woman and her family in seeking out
services when they determine there is a complication.

Women in this study area are not that distant from the referral hospital; approximately 42 percent are within 60 minutes of the hospital. Roads
are relatively good, and transportation is available. Thus, the use of services for women with maternal complications appears to be fairly normal
behavior, although uncomplicated births at home with a traditional birth
attendant is the common procedure in Quetzaltenango.

The interventions had more effect at the hospital. Patient satisfaction
(measured as the percentage stating they would return) significantly in-

creased. Delays between admission and treatment decreased significantly. A medical audit revealed that the case management in hospitals of newborns had improved over the life of the project. Most women admitted with prolonged labor from home were subsequently managed correctly in the hospital. But late referral by a traditional birth attendant or late recognition and decision making by the family, and to a lesser extent lack of hospital supplies (lack of oxygen during one of the project years), continued to plague the project (Schieber et al., 1995). Perinatal mortality also decreased, though the difference was not statistically significant.

Program for Reduction of Maternal and Perinatal Deaths, Brazil, 1975-1984

A program in rural Northeast Brazil was intended to reduce maternal and perinatal deaths by ensuring prompt referral of complicated pregnancies and deliveries to a teaching hospital in the city of Fortaleza. Mini maternity units were set up throughout the region and traditional birth attendants were trained, some of whom were chosen to work in the units. The 40 units varied in size, resources, and services: the largest had 8-10 beds and could offer a wide variety of services, including prenatal, delivery, and postpartum care; the smallest consisted of a single room adjoining traditional birth attendants' homes where services were limited to normal delivery and postpartum care. Training of all traditional birth attendants consisted of five 1-hour meetings and practical experience at a maternity unit to ensure that each could provide prenatal care, identify problem pregnancies, and assist in normal deliveries and postpartum care for mother and newborn. They were taught to refer women who had a prenatal problem, especially eclampsia or hemorrhage; a complicated labor, including placenta previa or abruptio; a malpresentation and cases of cord or limb prolapse; and to consider for referral women under age 19 or over 35. The program included supervision and instruction by the teaching hospital staff as well as local hospital staff.

In one of the program counties, Trairi, which is far from Forteleza with difficult transportation and impassable roads in the rainy season, four mini maternity units were established and 78 traditional birth attendants trained for a population of 30,000. In 1984 (10 years after the program was begun), 64 percent of deliveries took place at home, primarily with a traditional birth attendant, and 36 percent in hospitals. Of the 10 percent of all women with singleton births who suffered complications in labor, 93 percent delivered in a hospital, with 49 percent referred by traditional birth attendants and 51 percent self-referred (Bailey et al., 1991). The traditional birth attendant referrals were more often linked with a complication: 52 percent of their referrals were diagnosed by hospital personnel as having a complication, but only 18 percent of the "walk-ins" actually had a medically diagnosed complication (Bailey et al., 1991). This may have been because women who themselves identified a complication were more likely to go to a traditional birth attendant, who then referred them to the hospital (Janowitz et al., 1988). That trained traditional birth attendants could distinguish severity of conditions and refer appropriately is indicated by the prenatal pathologies referred: 10 of 15 women with hemorrhage or hypertension were referred, while only 1 of 12 women with fatigue, nausea, dizziness or vomiting was sent to hospital (Janowitz et al., 1988).

Assistance at birth did not have a significant impact on infant survival in home deliveries. However, the odds of dying for a baby delivered by a traditional birth attendant with a high caseload (>29 births per year) were 0.6 that of a home birth not delivered by a traditional birth attendant. Although there was also no significant association between survival and attendant or place of delivery, perinatal mortality was lowest for deliveries at the mini maternity units with trained traditional birth attendants.

The authors concluded (Janowitz et al., 1988:56):

> Providing one-bed obstetric units for the busiest traditional birth attendants appears to be an intervention that can reduce mortality. The construction of additional units would further concentrate deliveries and make supervision easier than overseeing the work of 78 traditional birth attendants, some of whom attend only a few deliveries a year.

While supervision may be made easier, mini maternities still do not attract many deliveries: even 10 years after the initiation of the program, only 1 in every 10 women delivered in the mini maternities. Although not statistically significant, mortality among deliveries to women with complications of labor or malpresentations was higher for home than for hospital deliveries. The authors concluded that the mortality could have been lowered with earlier and more frequent referral of problem cases, an improved transportation system, and possibly an improvement in the local hospitals so that they did not have to send out referrals for cesarean section (a little over 1 percent of births were referred from a local hospital to the teaching hospital) (Janowitz et al., 1988).

Other Training Efforts

In contrast to the Fortaleza experience, the Danfa Project in Ghana found that traditional birth attendants were reluctant to refer women to hospitals. The Danfa Project area is located 30 kilometers north of Accra, a busy metropolis with 6 hospitals and 68 maternity homes. Yet 93 percent of deliveries in the project area were assisted by traditional birth attendants, even 15 years after the project began with an emphasis on recognition of complicated cases and referral. While the trained traditional birth attendants could appropriately identify what constitutes a "high-risk" case (e.g., primiparas; short, previous cesarean section; twins; malpresentation) and stated they would refer them, many reported routinely performing such deliveries themselves. The only major complication which most (74 percent) stated they would refer directly was eclampsia, while bleeding during pregnancy or in the postpartum period would be first treated with herbs in two-thirds of the cases (Eades et al., 1993).

Reasons for women's preference for the traditional birth attendant even when midwives and physicians are available include not only the cost, distance, and lack of supplies and equipment at the center or hospital, but also fear of anticipated treatment in the hands of medically trained staff. Traditional birth attendants reported that patients feared painful and disrespectful treatment from hospital personnel.

In an urban study in Benin, Sargent (1985) found that clients and traditional birth attendants share similar beliefs, values, and ideas about the cause of illness; hence, even in a city, assisted deliveries were more the norm than the exception. The traditional birth attendants' duties included traditional healing activities, which patients found valuable. The perceived sociocultural similarity may explain many women's preference for a traditional birth attendant even when modern facilities are accessible.

STEP 3: REACHING CARE OF ADEQUATE QUALITY

Maternal mortality fell in Sweden in the eighteenth and nineteenth centuries, unlike in other European countries, apparently because of home visits by certified midwives (Hogberg and Wall, 1986). There have also been promising results of prenatal screening of demonstrated risk factors and identification of danger signs by joint efforts of midwives with traditional birth attendants at the health center or community levels in Ethiopia and Nigeria (Brennan, 1992; Poovan, Kifle, and Kwast, 1990). Several attempts have been made to bring services closer to women through midwifery outreach or to bring women closer to services through maternity waiting home located close to hospitals.

The Matlab Project, Bangladesh, 1987-1989

In Matlab, a rural subdistrict of Bangladesh, an effective community-based maternal and child health and family planning project was introduced in late 1977. The key service providers are the female village health workers. They offer a choice of contraceptive methods at the home of each woman, motivate and counsel mothers for family planning, monitor and manage adverse effects, administer vaccines, promote oral rehydration, distribute vitamin A capsules, provide nutritional education, detect and refer malnourished children, and distribute safe delivery kits and iron tablets to pregnant women. They refer severely sick mothers or children to one of four decentralized outposts staffed by female paramedics or to the central Matlab clinic where at least one female physician is always available.

In 1985, when the 10-year effects of this project were reviewed, the maternal mortality rate in the comparison area was roughly twice that of the treatment area (121 versus 66 per 100,000 women). However, differences in the maternal mortality ratio, which measures only the obstetric risk, were not substantial, remaining around 550 per 100,000 live births (Koenig et al., 1988). This result suggests that the most important reason for the difference in maternal mortality rates between treatment and comparison areas was the intensive family planning program. By 1985, the contraceptive prevalence rate in the Matlab treatment area had reached approximately 44 percent, while the level in the comparison area was close to the national average of 17 percent (Fauveau, 1991).

A community-based maternity care project with referral links and transportation to a local and district hospital was added to the Matlab Project in part of the treatment area in 1987. One trained nurse midwife was posted at each of the two health centers in the study area. Their duties were to attend as many home deliveries as possible and to complement activities of traditional birth attendants, manage obstetric complications at their onset, and accompany patients requiring referral for higher level care to the project's central maternity clinic. The community health and family planning workers identified pregnant women for the midwives, linked them for prenatal visits, and notified the midwives when labor began. The intervention also included arrangements for emergency transportation to the maternity center in simple "ambulances" (country boats dedicated to the project). A female physician was available 24 hours a day at the Matlab Maternity Center. This hospital was equipped to provide vacuum extractions and dilation and curettage and to manage pre-eclampsia and eclampsia, but cases requiring blood transfusion or surgery were referred and transported to the district hospital an hour away (Maine et al., 1996).

Outcomes were measured by comparing maternal mortality ratios in the maternity care intervention area and the rest of the treatment area (that is, both areas benefitted from the intensive home visit program started in 1977). During the 3 years prior to the maternity care intervention (1984-1986), there was no significant difference between the two areas in maternal mortality rates or ratios. During the 3 years after the expanded project was implemented (1987-1989), the maternal mortality ratio in the intervention area had fallen by 68 percent (which was statistically significant). The causes of death that were reduced by the program were, in order of importance, the complications of abortion, postpartum hemorrhage, postpartum sepsis, and eclampsia. Other causes of adult female mortality were constant over the project period. Although abortion was not a specific focus of the project, a decrease in abortion-related mortality may have been due to provision of early abortions by manual vacuum aspiration ("menstrual regulation," which is legal in Bangladesh) or early intervention in cases of abortion complications (Fauveau et al., 1991; Fauveau, 1991; Maine et al., 1996).

A common problem in evaluations of complex interventions is isolating the "active ingredients." The Matlab maternity care project included the posting of trained midwives to clinics. It also included using well-established family planning and health workers in the community, an ambulance service, a maternal and child health hospital staffed by physicians at all times, a district hospital capable of providing the range of obstetric services discussed in Chapter 5, and good referral links among all the providers. Its apparent success holds promise for the mixed strategy of community- and hospital-based efforts we have recommended, but a great deal of further work is required to determine how to adapt this model in other settings (Maine et al., 1996).

Indonesian *Bidan di Desa* Program

The government of Indonesia began training and posting certified midwives (*bidan di desas*) in each of the country's 64,000 villages in 1989. The *bidan di desas* have multiple functions: provision of health services for the community in the home including handling deliveries, family planning and screening for clinical contraception, provision of assistance to the traditional birth attendants, and detection of complications and referral. Following technical training, a 1-week orientation may be given at provincial level for the *bidan di desa* followed by a 1-4 month orientation at her assigned health center. The problems in large-scale implementation of this program have become apparent in its first 5 years.

One study found that the *bidan di desas* are often filling in on administrative tasks for understaffed health facilities. In addition, many of them expressed reluctance to be assigned to remote areas (Radyowiyati and Sequeira, no date). General acceptance of this new cadre into the fabric of village life remains an obstacle, especially for *bidans* who are not from the areas where they are posted. A successful posting also depends on the enthusiasm and receptiveness of village leaders, of both the men and their wives. Yet often there is little communication with villagers about the new health worker's role. Not surprisingly, there has been competition between *bidan di desas* and traditional birth attendants, who currently attend most deliveries in homes. The new *bidans* are finding it difficult to attract business: they are typically younger and less experienced than are traditional birth attendants; they charge higher fees; and the traditional birth attendants perform many additional valued services that the *bidans* do not, such as massage and participation in ceremonies and rituals (Radyowiyati and Sequeira, no date).

In a study with direct observation of 58 *bidan di desas*, they were found to spend most of their time providing care to children under 5 and first aid for adults in Central Java and prenatal care in South Sulawesi; very little of their time was spent attending births. They often had only a blood pressure gauge, stethoscope, and a room with a bed for examinations; only a few had any medications or injection sets needed for stabilizing or managing obstetric emergencies (Achadi et al., 1994). Some stated they did not feel competent to deal with complications of delivery or other emergencies, but their ability to treat minor health problems has opened doors to acceptance by the communities.

Many adjustments to the *bidan di desa* program are presently being planned, including changes in the initial technical training to incorporate a focus on how to approach communities and possible continuing education to increase skills in managing common diseases such as diarrhea and acute respiratory infections, as well as education to enhance midwifery skills and a rotation for training at an assigned health center or hospital to maintain skills.

Maternity Waiting Homes

Maternity waiting homes are designed to overcome the difficulties of emergency transportation over long distances by women experiencing life-threatening emergencies in labor, by bringing women within reach of a hospital before labor begins. A recent report from Attat in rural Ethiopia shows that, with community consultation and participation, women at high risk will come to stay in a suitable waiting home near the hospital in the last month of pregnancy (Poovan, Kifle, and Kwast, 1990). Of the 151 women who used the home in its first year, 111 were at high risk because of previous cesarian sections or poor obstetric histories, including ruptured uterus and other emergencies: over one-third came from more than 40 kilometers away. Hence, appropriate use was being made of the waiting home.

Another study of more than 5,600 women who delivered singleton full-term infants in a rural district hospital in rural Zimbabwe compared women who used a maternity waiting home with women who were referred by a traditional birth attendant from home (control 1) or from home or clinic directly (control 2). Women with obstetric risks (such as no births or more than six previous poor outcomes) made up 56 percent of the total study population. Among these women, the perinatal mortality rate of the maternity home group was nearly 50 percent lower than that of control group 1 and even lower compared with group 2 control. However, for all women who stayed at the home, the perinatal mortality rate was not significantly reduced (Chandramohan, 1992).

Financing Maternity Care

Fees for services may be a barrier to using services, especially for the poor. But fees can be manipulated to stimulate desired behaviors among both providers and clients. In Zimbabwe, for example, pregnant women are charged a flat fee for prenatal care, plus a regular delivery and in-patient per diem fee for an in-patient delivery. Kutzin (1993) reports that following intensification of these fee collections, one district hospital had an increase in the numbers of women arriving having just delivered. Staff assumed this was because mothers were waiting until the last minute in order to avoid additional bed fees. Yet in another municipal hospital in Zimbabwe, fees were "bundled" so that a woman paid a flat fee for prenatal care, delivery, emergency transport, if needed, and postnatal care. This scheme encourages women to seek prenatal care, to come to the maternity center when labor begins, and to follow up with postpartum checkups. The bundling of services for one fee is an incentive for women to use services appropriately and not to delay seeking care (Kutzin, 1993).

STEP 4: IMPROVING QUALITY OF CARE

Refresher training for medical providers, developing and implementing protocols for management of obstetric and neonatal care, and the institution of maternal and perinatal death audits within facilities have been the three primary interventions to improve the quality of maternity and newborn care.

Training Midwives in Life-Saving Skills, Africa

Between 1988 and 1994, midwives were given advanced obstetric training to upgrade skills needed in managing complications through a competency-based curriculum for midwives developed by the American College of Nurse Midwives in several sites in Ghana, Uganda, and Nigeria. The course consisted of 10 modules, covering essential care for obstetric complications (defined in Chapter 5), plus risk assessment during prenatal care and resuscitation. Typically, training lasts 3 weeks at a high-volume maternity hospital.

In Uganda, both trainees and tutors showed improvement in knowledge immediately after training. A longer term evaluation in 1994 (3 to 12 or more months posttraining) tested a 14 percent sample of midwives purposely selected to be representative of the sites and types of organizations that had participated in the training (Mantz and Okong, 1994). A skills tests on the use of the partograph showed continued understanding of its use by 75 percent of midwives. Fewer midwives passed a test of their ability to use a gestational wheel and the "Handbook for Midwives" as resources in determining how to manage an obstetric emergency. Inspection of facilities where the trained midwives worked revealed that the handbooks were scarce, even though they had been issued to the midwives during their training to provide them with up-to-date information on case management. A record review of partograph use in 36 facilities showed that midwives in most facilities carried out appropriate activities according to partograph guidelines more than 50 percent of the time. There was no real difference in midwives' activities whether they had been trained 3 or 12 or more months prior to the review.

Facilities where the trained midwives worked supported their work with the necessary equipment in 29 of 38 inventoried, but in only 7 was the revised handbook available, and in 7 there was no access to water (including one 100-bed hospital). Frequently, pressure gauges were unavailable or not functioning, and records were often lacking or locked up for safe-keeping. Trained midwives faced a number of other barriers as well, including lack of time to carry out tasks appropriately, especially in the prenatal clinics or labor and delivery wards when there were high numbers of patients and only one or two midwives on the ward (there is a chronic lack of staff); lack of support from the institutional authority to allow them to carry out tasks for which they are trained (e.g., start intravenous fluids, examine the cervix, or take any other active management measures); transferrals to new sites with staffs that were not oriented to the training; and chronic financial constraints that made it impossible for districts to provide continuing education and supervision.

A Nigerian facility that served as a site for similar training recorded nearly a doubling in the number of deliveries by the midwives during the year following the training, apparently due to the improved image and perceived quality of care.

Implementing Standards of Care and Protocols, Quetzaltenango, Guatemala, 1989-1993

The Western General Hospital San Juan de Dios in Quetzaltenango, Guatemala, is a general hospital with an obstetric department that delivers approximately 3,000 newborns per year. Prior to the start of the maternal and neonatal health project described above, the sanitary conditions in the sick baby nursery were poor, overcrowding of incubators was a problem, adequate temperature control was difficult to maintain, resuscitation facilities were suboptimal, and equipment, including oxygen, was in short supply.

In 1990 a neonatologist joined the hospital staff, and protocols and standards of care were developed for normal and abnormal obstetric and neonatal conditions by a specialist team of obstetrician-gynecologists and neonatologists. Training of hospital staff to use these norms took place in March 1991. Simultaneously, changes were made in the temperature control in the nursery with portable heaters, and cot nursing, guidelines for clothing sick neonates, infection control, and handwashing surveillance were initiated.

To evaluate the effect of these changes, a medical audit of case management through record review was carried out retrospectively in 1993 (Schieber et al., 1995). A random sample of cases was drawn from the early neonatal deaths for 1 year before implementation of the interventions and 2 years after. Avoidable factors were categorized as patient or home circumstances; referral by traditional birth attendant or others; service factors due to management by obstetric, pediatric, or nursing staff; or lack of equipment, facilities, and medications.

The hospital neonatal mortality rate decreased from 38.3 in 1989 to 25.9 in 1991, but it increased to 31.9 in 1992. This same pattern was seen in early neonatal mortality—a significant decrease from 32.9 per 1,000 live births in 1989 to 23.6 in 1991, and then an increase to 26.0 in 1992. The arrival of a neonatalogist and revision of standards of both obstetric and neonatal care by 1991 apparently had an effect. The rise in the mortality rates in 1992, however, may have been associated with the shortage of oxygen experienced in that year as determined by the medical audit. Most of the change was due to reductions in mortality due to sepsis and among low birth weight babies: 50 percent of deaths were within the first 24 hours of life throughout the study period, mainly due to asphyxia and hyaline membrane disease, which is associated with prematurity. In spite of intensive training in resuscitation, the low Apgar scores at births (0-3) changed only somewhat at 5 minutes. That the majority of these babies were at-term points to the need for urgent improvement of labor management both in communities (to ensure women go to appropriate facilities earlier) and in hospitals. But between 1989 and 1991, there was a remarkable drop in avoidable factors assigned to staff as contributors to early neonatal deaths, emphasizing the improvement in the pediatric staff in responding to newborn problems (Schieber et al., 1995).

Instituting the Medical Audit of Maternal and Perinatal Death

Institution of medical audits of maternal and perinatal deaths within facilities may be a powerful intervention to improve the quality of services. One report from India shows a decrease in errors in judgment or delays in treatment at the department level and an increase in the number of high-risk and emergency cases attended by consultant obstetricians, with consequent decreases in maternal deaths from eclampsia and from the development of obstructed labor after admission, 10 years after institution of the medical audit within one facility (Bhat, 1989). Records were designed to document clinical management of all deliveries, confidential records of all maternal deaths were created for review by a committee, and weekly rounds reviewed all emergency cases, maternal and perinatal deaths, operative deliveries, and complicated pregnancies. Since this was a referral hospital, a team of a consultant, a resident, and a technician began visiting the surrounding primary health care centers periodically to provide prenatal care and communicate the outcome of referred cases.

Prior to the institution of the medical audit, a review of maternal deaths revealed that consultants did not always attend the cases that resulted in death and that residents failed to diagnose early enough such problems as malpresentation and concealed accidental hemorrhage and did not always call a consultant at the time of surgery. There was also delay in performing cesarean sections. At times when staffing was inadequate, such as at night and on weekends or holidays, there were more maternal deaths.

REFERENCES

Achadi, A., E. Achadi, A. Kusdinar, D. Dachlan, A. Watief, B. Boer, Zahro, and H. Setwiawan
   1994   Village Midwife (Bidan Di Desa) in Central Java and South Sulewesi. A collaboration between Center for Child Survival, University of Indonesia, and Directorate of Family Welfare, Ministry of Health, Republic of Indonesia, Jakarta, Indonesia.
Bailey, P.E., R.C. Dominik, B. Janowitz, L. Araujo
   1991   Obstetrica e mortalidade perinatal em uma area rural do nordeste Brasileiro. *Boletin de la Oficina Sanitaria Panamericana* 111(4):306-318.

Bailey, P.E., J.A. Szaszdi, and B. Shieber
  1994   *Analysis of the Vital Events Reporting System of the Maternal and Neonatal Health Project: Quetzaltenango, Guatemala.* Paper #3 prepared for the U.S. Agency for International Development. MotherCare Project #DPE-5966-Z-00-8083-00. Arlington, Va.: John Snow, Inc.
Belizan, J.M., F. Barros, A. Langer, U. Farnot, C. Victora, and J. Villar
  1995   Impact of women education during pregnancy on behavior and utilization of health resources. *American Journal of Obstetrics and Gynecology* 173:894-899.
Bhatt, R.V.
  1989   Professional responsibility in maternity care: Role of medical audit. *International Journal of Gynecology and Obstetrics* 30:47-50.
Bower, B., and A. Perez
  1993   *Final Project Report: Cochabamba Reproductive Health Project.* Report prepared for the U.S. Agency for International Development. MotherCare, Arlington, Va.: John Snow, Inc.
Brennan, M.
  1992   Training traditional birth attendants. *Postgraduate Doctor Africa* 11(1):16.
Chandromohan, D.
  1992   Effectiveness of Maternity Waiting Homes in Reducing Adverse Perinatal Outcomes: Experience from Rural Zimbabwe. Unpublished master's dissertation. London School of Hygiene and Tropical Medicine, England.
Eades, C., C. Brace, L. Osei, and K. LaGuardia
  1993   Traditional birth attendants and maternal mortality in Ghana. *Social Science & Medicine* 36(11):1503-1507.
Fauveau, V.
  1991   Matlab Maternity Care Program. Review paper prepared for the Department of Population and Human Resources, World Bank, Washington, D.C.
Fauveau, V., K. Stewart, S.A. Kahn, and J. Chakroborty
  1991   Effect on mortality of a community-based programme in rural Bangladesh. *Lancet* 338:1183-1186.
Hessler-Radelet, C.
  1993   Lessons Learned About the Impact of the Regionalization of Perinatal Care Project. Field report prepared for the U.S. Agency for International Development. MotherCare Project #936-5966. John Snow Inc., Arlington, Va.
Hogberg, U., and S. Wall
  1986   Secular trends in maternal mortality in Sweden from 1750 to 1980. *Bulletin of the World Health Organization* 64(1):79-84.
Howard-Grabman, L., G. Seoane, and C.A. Davenport
  1993   *The Warmi Project: A Participatory Approach to Improve Maternal and Neonatal Health: An Implementor's Manual.* MotherCare Project. Arlington, Va.: John Snow, Inc.
Janowitz, B., P.E. Bailey, R.C. Dominik, and L. Araujo
  1988   TBAs in rural northeast Brazil: Referral patterns and perinatal mortality. *Health Policy and Planning* 3(1):48-58.
Koenig, M.A., V. Fauveau, A.I. Chowdhury, J. Chakraborty, and M.A. Khan
  1988   Maternal mortality in Matlab, Bangladesh: 1976-1985. *Studies in Family Planning* 19(2):69-80.
Kutzin, J.
  1993   Obstacles to women's access: Issues and options for more effective interventions to improve women's health. *Human Resources Development and Operations Policy.* Human Resources working paper no. 13. Washington, D.C.: World Bank.

Kwast, B.E.
1995   Building a community-based maternity program. *International Journal of Gynecology and Obstetrics* 48(Suppl.):s67-s82.

Maine, D., M.Z. Akalin, J. Chakraborty, A. de Francisco, and M. Strong
1996   Why did maternal mortality decline in Matlab? *Studies in Family Planning* 27:179-187.

Mantz, M.L., and P. Okong
1994   *Evaluation Report: Uganda Life Saving Skills Program for Midwives, October-November, 1994*. Report prepared for the U.S. Agency for International Development. MotherCare Project #5966-C-00-3038-00. Arlington, Va. : John Snow, Inc.

Poovan, P., F. Kifle, and B. Kwast
1990   A maternity waiting home reduces obstetric catastrophes. *World Health Forum* 11:440-445.

Radyowiyati, A., and T. Sequeira
no date *Bidan Desa: A Case Study of Two Javanese Villages in Yogyakarta*. Center for Women's Studies and Department of Health, Gadjah Mada University, Indonesia

Sargent, C.
1985   Obstetrical choices among urban women in Benin. *Social Science and Medicine* 20:287-292.

Schieber, B.A., M. Mejia, S. Koritz C. Gonsalez, and B. Kwast
1995   *Medical Audit of Early Neonatal Deaths: INCAP: Quetzaltenango Maternal and Neonatal Health Project*. Technical Working Paper #1 prepared for the U.S. Agency for International Development. MotherCare Project #936-5966. Arlington, Va.: John Snow, Inc.

Villar, J., U. Farnot, F. Barros, C. Victora, A. Langer, and J.M. Belizan
1992   A randomized trial of psychosocial support during high-risk pregnancies. *New England Journal of Medicine* 327:1266-1271.

Winnard, K.
1993   *Applying Social Marketing to Maternal Health Projects: The MotherCare Experience*. MotherCare Project, The Manoff Group. Arlington, Va.: John Snow, Inc.

APPENDIX
C

Estimating the Cost of Interventions: The Mother-Baby Package

The task of marshalling support for reproductive health care investments in reproductive health care is complicated by the resource constraints that face most developing country governments. Ideally, decisions about the mix and scale of reproductive health programs (like other public investments) should be guided by an enlightened form of cost-effectiveness analysis, with the costs being defined broadly so as to encompass all social costs, and effectiveness likewise defined broadly to include the dimensions of health, survival, and protection against unintended pregnancy. In practice, decisions have to be made with a great deal of uncertainty. As we have shown in the chapters of this report, there are large gaps in knowledge about the effects and costs of interventions and compelling reasons for thinking that results in different settings will vary widely.

In Chapter 7 we discuss results of an attempt by the World Bank to produce a set of cost-effectiveness comparisons for a broad range of health sector programs using a consistent set of estimates (World Bank, 1993). These estimates are useful, in our view, for highlighting areas where there are large differences between alternative forms of investment, rather than for detailed comparisons of narrowly defined interventions or for precise estimates of costs for a particular country. We called for further research on costs of interventions in different settings. In this appendix we illustrate one way in which the results of such research could be used in cost models for planning and budgeting in reproductive health. This exercise also illustrates important limitations of the approach, given the data currently available or likely to be available in the near future.

The cost model discussed below was developed for one set of reproductive health interventions, known collectively as the Mother-Baby Package. The costs considered here are only public-sector costs—for example, there is no cost estimate for patient travel time—and even these estimates are subject to considerable uncertainty and would vary among settings. Nevertheless, we believe that it is useful to show how costs may be affected by elements of program design and scale.

As noted throughout the report, interventions vary considerably in the degree to which their effectiveness in developing countries is known. All the interventions included in the package have at least passed a minimal test of plausibility, that is, they have been judged by experts convened by the participating agencies to reduce a substantial amount of maternal/neonatal deaths or disability. In other words, the interventions embedded in the package make good sense, to judge from the clinical record, but that record has not yet furnished the numerical estimates needed for precise ranking.[1]

The data available do support an examination of the public-sector costs associated with the package's interventions and activities and enable us to determine the likely sensitivity of the cost estimates to changes in key assumptions. We believe that such calculations are informative and suggest promising directions for future research.

Throughout, we present hypothetical cost estimates that are built upon a series of assumptions. Apart from the published international prices of various drugs and supplies, there are few numbers that are based on empirical data. This exercise is not unlike a population projection in spirit. It is, in the end, no more than an extrapolation of assumptions. Its value lies in highlighting those assumptions that appear to be most critical and that therefore merit closest scrutiny.

THE MOTHER-BABY PACKAGE: OVERVIEW

The elements of the intervention package, described by the World Health Organization (1994), do not span the full range of reproductive health discussed in Chapters 2-5. Rather, they are focused on the events

---

[1]Some global effectiveness estimates for maternal mortality and neonatal mortality (percentage of deaths averted) are presented in the World Health Organization (1994:Table 1, Table 5). The major compilation of effectiveness studies (Chalmers, Enkin and Keirse, 1989), contains an assessment of a number of the interventions considered in the Mother-Baby Package.

and complications that surround pregnancy, delivery, and the postpartum period.

This focus on one segment of the reproductive lifespan, and the treatment of mother and child as a unit, have been proposed by the World Health Organization (1994:Table 3; also p. 11). The rationale is essentially that many complications of pregnancy and delivery for the mother are paired with complications that affect the child, at least in the case of neonates (see Chapter 5; see also Alisjahbana et al. [1995:Table 8]). For example, hemorrhage may bring on shock and cardiac failure for the mother, and this in turn may bring about asphyxia and stillbirth for the child. Some reproductive tract infections may induce premature onset of labor, and may also cause neonatal eye infections, pneumonia and the like.

In terms of service provision during pregnancy and labor, the package assigns the leading role to midwives. The World Health Organization (1994:18) describes the role of the midwife in this way:

> The person best equipped to provide community-based, appropriate technology and cost-effective care to women during their reproductive lives is the person with midwifery skills who lives in the community alongside the women she treats. Midwives understand women's concerns and preoccupations. They accompany women through their reproductive lifespan, providing assistance at birth, then during adolescence, pregnancy and delivery, and providing family planning services when needed. Most interventions related to care of the mother and newborn are within the capacity of a person with midwifery skills.

Trained midwives are linked to other health personnel, and these personnel to each other, by a system of referral. Midwives and other first-stage health care providers diagnose the type of complication a woman is experiencing and gauge its severity. Depending on severity, they then direct her to the appropriate facility, which is either a health post, a health center, or a district hospital. The package as a whole is envisioned as a set of interventions to be undertaken within health districts, administrative units with average populations of 500,000.[2]

Care for neonates, in this package, consists of the following (World Health Organization, 1994:x):

> All health workers (including TBAs), wherever they perform deliveries, will be trained to provide basic newborn care. They will assure clean

---

[2]The World Health Organization (1994:12-13) provides the following rationale for the district focus: "The district has proved to be an effective unit for planning and implementation of public health programmes such as immunization, which scheduled services right down to village level and indicated the logistics and personnel support needed."

delivery, clean cord care and prevent ophthalmia neonatorum, ensure that the room in which the delivery takes place is warm, prevent hypothermia by immediately drying the baby and putting it in skin-to-skin contact with the mother, and initiate and support early and exclusive breast-feeding. Health workers will be trained to identify asphyxiated babies by assessing their breathing and heart rates and to resuscitate them by using appropriate equipment. Mothers and family members will be taught to care for their newborns at home (e.g., keep them dry and warm, protect them from cold and excessive heat, breast-feed them exclusively). For low birth weight babies, mothers will be taught the need for more frequent breast-feeding and the importance of keeping the baby warm. They will learn how to recognize newborn illnesses and where to seek help. Control of diarrhoeal diseases and of acute respiratory infections are important complementary strategies to reduce neonatal mortality.

Further discussion is provided in WHO (1994:51-56) on asphyxia, hypothermia, and ophthalmia neonatorum.

The other major form of intervention envisioned in the package is the delivery of family planning information and services on a postpartum basis and condom use for protection against AIDS and other STDs. Safe abortion services are not included in the package, although the treatment of abortion complications is considered. Postpartum family planning counseling includes support for breastfeeding (World Health Organization, 1994:57-59).

In sum, the heart of the Mother-Baby Package is a set of services including prenatal care, delivery care performed in most cases by trained midwives, treatment of complications for the woman or child or both, and the delivery of postpartum information on contraception and family planning services for the women who want them.

THE MOTHER-BABY COST MODEL

The public-sector costs associated with the Mother-Baby Package interventions have been estimated by Cowley and Bobadilla (1995), with further revisions by Cowley and Gamponia.[3] All costs are expressed in 1992 U.S. dollars. Estimates of the costs of vaccines; disposables; supplies; information, education, and communication campaigns; refrigeration; transport; and some salaries were drawn from the Indian Child Survival and Safe Motherhood Project (Nirupam, 1993). Data on drug costs

---

[3] Cowley and Gamponia created a Excel program, using linked spreadsheets, to calculate the costs of the intervention package. Their assumptions and data have been incorporated, with some modifications, in a Fortran program for the analyses reported here.

were provided by Management Sciences for Health (Management Sciences for Health, 1992; Rankin, Sallet, and Frye., 1993). Capital costs are based on estimates by Herz and Measham (1987) and Tinker and Koblinsky (1993).

Health Posts, Centers, and Hospitals

As noted above, the Mother-Baby Package links trained midwives directly or through referral to three levels of the district health care system: health posts, health centers, and district hospitals. (In some country settings, three levels of health service delivery might not be feasible.) The clinical staffing of these facilities is set out in Table C-1.

A health post is typically staffed by a midwife who has been trained in aseptic delivery practices, as well as basic antenatal and postnatal care, and a nurse auxiliary. In the baseline costs model, the post is assumed to be capable of seeing as many as 10 patients per day. Although the staff of the health post are meant to attend all deliveries in its catchment area, the deliveries are assumed to take place in the patients' homes or in the homes of their midwives.

A health center is staffed by a registered nurse as well as a midwife and nurse auxiliary, and has access to a pharmacist, with a doctor available during daytime hours. Some centers are assigned to be equipped with a laboratory that can do selected tests and staffed by a part-time technician. The center can treat as many as 18 patients per day. Among women who go to a center, most of their deliveries take place in the center.

A district hospital is staffed by full-time nurses and primary care doctors with specialists available on an as-needed or part-time basis. The hospital is equipped with X-ray and other equipment, most of the usual laboratories, has some microbiological capabilities, and employs a full-time lab technician.[4] It has 29 beds devoted to maternity care. Among women who go to the hospital, all deliveries are assumed to take place in the hospital.

As discussed above, the baseline model allows some members of the clinical staff, and all other personnel, to be available to address other health needs not included in the package. The assumption of the baseline model is that, apart from certain clinical personnel whose time is assumed to be fully devoted to the package (midwives, obstetricians, and nurse-

---

[4]The World Health Organization (1994:83-86,93-96) offers succinct descriptions of posts, centers and hospitals; a list of essential drugs and equipment is presented on pages 97-106.

TABLE C-1 Assumptions Regarding Clinical Staffing in Rural and Urban Baseline Models of Mother-Baby Package

Clinical Staff	Health Post	Health Center	Hospital
Nurse Auxiliary	1[a]	2[a]	6[a]
Pharmacist		1	1
Midwife	1[a]	2[a]	2[a]
General Physician		1	1
Obstetrician			1[a]
Lab Technician		0.25	1
Education Specialist			1
Registered Nurse		1	5
Nurse Anesthesiologist Respiratory Therapist			1
X-ray Technician			1
Pediatrician			1
Total	2	7.25	21

NOTE: The percentages assumed to be devoted to the package vary by type of facility: for health posts, 75 percent of time is devoted to the Mother-Baby Package; for centers, 50 percent, and for hospitals, 30 percent (see also Table C-4). In the case of health posts, all clinical personnel are fully devoted to the *Package*, but support personnel and other facility-level resources are not.

[a]Staff are fully devoted to the package.

auxiliaries), some 25 percent of health post staff time and other resources are available for other uses, as much as 50 percent of health center time and resources, and 70 percent of hospital staff time and resources.[5]

Diagnosis and Referral

Figure C-1 shows the system of diagnosis and referral that is envisioned in the Mother-Baby Package cost model. In this model, diagnosis and referral is dependent on a set of assumptions regarding probabilities of complications; these are presented in Table C-2 by type of condition.

The baseline model assures that most pregnant women contact a trained midwife who is linked to the local health post. Some women will go to the nearest health center as walk-in patients for prenatal care and delivery, and, likewise, a few will go directly to the district hospital. At

---

[5]The baseline model examined here departs from the Cowley-Gamponia model in assuming that the clinical personnel just mentioned are devoted full-time to the package activities; see Table C-1.

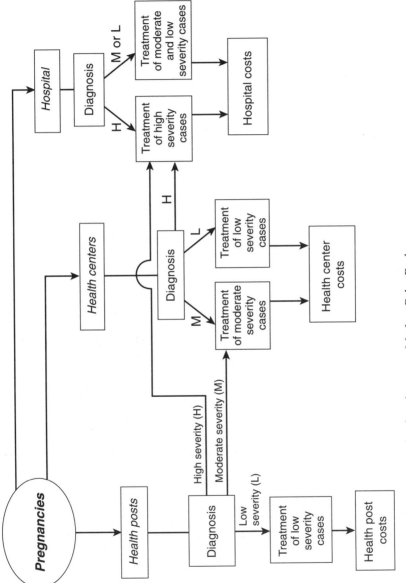

FIGURE C-1 Diagnosis and referral system; Mother-Baby Package.

TABLE C-2 Assumptions Regarding Conditions, Severity, and Referral
in the Rural Baseline Model: in percent

| Type of Condition | Pregnancies with the Condition | Of those with condition, severity level | | | |
| | | Low | Moderate | High | |
				No Surgery	Surgery
Abortion complications	2	90	0	7.5	2.5
Anemia	30	50	30	20	0
Reproductive tract infection	2	50	30	20	0
Eclampsia or hypertensive disorder	5	20	50	22.5	7.5
Hemorrhage	10	20	50	22.5	7.5
Obstructed labor	5	20	50	22.5	7.5
Sepsis	8	20	50	30	0

NOTE: Low severity cases are treatable at all levels; moderate severity cases are treatable at
a health center or hospital; high severity cases are treatable only at a hospital.

all facility levels, the existence of a potentially threatening condition for
the woman is diagnosed, and an assessment made as to the severity of the
condition. Mild severity conditions can be treated at any level of the
system; moderate severity conditions can be treated only at the health
center or hospital; and high severity conditions (some of which demand
surgery) require treatment at the hospital. The diagnosis that decides
such referrals is based on clinical observation only. For simplicity, the
baseline model does not include an allowance for inappropriate referrals
or for women who do not show up at the facility to which they have been
referred, but these complexities can be added without changing basic
results.

The assumptions about family planning information and service delivery are also somewhat artificial. As shown in Tables C-3 and C-4, the
baseline model assumes that 15 percent of pregnant women will want to
space or limit their next births. This figure is taken to be a constant and is
not linked directly to the expenditures in the Mother-Baby Package on
information, education, and communication efforts. The method mix is
assumed to vary among facilities, with more clinical methods being delivered in the higher level facilities. In view of the leading role played by
trained midwives in the Mother-Baby Package, it would be particularly
important to refine estimates of training costs. Those used in the baseline

TABLE C-3 Assumptions Regarding Family Planning Use in the Rural Baseline Model: in percent

Of women wanting to space or limit births and presenting to	Condom	Oral Contraceptives	IUDs	Injectable	Tubal Ligation
Health Post	25	50		25	
Health Center	10	50	25	15	
Hospital	5	50	25	10	10

NOTE: Of all pregnant women, 15 percent are assumed to want to space or limit births, following information, education, and communication exposure; see Table C-4.

model are derived from cost studies by the MotherCare Project in two Nigerian states (Koblinsky, personal communication). All these simplifying assumptions would have to be modified in a rigorous analysis of cost-effectiveness for a particular setting.

Allocating Facility-Level Costs Across Activities

A key task for cost models is the distribution of costs of fixed inputs across various program outputs and services. For this model, these shared costs include salaries of clinical and support staff, infrastructural services, management, and transportation.

We can illustrate the approach using the example of a woman who appears at the health post and is not referred to the health center or hospital. Let k index the type of service required by the patient. A woman may require more than one type of service, such as delivery care plus treatment of complications plus postpartum family planning services. Let

Y^k = the number of patients of type k treated at the post;
c^k = clinical personnel contacts needed per patient of type k.

Further, let

C = post capacity, that is, the total number of contacts of all types that can be made by one post's (clinical) personnel.

Then for a post operating at full capacity,

$$\sum_k \rho^k c^k = C.$$

TABLE C-4 Major Miscellaneous Assumptions in the Rural Baseline
Model (Not Otherwise Presented in Tables C-1 to C-3)

Factor	Assumptions
Information, Education, and Communication	Advertising undertaken by both posts and centers; this plus outreach and audiovisuals occur at the district hospitals. To each health post some $6,010 is devoted; to each center, $4,250; and to each hospital, $5,500.
	These expenditures do not affect the demand for family planning or other services at a particular facility.
Demand for Services	The crude birth rate (CBR) = .042; the crude pregnancy rate is 10 percent higher than this.
	Some 15 percent of pregnant women wish to space or avert entirely their next birth. No explicit link is made between the CBR and the demand for family planning or between the CBR and actual family planning use by method.
	80 percent of pregnant women are attended (covered) by package-supplied personnel and services. Of these, 85 percent present to health posts for prenatal care and normal (uncomplicated) delivery; 12 percent present to centers and 3 percent to hospitals.
Diagnosis and Referral	Diagnosis is on the basis of clinical observation only; no other resources are involved.
	The existence of a condition and its severity level are correctly diagnosed; no inappropriate referrals occur. Referred patients always arrive at the facility to which they were referred.
	Some 12 percent of births require neonatal management.
Initial Staffing and Resource Levels	None of the resources required for package are treated as sunk costs. Assumption is that long-run average costs equal marginal costs (whether supplies, clinical and support personnel, or additional infrastructure, management and transportation).
Training	All training costs are allocated to the district as a whole, not separately to hospitals, centers, or posts.
	District-level site preparation, cost of $16,000, one-fifth of the estimated total cost. Training will take place at the provincial level, each province having five districts. The depreciation period is 10 years.
	The total number of midwives required in the district is calculated, then the number of master trainers is derived on the assumption that 10 midwives can be trained by each master trainer. Training costs are $500 per master trainer and $125 per midwife. The depreciation period is 5 years.
Facility Capacities	One health post can engage in a maximum of 10 patient contacts per day, for 240 days per year. Effective capacity, however, is only 82 percent of this maximum.

TABLE C-4 Continued

Factor	Assumptions
	One health center can provide a maximum of 18 patient contacts per day, for 240 days per year. Effective capacity is 85 percent of the maximum.
	One district hospital can accommodate 29 beds per day, for 365 days per year. Effective capacity is 95 percent of the maximum.
Transportation	Each health post has a bicycle; each center, two-way radios, bicycles, a motorbike, and a claim on one-fourth of a jeep and driver; four centers will share the vehicle; each hospital has radios, bicycles, a jeep, and an ambulance, plus $2,500 per year in transportation subsidies.

Let W = total clinical salaries at the post. Now since it is identically true that

$$\sum_k \rho^k \left(W \frac{c^k}{C} \right) = W,$$

it seems reasonable to apportion total clinical salaries W into components a^k that are specific to types of patients, where

$$\omega^k \equiv \frac{Wc^k}{C} .$$

We can then view the product $Y^k a^k$ as the clinical salary costs associated with all patients of type k at a given post. This amounts to an allocation rule whereby (short-run) fixed costs, such as salaries, are allocated across patient types in proportion to the number of clinical contacts required. Similar expressions, differing only in what is assumed about the required clinical contacts c^k and capacity C, apply to centers and hospitals. For costs of nonclinical staff, infrastructure, and services, costs are distributed across patients of various types in proportion to the required clinical contacts.

   The baseline cost model provides estimates of total costs assuming that posts, centers, and hospitals operate at their full effective capacity (Table C-4). In determining the required number of posts, centers and hospitals, the model takes into account only the number implied by the Mother-Baby Package in conjunction with the assumed demographic characteristics of the district.

HYPOTHETICAL COST ESTIMATES

We begin by describing the implications of the baseline model of a low-income rural area and vary the parameters of that model to explore the impact on total costs. We then turn to a second baseline model that is meant to represent a middle-income and more urbanized area.

Total Costs: Rural Baseline Model

The baseline cost estimates suggest that for a district of 500,000 population, with 80 percent of pregnancies covered by the package services, annual total costs would be $1,500,000 (in 1992 U.S. dollars). Of this total, some $740,000 is expended at the health post level, $360,000 at the health clinic level, and $420,000 at the level of district hospitals. The total estimated costs for the Mother-Baby Package are thus just over $3 per person per year. Given a total of 23,100 total pregnancies, 80 percent of which are covered by the package, the cost per pregnancy is $66. The cost per attended pregnancy, of which there are 18,480, is $83. The package is supported by training activities for midwives; on an annual basis this requires $4,600 per district. The required number of health posts is 59; some 11 centers are required, and a total of 3 district hospitals.

Figures C-2 and C-3 provide breakdowns of costs according to type of cost and patient condition. Figure C-2 shows that the two largest areas of expenditure are clinical salaries, 27 percent of the annual budget, and information, education, and communication 22 percent. Infrastructure is also an important item, accounting for 18 percent. This percentage reflects assumptions about the lifespan of infrastructure: straight-line depreciation is used to convert initial construction or purchase costs into annual figures.

Figure C-3 shows the use to which these services are put: some 42 percent of expenditures for prenatal care, 10 percent for normal delivery care, and 9 percent to normal neonatal care. These services are supplied for all pregnancies and births. Postpartum family planning services take up 5.5 percent of the budget. The remaining service costs shown in Figure C-3 reflect the incidence and severity of pregnancy-related complications as well as the clinical and variable resources required to treat such complications. For example, anemia treatment occupies just over 10 percent of the annual budget, and treatment of hemorrhage some 8 percent.

Sensitivity Analyses

Figures C-4 and C-5 show how the incidence of particular conditions affects total costs. Here the baseline level of total costs, $1.5 million, is the

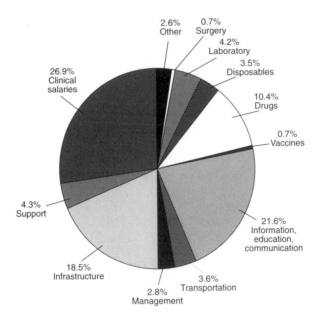

FIGURE C-2 Distribution of costs by type.

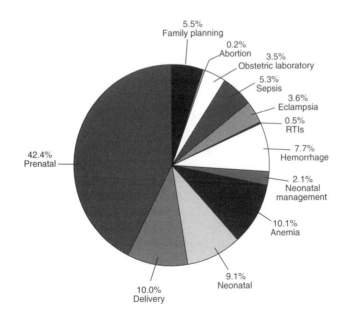

FIGURE C-3 Distribution of costs by condition service.

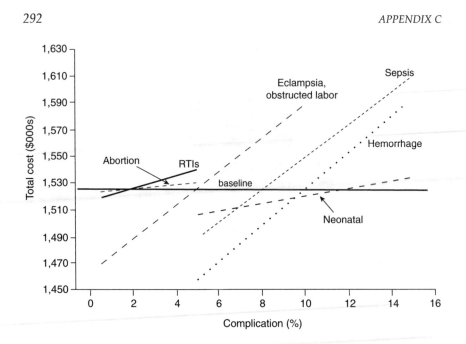

FIGURE C-4 Total costs by prevalence of complication.

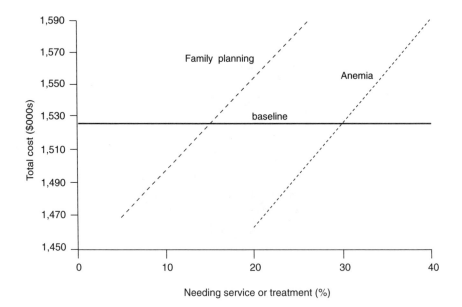

FIGURE C-5 Total costs of family planning services and anemia.

horizontal line. For each condition, the probability of occurrence is varied in a range around the baseline value given in Table C-3. For example, in the baseline the percentage of pregnancies with hemorrhage is assumed to be 10 percent. We assess how total costs vary as this percentage is varied over the range from 5 to 15 percent. The result is shown in the dotted line in Figure C-4. Note that the distribution of hemorrhage severity is not altered during the calculations, only the likelihood that a hemorrhage occurs.

Changes in the incidence of abortion complications, RTIs, and neonatal complications appear to exert rather modest effects on total costs. By contrast, changes in the incidence of eclampsia and obstructed labor, hemorrhage, and sepsis have much larger effects on costs. This is important for projections of costs of safe pregnancy and delivery care because, as Chapter 5 shows, there is considerable uncertainty about the incidence and prevalence of these conditions.

Figure C-5 shows the result of similar calculations for the incidence of anemia and also presents the cost implications of changes in the level of demand for family planning. Changes in anemia incidence and family planning demand exert considerable influence on total costs.

The role of assumptions about joint costs is explored in Figure C-6. Recall that in the rural baseline model, it is assumed that certain staff—

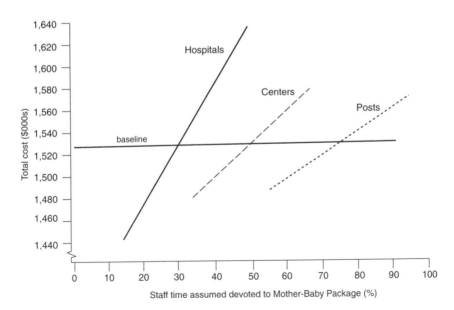

FIGURE C-6 Total costs by joint cost assumptions.

obstetricians, midwives and nurse auxiliaries—are devoted full time to package activities. Support staff, however, and services such as transport and infrastructure, are not fully charged to reproductive health care and are available for other health care needs. At the health post level, the assumption in the baseline model is that 75 percent of support staff, transport, and infrastructure are devoted to package activities; at the center level, 50 percent; and at the hospital level, 30 percent. These assumptions about joint costs prove to be critical in estimating the total costs of the Mother-Baby Package since the costs shared with other health care needs are a large proportion of the total. Especially at the hospital level, assumptions about joint costs have a strong impact on the total estimated costs of the Mother-Baby Package.

Model for an Urban Population with Lower Birth Rate

The rural baseline costs can be compared with estimates for a moderate-income urbanized area. The principal differences in the urban model are in the following assumptions: the crude birth rate is 30 per thousand, as compared to 42 in the rural baseline; the proportion of postpartum women wishing to use family planning is 25 percent, compared with 15; and the prevalence of RTIs is 5 percent rather than 2 percent; see Table C-5. In addition, a higher proportion of women are assumed to use centers and hospitals for prenatal and delivery care, 40 percent, compared with 15 percent in the rural model. Personnel costs, however, are assumed to be the same as in rural areas; this assumption would not hold in many health services. We also incorporated lower costs for vehicles, assuming that clinics in densely populated areas would rely less on mobile services.

These differences in assumptions have clear implications for total costs. For an urbanized district of the same population size, 500,000, as

TABLE C-5 Urban Baseline Model: Differences in Assumptions

Factor	Assumptions
Demand for Services	The crude birth rate = .030. Some 25 percent of pregnant women wish to space or delay their next birth. As with rural model, some 80 percent of pregnant women are attended by package-supplied personnel and services; but of these, 60 percent present to health posts for prenatal care and (uncomplicated) delivery, 30 percent to health centers, and 10 percent to hospitals. 5 percent of pregnant women have RTIs or STDs.

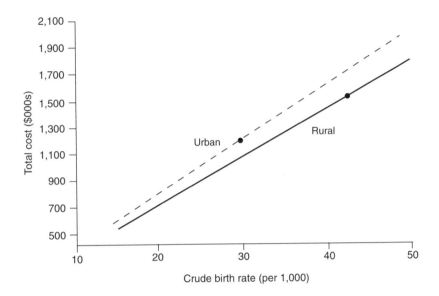

FIGURE C-7 Total costs by crude birth rates, rural and urban.

the rural district modeled above, the total costs of the package are estimated to be $1.2 million, about 80 percent of the costs for the rural district.
On a per capita basis, the urban costs are $2.46; this translates to $75 per
pregnancy and $93 per attended pregnancy. The urban-rural cost differ-
ences are mainly attributable to the smaller number of pregnancies. The
difference in crude birth rates is partly offset by a greater demand for
family planning services in urban areas, by greater incidence of RTIs and
STDs, and by the greater use of centers and hospitals.

These urban-rural differences are depicted in Figure C-7, which indicates that at a given level of the crude birth rate (on the horizontal axis),
urban total costs exceed those for rural areas. The baseline urban and
rural cost estimates, which use different crude birth rates, are shown in
the two dots.

REFERENCES

Alisjahbana, A., C. Williams, R. Dharmayanti, D. Hermawan, B. Kwast, and M. Koblinsky
    1995   An integrated village maternity service to improve referral patterns in a rural
            area in West Java. *International Journal of Gynecology and Obstetrics*
            48(Supplement):Table 8.
Chalmers, M.E., M. Enkin, and M. Keirse, eds.
    1989   *Effective Care in Pregnancy and Childbirth.* Oxford, England: Oxford University
            Press.

Cowley, P., and J.L. Bobadilla
  1995   Costing the Mother-Baby package of Health Interventions. Population, Health, and Nutrition Department, World Bank, Washington, D.C.
Herz, B., and A. Measham
  1987   The safe motherhood initiative: Proposals for action. *World Bank Discussion Paper* No. 9. Washington, D.C.: World Bank.
Management Sciences for Health
  1992   *The International Price Indicator Guide, 1991.* Boston: Management Sciences for Health.
Nirupam, S.
  1993   *Child Survival and Safe Motherhood Project Costs in India.* Geneva, Switzerland: World Health Organization.
Rankin, J.R., J.P. Sallet, and J. Frye
  1993   *International Drug Price Indicator Guide, 1992-93.* Arlington, Va.: Management Sciences for Health.
Tinker, A., and M. Koblinsky
  1993   *Making Motherhood Safe.* World Bank Discussion Paper No. 202. Washington, D.C.: World Bank.
World Bank
  1993   *World Development Report 1993: Investing in Health.* Washington, D.C.: World Bank.
World Health Organization
  1994   *Mother-Baby Package: Implementing Safe Motherhood in Countries.* Geneva, Switzerland: The World Health Organization.

Biographical Sketches

AMY ONG TSUI is professor in the Department of Maternal and Child Health of the School of Public Health at the University of North Carolina, Chapel Hill. She also directs the EVALUATION Project of the Carolina Population Center, funded by the U.S. Agency for International Development. She was previously associate director of the Community and Family Study Center at the University of Chicago and assistant research officer for the U.N. Economic and Social Commission for Asia and the Pacific. Her research has dealt with a wide variety of topics related to family planning programs, contraceptive use, child health, and family formation in Asia and Africa. She received B.A. and M.A. degrees from the University of Hawaii and a Ph.D. degree in sociology from the University of Chicago.

JUDITH N. WASSERHEIT is the director of the Division of STD Prevention in the National Center for HIV, STD, and Tuberculosis Prevention of the Centers for Disease Control and Prevention. She has worked extensively in Asia, as well as in selected countries in Africa and Latin America. She is a member of the executive board of the American Venereal Disease Association and the board of the International Society for STD Research. Her research has included clinical and epidemiological aspects of sexually transmitted diseases and HIV prevention, particularly in relation to women's health. She has a B.A. degree from Princeton University, an M.D. degree from Harvard Medical School, and an M.P.H. degree from the Johns Hopkins University School of Hygiene and Public Health.

ALAKA MALWADE BASU is senior research associate at the Division of Nutritional Sciences at Cornell University. Her major research work is in the social and cultural context of demographic behavior and the political context of population research and policy, especially the interrelationships between women's status and demographic behavior. She has done extensive field research in India. She served as the chair of the Scientific Committee on Anthropological Demography of the International Union for the Scientific Study of Population. She earned B.Sc. degrees in biochemistry from the Universities of Bombay and London, and an M.Sc. degree in medical demography from the London School of Hygiene and Tropical Medicine.

JOSE LUIS BOBADILLA was principal health specialist at the Inter-American Development Bank (IADB) before his death in October 1996. Before joining the IADB, he had been senior health specialist at the World Bank, a center director at the Instituto Nacional de Salud Publica in Mexico City, and professor in the medical faculty of the Universidad Nacional Autonoma de Mexico. His recent work included helping developing countries use analyses of disease burden and cost-effectiveness of interventions to plan health programs. His research interests included the epidemiologic transition in Latin America and the effectiveness of obstetric and perinatal services. He completed his medical studies at the Universidad Nacional Autonoma de Mexico, and earned an M.S. degree in community medicine and a Ph.D. degree in health care epidemiology from the London School of Hygiene and Tropical Medicine. (Please see Dedication to this volume.)

WILLARD CATES, JR., is senior vice president of Biomedical Affairs, Family Health International (FHI), North Carolina, and visiting professor of epidemiology at several universities. Prior to joining FHI, he was at the Centers for Disease Control and Prevention (CDC), where he served as Director of the Division of STD/HIV Prevention for 9 years. While at CDC, he also directed the Division of Training, overseeing the Epidemic Intelligence Service and Preventive Medicine Residency. He is past president of the Society for Epidemiologic Research and co-author of two major reproductive health textbooks. He received an undergraduate degree from Yale University; a masters degree in history from Kings College, Cambridge University, Cambridge, England; and a combined M.D.-M.P.H. degree from Yale School of Medicine. He trained clinically in internal medicine at the University of Virginia Hospital.

CHRISTOPHER J. ELIAS is a senior associate in the International Programs Division of the Population Council and serves as country representative for the Population Council in Thailand, responsible for activities in

Thailand, Myanmar (Burma), and Laos. His interests include reproductive health, family planning operations research, expansion of contraceptive choice, gender and development research, and institutional strengthening. In conjunction with the Population Council's Center for Biomedical Research, he also coordinates efforts to develop woman-controlled vaginal microbicides. He received an M.D. degree from Creighton University, completed postgraduate training in internal medicine at the University of California San Francisco, and received a M.P.H. degree from the University of Washington, where he was a fellow in the Robert Wood Johnson Clinical Scholars Program.

JOHN G. HAAGA is the staff director for the Committee on Population of the National Research Council. Previously, he directed the MCH-Family Planning Extension Project at the International Centre for Diarrhoeal Disease Research in Bangladesh. He has also been a policy analyst in the Social Policy Department of RAND, working on health care, immunization, and demographic surveys in the United States, Malaysia, and Indonesia. From 1982 to 1985 he was Deputy Director of the Nutritional Surveillance Program at Cornell University, working on nutrition surveys and nutrition policy research in Africa. He received master's degrees in modern history from Oxford University and in international relations from Johns Hopkins University, and a Ph.D. degree in public policy from the RAND Graduate School.

MARJORIE A. KOBLINSKY is director of the MotherCare Project with John Snow, Inc. Her interest and work in women's reproductive health began with her biochemical research and has included positions with the Ford Foundation, the Asia Regional Office of International Development Research Centre, and the International Centre for Diarrhoeal Disease Research, Bangladesh. Her current research interests include maternal mortality and morbidity and measurement issues. She was awarded a B.S. degree in chemistry by Simmons College and a Ph.D. degree in biochemistry by Columbia University.

PIERRE MERCENIER recently retired as professor at the Institute of Tropical Medicine in Antwerp, Belgium. He had previously served as a medical officer for the World Health Organization, working on the national tuberculosis control program in India; as a physician in Rwanda, Burundi, and Zaire; as a researcher at the Scientific and Medical Centre of the Free University of Brussels in Kasongo, Zaire; and as a consultant for the World Health Organization and several bilateral aid agencies in Africa, Asia, and Latin America. His research has focused on the organization and evaluation of health services. He holds the Licence Speciale in public health and a medical degree from the Free University of Brussels, the Diploma of Tropical Medicine from the Institute of Tropical Medicine in Antwerp, and certificates and aggregation in pneumophtisiology from the Faculty of Medicine in Paris.

MARK R. MONTGOMERY is associate professor of economics at the State University of New York, Stony Brook, and associate at the Population Council. He has also served as senior fellow in the Department of Geography and Planning at the University of Lagos, Nigeria, and as assistant professor at the Office of Population Research, Princeton University. He is a member of the National Research Council's Committee on Population and of the Institute of Medicine's Committee on Unintended Pregnancies. His published research includes economic analyses of marriage, contraception, and fertility, studies of child health, and work on urban growth and migration in Africa. He earned a B.A. degree from the University of North Carolina and a Ph.D. degree in economics from the University of Michigan.

SUSAN E. PICK is president of the Mexican Institute for Family and Population Research (IMIFAP) and professor of social psychology at the National Autonomous University of Mexico (UNAM). As founder and president of IMIFAP, she has directed the development, implementation, and evaluation of integrated sex and family life education programs for children, adolescents, parents, and health and education professionals, as well as programs in AIDS prevention, advocacy and policy, teacher training, public opinion and educational materials in nine Latin American countries, Greece, and with Latinos in the United States. Since 1984 she has held the title of National Researcher in Mexico, and in 1991 she received the National University Award for Young Academics in Social Science Research from UNAM. She has a B.Sc. degree in social psychology from the London School of Economics and Political Science of the University of London and a Ph.D. degree from the University of London.

ALLAN ROSENFIELD is DeLamar professor and dean of the Columbia School of Public Health. An international expert in women's reproductive health, family planning, population, and international health, he is a member of the Institute of Medicine, diplomate of the American Board of Obstetrics and Gynecology, and a fellow of the American College of Obstetricians and Gynecologists. He serves on the boards or committees of a broad array of population, health, and science organizations, including the International Bank for Reconstruction and Development, the U.S. Agency for International Development, the World Health Organization, the Institute of Medicine, the National Council on International Health, the New York State and New York City Departments of Health, and several local New York City and State non-profit organizations. He has served as president of the New York Obstetrical Society and chair of the executive board of the American Public Health Association and is currently chair of the Alan Guttmacher Institute and president of the Association of Schools of Public Health. He holds undergraduate degrees from Harvard University and an M.D. from Columbia University.

HELEN SAXENIAN is senior economist in the Population, Health, and Nutrition Department of the World Bank. She has worked on health policy and agricultural projects in Latin America and was a coauthor of the 1993 World Development Report, *Investing in Health*. She has written both research reports and sectoral reviews of women's reproductive health and child nutrition in Brazil and Venezuela. She holds a B.A. degree in economics from the University of California, Berkeley, and a Ph.D. degree in applied economics from Stanford University.

JAMES TRUSSELL is professor of economics and public affairs, director of the Office of Population Research, and associate dean of the Woodrow Wilson School of Public Policy and International Affairs at Princeton University. His research deals primarily with demographic methodology and reproductive health. In recent years he has published extensively on contraceptive technology, including the safety and efficacy of emergency contraceptives. He is a former member of the National Research Council Committee on Population and was co-chair of the Panel on Data and Research Needs for AIDS in Sub-Saharan Africa. He is a research associate of the National Bureau of Economic Research and a member of the board of directors of the Population Association of America and the Alan Guttmacher Institute. He has a B.S. degree in mathematics from Davidson College, a B.Phil. degree in economics from Oxford University, and a Ph.D. degree in economics from Princeton University.

HUDA ZURAYK is senior associate in the Population Council Regional Office for West Asia and North Africa in Cairo. She is responsible for the reproductive health program and coordinates the Reproductive Health Working Group (RHWG), a regional interdisciplinary network of research scholars in reproductive health. Members of the RHWG in Egypt undertook the Giza Morbidity Study, which has contributed to drawing attention to the magnitude of gynecological and related morbidity in developing countries. She is currently member of the Council of the International Union for the Scientific Study of Population. She is also visiting professor at the Faculty of Health Sciences of the American University of Beirut, where she served as full-time faculty member from 1974 to 1987. She holds a Ph.D degree from the Johns Hopkins University School of Public Health.

Index

Selected Publications,
Committee on Population

Available from the National Academy Press (2101 Constitution Avenue, N.W., Washington, D.C. 20418; 1-800-624-6242 or 1-202-334-3313); available on-line at http://www.nap.edu.

Preventing and Mitigating AIDS in Sub-Saharan Africa: Research and Data Priorities for the Social and Behavioral Sciences. J. Trussell and B. Cohen, eds. 1996.

Social Dynamics of Adolescent Fertility in Sub-Saharan Africa. C.H. Bledsoe and B. Cohen, eds. 1993.

Effects of Health Programs on Child Mortality in Sub-Saharan Africa. D.C. Ewbank and J.N. Gribble, eds. 1993.

Factors Affecting Contraceptive Use in Sub-Saharan Africa. Working Group on Factors Affecting Contraceptive Use. 1993.

The Epidemiological Transition: Policy and Planning Implications for Developing Countries, Workshop Proceedings. J.N. Gribble and S.H. Preston, eds. 1993.

Developing New Contraceptives: Obstacles and Opportunities. Institute of Medicine, L. Mastroianni, Jr., P.J. Donaldson, and T.T. Kane, eds. 1990.

Contraception and Reproduction: Health Consequences for Women and Children in the Developing World. Working Group on the Health Consequences of Contraceptive Use and Controlled Fertility. 1989.

Contraceptive Use and Controlled Fertility: Health Issues for Women and Children. A.M. Parnell, ed. 1989.

Available from the Committee on Population (National Research Council, 2101 Constitution Avenue, N.W., Washington, D.C. 20418; phone: 202-334-3167, fax: 202-334-3768, email: cpop@nas.edu. Also available online at http://www.nap.edu.

Data Priorities for Population and Health in Developing Countries. C.E. Malanick, and A.R. Pebley, eds. 1996.

Reproductive Health Interventions: Report of a Meeting. J.G. Haaga, A.O. Tsui, and J. Wasserheit, eds. 1996.

Resource Allocation for Family Planning in Developing Countries: Report of a Meeting. J.G. Haaga and A.O. Tsui, eds. 1995.

Organizing for Effective Family Planning Programs. R.J. Lapham and G.B. Simmons, eds. 1987.

Available from Plenum Press (233 Spring Street, New York, N.Y., 10013-1578):

Demographic and Programmatic Consequences of Contraceptive Innovations. S.J. Segal, A.O. Tsui, and S.M. Rogers, eds. 1989.